New Paradigms in Healthcare

In the first two decades of this new millennium, the self-sufficiency of Evidence-Based Medicine (EBM) have begun to be questioned. The narrative version gradually assumed increasing importance as the need emerged to shift to more biologically, psychologically, socially, and existentially focused models. The terrible experience of the COVID pandemic truly revealed that EBM alone, while being a wonderful scientific philosophy and containing the physician's paternalistic approach, has its limitations: it often ignores both the patient's and physician's perspectives as persons, as human beings; it pays relentless attention to biological markers and not to the more personal, psychological, social, and anthropological ones, removing the emotions, thoughts, and desires of life, focusing on just the "measurable quality" of it.

Health Humanities, Medical Humanities and Narrative Medicine are arts intertwined with sciences that allow to broaden the mindset and approach of healthcare professionals. helping them to produce better care and more well-being.

Aim of this series is to collect "person-centered" contributions, as only a multidisciplinary and collaborative team can meet the challenge of combining the multiple aspects of human health, as well as the health of our planet, and of all the creatures that live on it, in a common effort to stop or reverse the enormous damage committed by humans during our anthropocentric era: a new paradigm of healthcare, education and learning to create a sustainable health system.

Jonathan McFarland • Susana Magalhães
Jacek Mostwin • René Génadry
Editors

Humanism in Surgery

Reflective Dialogue across Arts, Humanities and Health Sciences

Springer

Editors
Jonathan McFarland
Faculty of Medicine
Pompeu Fabra University
Barcelona, Barcelona, Spain

Faculty of Medicine
Autonomous University of Madrid
Madrid, Spain

Jacek Mostwin
Department of Urology
Johns Hopkins Medical Institutions
Baltimore, MD, USA

Susana Magalhães
Institute for research and innovation in health (i3S)-University of Porto
University Fernando Pessoa
Porto, Portugal

René Génadry
Carver College of Medicine
University of Iowa
Iowa City, IA, USA

ISSN 2731-3247 ISSN 2731-3255 (electronic)
New Paradigms in Healthcare
ISBN 978-3-031-86017-1 ISBN 978-3-031-86018-8 (eBook)
https://doi.org/10.1007/978-3-031-86018-8

This Springer imprint is published by the registered company Springer Nature Switzerland AG
The registered company address is: Gewerbestrasse 11, 6330 Cham, Switzerland

This book is dedicated to John Bryan McFarland

Foreword

Surgery is for many effectively a calling in which individuals can express the links between their intellectual and academic abilities and hand/eye co-ordination for the benefit of the patient. The surgeon should always respect the person entrusting their body to the professional since this is a sacred bond linking the patient, their illness and the clinician.

Hospitals are of course for ill people and the staggering technical and therapeutic advances that all clinicians witness over a working lifetime of 30 or 40 years means that often the patient entering the clinical environment has a very high expectation of a successful outcome. And this is where the humanity of the clinician becomes so important; the care and alleviation of the patient's problem may not always result in a cure, permanent or even temporary. The inevitability of continuous suffering, or even death, must then be faced. In these circumstances the humanism of the surgeon and others delivering the care can considerably ease a distressing progression. The caring for the patient's condition should always require caring for the patient, which acts as a commitment to the shunning of inappropriate or futile therapeutic options. Herein lies the basis of the skill and restraint of the enlightened surgeon.

In this context all forms of surgery carry one extra dimension to other less physically demanding disciplines as the result of a surgical intervention often leads to irreversible anatomical and physiological changes to the patient. Therefore, the surgeon should always understand that the basis of caring for the patient requires seeing the individual as a whole person and not just a limited technical problem. Moreover, to fail to do so results in an uncaring professional in whom the patient rapidly loses trust, and trust is at the centre of medicine, or is even perhaps its essence. This book, from my knowledge the first of its kind, tries to tease out and explain this fundamental tenet.

The narrative exposition of the principle related by many practicing exponents of these issues and the telling description of the three Liverpool surgeons, one of whom was my own guide and mentor, and who were the original inspiration behind Humanities, Humanism and Surgery provide a strong beacon for all who follow the advancement of medicine for the benefit of all.

Former President of RCS(Ed) and BMA
Birmingham, West Midlands, UK

Sir John Temple

Preface

'The part can never be well unless the whole is well'

'…And this is the reason why the cure of many diseases is unknown to the physicians of Hellas [Greece], because they are ignorant of the whole, which ought to be studied also; for the part can never be well unless the whole is well.' Plato in Charmides narrated by Socrates

Surgery is a highly technical field, often presented to the world as devoid of the kind of humanism and human qualities that we associate with other medical fields such as paediatrics, internal medicine, psychiatry and nursing. Surgery may too often be seen as attending to the part while disregarding the whole, leaving its practitioners described as 'technicians'. Some traditions have separated the medical and surgical aspects of medicine even more, limiting the term 'doctor' to physicians while addressing their surgeons as 'mister', a term that has become in recent years a kind of badge of honour. While there can be no question that technical features of medicine and surgery are supremely important, especially to those whose lives are at stake during their application, we wish to offer a broader perspective on the field, looking at the intrinsic humanism in surgery, the role of humanities in supporting it and the humanitarian efforts that surgeons take up by virtue of qualities that go far beyond technical interest in the mechanics of the body. In this book we consider some of the theory and experience that reflect this perspective and the resources available for the education of humane and humanistic surgeons. We have integrated this wide range of perspectives with transcripts of interviews, conversations really, with surgeons who are active in their field. These conversations provide insights into their personal and professional development, their perspective on life and medicine, their commitment to their work and the people they serve, and the trajectories that led them to become humane, humanistic, and sometimes, humanitarian, breathing life into the more theoretical chapters which provide scholarly perspective and resources.

The 'whole' of a patient includes many contextual dimensions in which surgical needs are embedded: physical, emotional, familial, social, intellectual, and economic. Listening to the patient intently with a caring attitude and accepting him or her in their 'wholeness' expands surgery from a merely technical craft to a more humanistic one. In his presentation before the Porto conference, Patrick Walsh (Ch. 12) cited Francis Peabody's well-known conclusion before medical students at Harvard in 1926:

> 'Time, sympathy, and understanding must be lavishly dispensed, but the reward is to be found in that personal bond which forms the greatest satisfaction of the practice of medicine. One of the essential qualities of the clinician is interest in humanity, for the secret of the care of the patient is in caring for the patient.'

Interest in Humanity and Caring for the Patient

For the surgeon, 'caring for the patient' may be reflected in attention directed towards a part of the body without necessarily seeing or even attempting to care for the whole, believing that the part is affecting the whole, and that alone is something of singular value. But we wish to advance a model of surgeons that embody what Peabody called that greater 'interest in humanity' in their work and attitude, not only in the other dimensions of the life of the whole person but also in the broader cultural, historical and artistic context of the world. We are suggesting that surgery contains within its work, and in the interests of its practitioners, a generosity of spirit that is embedded in its technical gesture but is less likely to be recognized in academic assemblies or medical schools. One could argue that the care of the surgical patient is expressed in the technical focus of the profession, in attention to detail, but we believe there is more to surgery than that, and that this theme of humanism in surgery deserves to be brought to the fore and presented to a wider audience so that students and educators might see opportunities that are less obvious, and in which experienced practitioners might find reinforcement of beliefs long held in quiet, beliefs that seem to find no venue for expression save in private conversation, informal gathering, or that 'personal bond which forms the greatest satisfaction.'

The Conference on Humanism and Surgery, 2022

This book grew out of a conference on Humanism and Surgery which took place at the i3S Research and Innovation in Health Institute in Porto, Portugal, in October 2022. At the time, we believed it was an unusual conference, as most such conferences address the role of humanities in medicine in general; this one did as well but was unique in its special attention to the surgical disciplines that represent so much of the work that medicine does. Originally it was our idea to assemble many of the presentations from that conference so that they could be codified and shared with a broader audience. As the project developed, however, we became interested in adding *conversations* with living surgeons to balance some of the more academic papers that had been presented to the Porto audience. As a result, we found we had assembled a very large and diverse collection of materials under a 'big tent' for a 'big' audience. And it seems fitting that we have done so, for medicine belongs to a wider world, not just to the specialties which practice their skills within it.

In the pages that follow, readers will encounter an eclectic approach with a wide variety of styles representing different perspectives. Some are personal, others scholarly. Some resemble lectures, or even manifestos, others provide recorded conversations. Some address humanism in medicine in general and sometimes more specifically, and especially in the conversations, in surgery. This underscores our belief that medicine and surgery are not as separate as they may sometimes be represented. The medical world is enmeshed in verbalism, but it also bristles with silent action. We are looking for common ground, yet we wish to preserve the special qualities that are imparted to surgery by its attention to the body and the physical interventions that surgery has developed to help it. The body is the person's infrastructure. Without it, we have no life as we know it. Yet, as Gilbert Ryle has argued, the separation of mind and body that grew out of the Enlightenment left us with a sense of the 'person' as a 'ghost in the machine'. Surgeons may thus be assigned the role of mechanics while others retain the claim to be the proper custodians of the person, or Ryle's 'ghost', in medicine. We prefer a different paradigm, as we cannot imagine a person without a body, and by definition, we cannot imagine a surgical perspective that does not in some way recognize the embodiment of that person, even if that recognition is subliminal. To us, it is apparent and is worth bringing to the foreground. Hence the conference in Porto, and hence this book.

The reflective dialogue to which we refer occurs not only across the disciplines of arts, humanities and health sciences but also across a wide variety of people who represent these disciplines and practices. And although patients themselves have not directly contributed to this presentation, their voices are still to be heard in some of the biographies and memoirs that are cited within these pages, and in the memories carried by some of the interviewed surgeons as revealed in conversation. Consequently, we have taken a very democratic approach to including some of the many voices that have a vested interest in the conduct of medicine and surgery and their shared role in the world.

Conversations with Surgeons

We have dedicated this book to John Bryan McFarland, a surgeon from Liverpool whose son Jonathan is one of the four editors. It was his legacy that inspired the creation of the organization we now call The Doctor as a Humanist, co-organizers of the Porto Conference with i3S. Jonathan was one of its founders in 2017 and remains active as its president. It was the relationship his father had with his patients and colleagues, as well as his whole approach to medicine and surgery, that gave rise to this desire to support what DASH calls 'the heart and soul of medicine' so that such things should not be lost as scientific progress continues. Jonathan's father was immersed not only in technical surgery, and medical education, but also wrote poems about his experience, loved the sea and the arts, and loved the people that he took care of and worked with. For him, Surgery was a way of life, for above all he loved life. None of this was lost on Jonathan as he developed DASH out of reverence for his father's memory and a love for the people who carry on this kind of medical tradition. In keeping with this dedication, Jonathan has written an introductory letter to the readers to reveal something of his father's life and the lives of his two grandfathers, both of whom were surgeons. It is our belief that to find humanism in surgery we must look for it in the people who perform it and who live in it. This introductory letter gives us such an opportunity.

After the introduction, the reader will find the first of 12 transcripts of interviews (or conversations, as we decided to call them) recorded with living, practicing surgeons in conversation with the editors. Surgeons tend to be busy people, and although they may need to write academically or create scientific publications, they also carry with them a rich treasury of lore, perspective and personal values that they are less likely to write about but will readily speak about. This may not be as apparent to the general audience and to their patients as we think it could be, yet many times it is exactly this that students and other interested parties wish to hear more about. In our conversations we have used some simple prompts or have followed the conversation wherever it will go so that these individuals can reveal what matters to them in their daily work and in their life's pursuit. For these individuals, surgery is a way of life. It should go without saying that their selection by the editors was not random. We selected individuals that we believed would support the general theme of humanism in medicine. If one were doing a quantitative analysis, this would hardly count as a representative sample. Yet each conversation carries with it many grains of truth that cannot fail to reach a sensitive and intelligent reader, especially students and younger physicians who may be looking for role models beyond the limits of their own educational systems.

In the first conversation, Dr Sohier Elneil recognizes the critical role of her familial environment that helped shape her development into a compassionate and caring physician and surgeon and deplores the absence of the appreciation of such important qualities as empathy, compassion within the industrialization of medicine.

Dr Manuel Pera speaks on the centrality of the patient and the importance of language and respect in caring for the individual patient. He reflects on the people who modelled these important qualities for him, especially his father, Cristobal Pera.

Dr William Reiner specialized in paediatric urology. Listening to his patients' concerns about gender and human identity he tried in psychiatry to further help his patients and their families by studying their identity challenges through a psychiatrists's eye.

Dr Christopher Wolfgang, raised on a farm, recognized the importance of working with commitment, passion and the highest work ethics. He followed in the footsteps of his maternal grandfather in science and problem solving, taking up the most difficult problem of pancreatic cancer requiring solution and perfecting his surgical technique. 'I think that your hands are a manifestation of what goes on inside your mind.'

Dr Wilkerson recognized early on his interest in working with the underserved. He shares his journey eventually leading him to Malawi where he helps solve the problems generated by obstetrical fistulas with its debilitating personal, social and societal effects. He deplores the mistaken perception of a 'sacrificial' nature of humanitarian work which he recognizes as a privilege and is actively involved in solving systemic problems in the delivery of care with passion and humility.

Dr John Tarpley wanted to blend the lives of Albert Schweitzer and William Halstead, eventually finding a way by taking his surgical training into Sub-Saharan Africa to build programs and educate local surgeons. He is retired from performing operations but remains active in medical education and program development for African countries.

Dr Handa explores his humanitarian involvement with the people of the island of Palau for whom he delivers much needed eye care and reflects on what it takes to manage successfully a sustainable and committed programme for over 27 years while maintaining his teaching and research commitments.

Dr Goh shares her journey into her involvement in humanitarian work on many continents and recognizes the innate nature of interest in humanitarian work. She also appreciates the importance of early exposure to such an opportunity along with nurturing the qualities of empathy, adaptability, flexibility and cultural adjustment.

Dr Breen acknowledges the importance of his Christian education and shares the circumstances that led to his life in Africa. He describes himself as a 'simple guy trying to do some good'.

Dr Arrowsmith insists on the 'covenant relationship' and personal investment that should exist between the surgeon and the patient. He shares his journey and his insights into mentoring, role modelling and teaching by example.

Dr Pastor also stresses the importance of a 'love relationship' with patients. Her interest in medicine was 'innate' and she developed a passion for the brain. 'Medicine is a philosophy of life' and she deplores the loss of empathy as well as the hardship women encounter in specializing in neurosurgery.

Dr Varallo shares the role of his Jesuit schooling and family circumstances that led him to develop empathy, a spirit of community and a keen engagement in social justice. He sees his humanitarian function as an innate 'calling' to be met with compassion, 'cultural humility', connectedness and flexibility to build sustainability and scalability.

The Chapters

Susana Magalhães reviews the theory and practice of narrative medicine and its value for education and practice as seen by a literary scholar. Indeed, the 12 conversations with surgeons can be thought of as a form of narrative practice, but instead of listening to patients, we are listening to our professional colleagues. They too have something to say. Their stories belong to the narrative tradition.

José Poças provides a philosophical reflection on the nature of human relationships in medicine and how they are affected by emerging technology. Ana Cardoso follows with a nurse's practical perspective on narrative medicine and the personal qualities of medicine. Ana Zhao reviews the role of studio and musical arts as therapeutic tools for patients, a well-known but still somewhat peripheral field generally not considered as a serious form of therapy compared to surgical intervention and pharmaceutical management, but viewed from the patient's perspective, a welcome, healing contribution to their welfare.

Margarida Lobo Antunes reviews the role of medical humanities, narrative medicine, literature and the arts in developing a broad literacy for physicians through disciplines that are not considered part of the scientific canon of medicinal education and practice but belong to the awareness of culture and civilization that fosters a more finely developed sense of the person who has the illness, to paraphrase William Osler.

'In Humanism and the Arts: Quo Vadis, where are you going?' Jacek Mostwin raises questions about the direction of humanism in education and the resources that are available to us to bring it to life, suggesting that the humanism is already in the medicine and what is needed are better ways of searching for it within the experience of its practitioners and patients. The role of the humanities, he suggests, is to support and lead that search.

Following on the theme of gestures of the hand, Jonathan McFarland and Manuel Pera reflect on the role of the word, silence and touch in medical encounters, reminding us that not all that matters can be expressed in language, paraphrasing Albert Einstein, and not everything that can be expressed in language matters. The world of surgery tales place in a silent realm of concentration and manual engagement with the patient's body. Language is part of the encounter, but the surgeon's toolkit extends beyond that. How can we best express an appreciation of those needs, skills and resources?

Joao Silva reviews the complex matter of shared decision making and guidance of patients towards surgery or away from it. In doing so, he approaches the delicate issues of utility: utility for the patients, as in 'will this operation improve my quality of life' and utility for society which must sometime struggle to make decisions about scarce resources.

Paulo Casella provides a personal reflection on the evolution of surgery as an internalized personal discipline and way of life. Then Mark Mekelburg provides gentle comic relief by reviewing his experiences a clown on a paediatric surgical service, solving difficult interpersonal problems, relieving stress and reminding us that, at least in medieval times, the jester was often the wisest in a room of kings and princes. The clown may well be the person amongst us who has the best developed skills in 'people whispering'.

Pia Sorto and her colleagues reflect on the aesthetics of surgery, suggesting that beauty, as seen in the human form, and the aesthetics of the surgeon's artistry, can be an end in itself, and one which can serve as a unifying force across the nations. Surgery is presented as a philosophy of life, a way of approaching life in a world where scientific progress is usually viewed as the common language of medicine. Few will remember that John Keats trained as an apothecary and wound dresser in London before moving to Italy for the remainder of this short life. But few can forget the final words of his *Ode on A Grecian Urn* which encourages us to link the grace of aesthetics and the arts to the rest of life:

> 'Beauty is truth, truth beauty,—that is all
> Ye know on earth, and all ye need to know.'

Patrick Walsh, one of the most distinguished urologists of his generation, offers a very personal reflection on the deeply held religious and spiritual motivation that has guided his work. When humanities emerged during the Renaissance, they were initially seen as a secular alternative to religious views of man. But over time, it appears that humanism and religion have been travelling in a common direction along parallel paths aligned to support a shared belief in the dignity of man, seeking understanding beyond empiricism and materialism.

Finally, Jacek Mostwin offers an extended presentation on the role of biography and memoir in understanding patients, physicians and surgeons in the final chapter entitled 'Learning from the Human Experience of Patients and Practitioners'.

This book is intended for a broad audience: educators, academics, practitioners, medical and healthcare professionals, students and trainees and anyone with an interest in the surgical world. We believe there is something in these pages for all of them, whether they are working to shape educational programs, seeking to find their way in the professional world or simply looking for reassurance that they are not alone in their search and recognition of humanism in surgery.

Final Introductory Thoughts

> 'We shall never be wholly free from magic in medicine, and we never should be, for the human body is not a test tube, but a mystic thing. And where there is life there is mystery.' (Oliver St. John Gregory)

In keeping with the words of Oliver St. John Gregory, an Irish writer and surgeon both friend and contemporary of James Joyce, we believe that surgeons, perhaps more than any others, see and understand the 'magic' and 'mystery' in medicine, the magic and mystery in the human body. In this book we have expanded on this view with a series of diverse chapters intertwined with conversations with surgeons whose words reveal the humanism in their work. Many surgeons express Peabody's 'care for the patient' in a variety of ways, whether in attention to technical details, focusing on the way in which they engage patients in conversation or examination or in broader ways of considering the richness of the human family as expressed in its arts and humanities alongside its science and technical progress.

More than ever, the world needs skilled, humane surgeons with a broad sense of the personal and social context of their work, surgeons who can blend the skill and awareness of their role with genuine care for the welfare of the person, whether they are consciously aware of it or not, surgeons who appreciate the arts and sciences in appropriate measure as contributors to a learned and skilled profession and a mature society. For such people, surgery can indeed become a way of life, and we hope that this book will offer some resources and inspiration to help them.

Barcelon, Spain — Jonathan McFarland
Porto, Portugal — Susana Magalhães
Baltimore, MD, USA — Jacek Mostwin
Iowa City, IA, USA — René Génadry

A Personal Letter to the Readers: The Lengthened Shadows

Surgeons must be very careful
When they take the knife!
Underneath their fine incisions
Stirs the Culprit-Life
(Emily Dickinson)

Deus Machina [1]

"An old, old man sat on a gate swinging his legs in space. It was autumn and the gate led to the winter woods. In front of the old man the hill sloped down for a long, long way. The old man said (Fig. 1),

> 'I can see the beginning and end of life spread out before me like a vast ocean with thousands of islands and great cities on these islands. I can see my life and your life, and all the world's lives, and all the world's follies and fears, and all the little forgotten kindnesses, for I am very, very old. If you call this knowledge I have supreme knowledge. If wisdom rests on supreme knowledge and understanding I have absolute wisdom. I have an infinite compassion for so was I blessed. Of course you want advice; you want me to impart my knowledge and my wisdom to you who are very young. For as you know I am very old, and you ask what use knowledge and wisdom are to one who is so soon to die. But you are so young that you think these things can be given. Knowledge and wisdom you should gain ere you are fit to die. May the gods give you compassion."

Dear Reader

We all carry stories on our backs, in our minds, our hearts; some painful, some not, some beautiful, some not, some pleasing, some not, and this chapter is the story of three surgeons, and why they have inspired me in more ways than is possible to describe. But I will try.

We are, of course, a complicated and complex entanglement of genes, upbringing, and education but perhaps the biggest influence on who we are or become is ingrained by our parents and family. I am no different, and the influence of my mother and father was tremendous; I was extremely lucky to be brought up by two highly intelligent and loving people who instilled the values I carry with me. It was

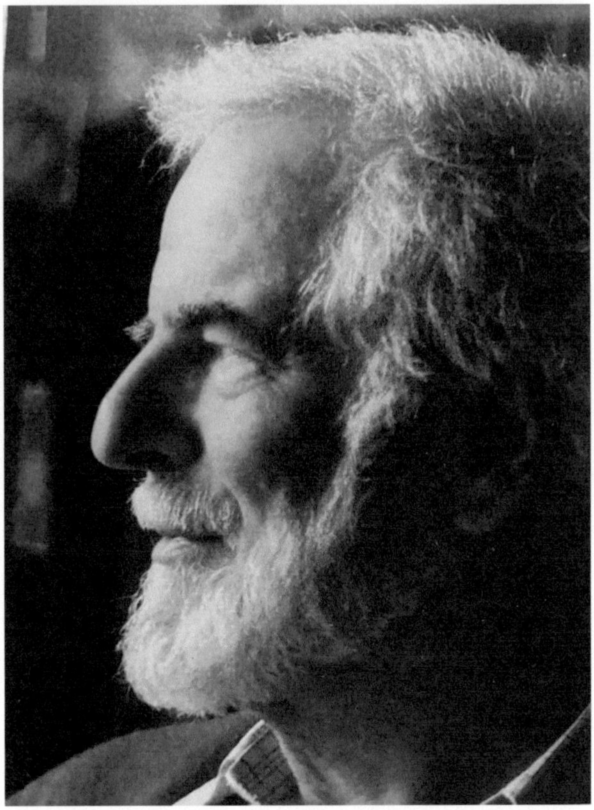

Fig. 1 A photograph of John Bryan McFarland

not without its particular difficulties but as I grow older, I begin to understand just how important they have been, and, even though both long dead, *still* are in my life. My father is the overriding reason for my interest in this intersection between medicine and the humanities and humanism, which we can call Medical Humanities he was a man who loved life, and who went into medicine, not because both his parents had been doctors, but because, as he once told me, he was interested in people, and wanted to understand them better, and what finer way to do so than to go into medicine and surgery, in particular, for how better to delve into the body of another person, literally. However, what really interested him was the *person within the patient*. In his own words, in a video-interview filmed in Soller, Mallorca, in 2009 by Daniel Lopez, he said,

> 'I chose to be a doctor, I stayed in Liverpool, I worked my way through the Liverpool system and eventually became a surgeon in my teaching hospital [2].')

Like his father and mother before him he trained at Liverpool University and worked as a surgeon in his city throughout his professional life with some specific exceptions. After qualifying in Medicine in 1954 he did his military service, where he was sent to Kenya, during what was then called the 'Mau-Mau insurgence', (see Appendix 1) where curiously enough he worked as an anaesthetist, 'which might explain why he was always kinder to and more tolerant of his anaesthetic colleagues than many others with a surgical leaning' [3]. A decade later, from 1962 to 1963, he trained under the great American surgeon Dr Curtis Artz, a renowned trauma and burns expert, in Jackson, Mississippi, where much of the research for his MD thesis on 'The Treatment of Duodenal Ulcer by "Gastric Freezing"' was carried out (under Dr Artz's guidance). His Doctoral Thesis in Surgery—'The Treatment of Hematemesis by Gastric Cooling'—was written two years later. In April 1963 he spoke at the History of Medicine Society of the University of Mississippi, and began by quoting Cicero,

> 'To be ignorant of what happened before you were born is to be ever a child. For what is man's lifetime unless the memory of past events is woven with those of earlier times [4].'

In his talk, he spoke about four men, all of whom he had some connection; Charles Darwin, my father attended the same school; James Paget, one-time president of the Royal College of Surgeons in London, where my father studied and later became an examiner; Joseph Lister, who was Chair of Surgery at Edinburgh University; more or less one hundred years later my father was house-surgeon to John Bruce, then the Chair of Surgery at Edinburgh University; and the last man was Hugh Owen Thomas, a pioneer in orthopaedic surgery and notable figure in the history of medicine in Liverpool. He ended his speech quoting from a Greek politician, Pericles, 'The whole world is the sepulcher of famous men, and their story is not engraven only on stone above their native earth, but lives on far away without visible symbol, woven into the stuff of other men's lives' [4].

He and my mother lived in Mississippi amidst the civil rights struggles and were acutely aware of the volcano bubbling below day-to-day life. During their time in Mississippi, my mother and father travelled to Mexico on a Greyhound bus and spent three days with another passenger, later to become famous or infamous; Lee Harvey Oswald, who told my mother that he was travelling to Cuba. My mother and father had to curtail their stay in Jackson, Mississippi, early due to my grandfather's terminal illness. Back in Liverpool my father worked as a consultant surgeon, in the Royal Southern Hospital and Northern Hospitals, both of which were closed to make way for the 'new' Royal Liverpool Hospital, which opened in 1978.[1] He was a general surgeon with a special interest in gastric surgery and breast cancer.

> 'The surgeon said "It's an ulcer.
> But you're fortunate, we can cut it away".
> They laid me on my back.
> The knife was clean, I suppose, unforgiving.
> and afterwards, there was great pain
> and someone else's blood dripping into me.
> I thought of you and my heart turned.
> I wished to see you sitting in the sun,
> to run my hand lightly down your back
> and think those things that one thinks

[1] The Royal Liverpool Hospital, where my father worked from its inauguration in 1978 until his retirement in 1991, was closed in 2022.

in the warm afternoon.
There were those days walking together,
you will remember them,
when it was you and the sky
in those warm us-days
and we crossed the clear, pebbled streams,
always your hand in mine.
The microscope confirmed the diagnosis.
But there's no need to worry,
they have cut it all away.'
(Crab—J.B. McFarland)

He later became a fellow of the Royal College of Surgeons of Edinburgh founded by King James IV in 1505. King James IV was a man of diverse intellectual pursuits, with science, medicine and surgery among them. In 1976, my father became a James IV Traveling Surgical Fellow; most fellows travelled west to the United States but, never one to take the easy route, he decided to travel east. A decision which influenced the rest of his life. He worked his way through Thailand, Singapore, Malaysia, Brunei, Hong Kong, Sri Lanka, India, Nepal, Afghanistan (a country and people he later always spoke very highly of) and Iran, even taking time to sail the South China seas in a small freighter 'a la Conrad', playing chess with the captain. At the end of his travels, he wrote,

'When we landed in London and took the train to Liverpool the same evening, I had been away for eighty days. My traveling was over, but my journey was not completed, nor is it yet and it may never be. It was all so different from what I had anticipated. For one thing, I was much more tired at the end than I had expected. That took some getting over, but I did become, and still am, a different person, asking different questions and, perhaps, finding different answers [5].'

It changed his life, leading him to have extraordinarily strong ties, both professionally and personally, with India for the rest of his life. This connection, which was not only surgical and medical but also cultural, resulted in him becoming an Honorary Fellow of the Association of Surgeons of India in 1981. Throughout the rest of his life, he travelled widely across the sub-continent; even trekking in Sikkim with Professor Robert Roaf, a Tibetan expert as well as my grandfather's successor as Chair of Orthopaedic Surgery at Liverpool. Robert Roaf was an exceptional man since as well as being one of the world's leading spinal surgeons he was also one of the few pre-war Himalayan climbers to reach Tibet when it was still independent from China. Marco Pallis who led the expedition allowed Roaf to travel in the team as the medical officer on condition he learnt Tibetan, which he duly did.

Growing up I was aware that my father's life centred around medicine, and never the other way around and even though I was interested, I only saw him operate twice in the Royal Liverpool Hospital in the early 1980s. I was 17 years old, and the operations made such an enormous impact that more than 40 years later the images of the patients on the operating table are clear; the first was a woman with breast cancer, her arms outstretched like a female Christ on the cross. A biopsy sample was sent to the pathology laboratory. Sometime later the results came back, obviously bad since the surgeons had to perform a radical mastectomy; more than 40 years later this operation remains vivid in my mind. Some years later, I saw my father operate under hugely different circumstances; off the west coast of Ireland in the North Atlantic Ocean where we were fishing with friends. Sudenly, there was a call for help from a nearby professional shipping boat via radio,

'Do you have a doctor on board? One of our crew has had an accident.'

Our captain responded affirmatively. Their boat came aside ours; the sea was quite choppy, but the injured man, a short but sturdy and strong Irish fisherman had no problems jumping on board our moving boat.

'I have a problem, Doc'

Indeed, he did, a large fishing hook had gone straight through his thumb, the barb gleaming with blood.

My father put his spectacles on and asked the captain of our ship whether he had any instruments and any whiskey on board. Irish whiskey and some pliers were delivered, and the fisherman was given the whiskey bottle, from which he rapidly drank down a quarter of the bottle in a few gulps, sat down, my father applied the remaining whiskey to where the hook had gone through the thumb, cut the barb, pulled the barbless hook through, bandaged the fisherman's thumb, and gave him another dram. The fisherman unflinching throughout, no word, nor sound emitted from his mouth, his face grittily determined, stood up immediately, thanked the surgeon, and jumped back onto his boat.

'Take the bottle with you and go to the hospital when you get to port'.

Five minutes later, a message came through the radio confirming that they were heading for port, and all was well.

As my knowledge of my father as a surgeon and doctor is limited and slightly subjective, I asked two of his colleagues to comment on him as a surgeon and man. Professor Averil Mansfield, who worked alongside him as a consultant in the Royal Southern Hospital in the early 1970s, told me that he was gentle and polite in the operating theatre and a skilled technician. She also mentioned that he was always kind and considerate with his patients and that he was wonderful with students and never sought to embarrass or demean them and they were remarkably high on his list of priorities. One of the things that she stressed was that he was a good colleague, watching her operating in a new branch of surgery at that time; vascular surgery, and she felt fortunate to have had him as her nearest surgical colleague.

One thing she highlighted was when she met him in India, near New Delhi, he made a 'dramatic appearance at dinner one night when I was visiting India, and he had a god-like appearance with long beard and long gown as he swept in from the hills'. This fits my image of him perfectly.

When I asked Sir John Temple,[2] he told me the following,

"I first came across him when I had been appointed registrar and John was the senior Lecturer (honorary consultant)

[2] https://www.bristol.ac.uk/graduation/honorary-degrees/hondeg14/temple.html

On a Friday during the ward round with Jim Kane, the Senior registrar, John popped his head around the door and indicated he was taking off for the weekend. After the round had finished, I also asked permission to go off as I was not on duty for the coming weekend. I drove with my family to Trearddur Bay, a small village on the coast of Anglesey, a small island off the northwest of Wales.[3] In the afternoon we went to the far side of the main bay and parked. Almost immediately another car came up and parked so that the driver's door was alongside my driver's door, and I wound the window down and to my surprise, the driver of the other car was my boss, John. On my part, an embarrassing second passed followed by silence, and then we both burst out laughing. This was the start of what became a happy friendship.

Our paths crossed several times afterwards and I became a Senior Registrar at the Royal Southern Hospital to Dad and Averil. He obviously trusted me a lot as he often left me with the firm to run when he was off examining for the Royal College of Surgeons (London), or the Moynihan Surgical Travelling Club[4], to which in the fullness of time I also became a member.

It is a long time ago, so I have few memories of working together. He was of course a very competent and respected surgeon with a kindly and interested concern for his patients. When necessary, he was a good teacher, but he often left me to get on with things. I think with Averil also it was a very happy team (or firm). Unbeknown to me he was also the internal examiner of my Mastership thesis, and he kept asking me, 'have you heard anything yet?' I would go on about 'those lazy examiners' who were so slow to give a verdict. Later, he eventually admitted his role, and the thesis was accepted!

On the social side there is much more to recall.

I captained the Royal Southern Hospital cricket team and in true 'Lancashire League' style he played as the 'senior professional', which was a tradition in the Lancashire League with noted overseas professionals playing, as a way of acclimatizing to English conditions."

Around this time, he was the editor of a book called 'Basic Clinical Surgery', [6] in which he wrote,

> 'There are, however, two final points which should be emphasized. Firstly, hospitals are for ill people. All of us who work in them have one common aim: it is to relieve suffering. Secondly, although we work very hard to save life there must eventually be an end. Death may be dreaded, hoped for or simply accepted, but everyone will die. It is his right to be allowed to do so with dignity.'

This sentiment and way of feeling about fellow humans was instilled in me, and reminds me in the first instance of Sir Francis Peabody,

---

[3] My father spent the war years in Anglesey with his two younger brothers and went to school at Trearddur Bay House school. These years were extremely important ones for him, as was the island itself.

[4] https://moynihan.org.uk/

"One of the essential qualities of the clinician is an interest in humanity, for the secret of the care of the patient is in caring for the patient" [7]. It is not often realised that Peabody when he wrote these words was himself suffering from cancer and died a year later. And, in the second instance, Iona Heath,

'Michel de Montaigne (1533–1592) owned a copy of Lucretius' verse essay, On the Nature of Things, and he quotes from it more than 100 times in his own essays. In the margin of his 1563 edition of Lucretius' poem, he wrote: 'Fear of death is the cause of all our vices' [8].

And this seems particularly true of the vices of modern medicine that allow doctors and other healthcare professionals to pretend that, to a very great extent, death is nothing to do with them. This leads directly both to the imposition of inappropriate and futile treatments, particularly at the end of life, and to what we might call the pharmaceiticalisation of death' [8].

I always wondered why my father did not want to follow in the footsteps of his father and become Professor, but he was quite adamantly against the idea, and he said, "Because my father was a Professor, and I saw what it did to him. I observed him latterly killing himself" by working an NHS practice, a Professional practice and his private practice'.

Apart from medicine, among his other lifelong passions were the sea and the arts. The former began at an early age, as he says in the same interview,

> 'It's important because always there has been the sea around me, even when I was evacuated in the Second World War, and I went to a cottage in Wales where we were in Anglesey and of course, surrounded by the sea. It was then that I first became, I think, seriously interested in boats. It's true that my father, when I was aged two, balanced me on the bow of his kayak and paddled around into the sea and my mother was not best pleased' [4]. Even during his professional career, the sea played its part, and as a medical student, no more than 20 years old, he served as a sick bay attendant on board the Queen Mary. He recounts his experiences,
>
> 'So, I travelled on the Parthia, the Samaria and even the Queen Mary to New York and had an extremely interesting time but never lost my interest basically in sailing ships. A privilege that the medical students in Liverpool, if they are assiduous in attending the Cunard headquarters, a privilege that they can obtain occasionally is to work in an assistant capacity on one of the big Cunarders. That is in the days about up to 1950. Then it all changed. So, my experiences in the Cunarders are now, is unique and the Queen Mary was, of course, the most special and my job was to attend to sick patients, that's to say I was a sick berth attendant down, down, down, down in the Queen Mary……... When you're a doctor, you're practically, in fact, in order of seniority, you're next to the captain. And the wise old travellers on the Cunard come up to the top of the steps and they ask the purser, and they say, "any seats at the captain's table?" Because that's where they want to be. "No, madam or no, sir."
>
> "Well then, is the doctor young and good-looking?"
>
> "And if he is, are there any seats at his table?" [4]
>
> And so, I had a rum group of people round my table, and we had a very good time. You're expected to be very host-like, the doctor. I may say that not many people ill, so it's not very medical, but you're expected to be very host-like.'

John had a love of literature and, especially, poetry throughout his life; this love was sparked at a very young age.

'Thus began John's first love affair with a book……….the war came, and many other things came into his head, but the book never left him, nor the characters and especially Ortho Penhale' [9]. The Owl's House was to remain a constant during his life to such an extent that he named our house in Mallorca after this book. I cannot help but think that he would be in complete agreement with a saying famously attributed to Ernest Hemingway that there is no friend as loyal as a book. This is true of John for he was a true bibliophile, and perhaps one who appreciated the benefits of Umberto Eco's 'AntiLibrary'. 'Read books are far less valuable than unread ones. ……….. You will accumulate more knowledge and more books as you grow older, and the growing number of unread books on the shelves will look at you menacingly. Indeed, the more you know, the larger the rows of unread books. Let us call this collection of unread books an *antilibrary*.' Eco could even be seen as one of the precursors of Bibliotherapy, 'we understand that it is good to have many at home rather than a few: when you want to feel better, then you go to the "medicine closet" and choose a book. Not a random one, but the right book for that moment. That's why you should always have a nutrition choice!' [10].

His connection with the Arts, visual arts, and literature was a constant throughout his life and started when he was a medical student where he went to drawing classes under Austin Davies at the Liverpool School of Arts as well as studying medicine at Liverpool Faculty of Medicine; at least for the first two years. He was perhaps one of the first to see the vital role that the Visual Arts could play in Hospitals, and in the early 1980s he managed to obtain a large grant from the Arts Council to commission artists from the northwest of England (Don McKinlay, Adrian Henri and Clement McAleer) as well as Bridget Riley from London, who later went on to paint many murals in different hospitals (Fig. 2).

Unfortunately, the idea was ahead of its time, and the murals were either removed or painted over in 1990. No more 'light and sun' for patients and healthcare workers. Goose Girl was actually vandalized and only in 2024 was it repaired and is now on permanent display in the John Moore's University School of Art. Nowadays, however, it is customary to have murals in hospitals around the world. He retired early, at the age of 61, highly aware of his father's plight, and the day after his retirement he and I sailed down the River Mersey towards the Irish Sea, and eventually reaching the port of Gibraltar. The year, 1991, has stuck in my mind since we often listened to the BBC World Service at sea, and, in the middle of the Bay of Biscay, we heard of the failed coup d'etat against Gorbachev. When my father retired, however, he did not disconnect himself completely from his medical and surgical career and he spent two consecutive winters in the Cortina Hospital, a small missionary hospital run by Catholic nuns, near Cochin in Kerala, India. There was no operating theatre and few medicaments, and he worked as a general doctor attending to the fishermen and their families; he later told me that many of them had respiratory problems, which he thought might be an interesting thing to follow up on (see Appendix 2).

When asking my daughter Aina about her grandfather she said, 'I remember one of the last conversations I had with him. I was only 12 and was very curious as to why he was always rubbing his hands together as though he was washing them, at different times of the day. He explained that it was because he had been a surgeon before retiring and that he did it unconsciously. I realised that despite having retired

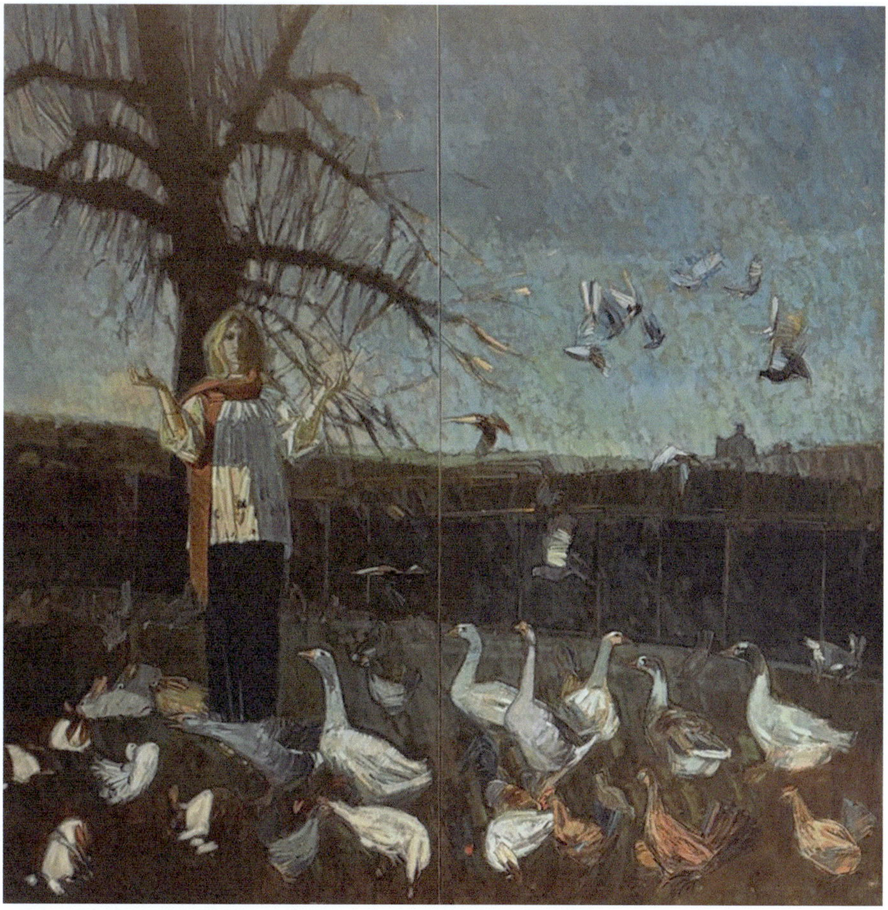

Fig. 2 Goose Girl by Don McKinlay (originally one of the murals in the Royal Liverpool University Hospital)

he was still a surgeon at heart and perhaps for that reason he always had an ability with his hands that few have. He would always be teaching my sister, Bianca and I how to be creative with our hands, whether it was painting, writing, making ceramics, or even making ice cream! He would also tell us that no matter your age, you still needed to be creative and curious, and perhaps that is perhaps why even to his last days he was still learning Spanish in bed. Years later I realised that this curiosity for life, and willingness to learn at 83 is not very common, and perhaps this was because he had found his true passion in life that he showed us how anything is possible. How you can be 20 or 80 and still be learning, and he is the perfect example of that'.

It is interesting that Aina noticed that habit, which combined with his 'party-trick' of writing with his left hand and signing cheques with his right hand, a result of his being left-handed but being physically forced to 'convert' to right-handed at school, was embedded in his character since his ambidextrousness was an obvious advantage for a surgeon.

These words written at the end of his obituary catch my father well (Fig. 3),

> There are many anecdotes involving such a colourful character, but John will be best remembered for his generosity of spirit, both ethereal and actual, his knowledge, skill and humanity as a general surgeon, his gifts as a teacher, his genuine pride and pleasure in the success of those he helped to train, and his unfailing courtesy and friendship to the many he encountered during a long life [3].

Nevertheless, my connection to surgery goes back even further since both my grandfathers were leading surgeons; contemporaries who often sat on the same Hospital boards. It is very different to write or speak about those you never knew; my paternal grandfather, Bryan McFarland died one year before I was born, but I have his writings and especially his speeches that say much about the man and both my father and my grandmother, who outlived him by 30 years, recounted many

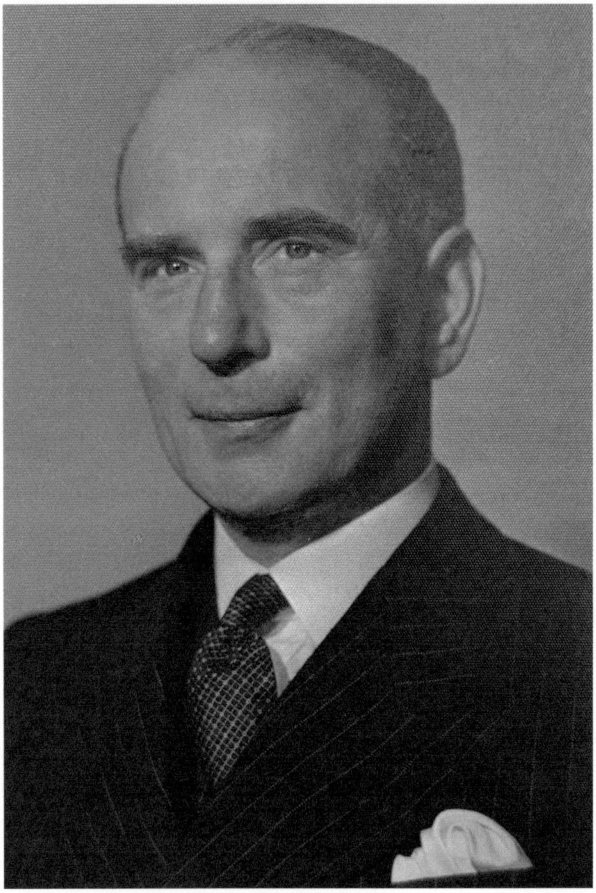

Fig. 3 McFarland family personal collection. (Bryan Leslie McFarland (1900–1963))

stories, and he was from all accounts 'larger than life', a fine, dedicated and extremely hard-working orthopaedic surgeon. Also, a raconteur, and after-dinner of some distinction. I will do my best to portray the man. My grandfather was born at the turn of the century in 1900, by all accounts a brilliant student, who qualified as a doctor from Liverpool University in 1922; and contributed to continuing to establish Liverpool as a world centre for orthopaedic teaching, being part of a long line of orthopaedic surgeons whose origins came from the bonesetters of Anglesey in North Wales. Bone setting in its time was considered,

> 'The art, it is true, may not be taught in schools, but it is as old as Hippocrates'.

Sir Robert Jones, the founder of the Liverpool school and often referred to as the father of orthopaedic surgery was the great great grandson of Evan Thomas (1804–1884), a renowned bone setter, was my grandfather's teacher and mentor, 'indeed the inspiration and magnetic personality of Robert Jones shone through many of his own qualities. He had the same happy, twinkling eyes, warm heart, deep sense of friendship, love of children, gift of humour and fund of anecdote. He too showed open honesty with disdain of pomp and arrogance. His intuitive simplicity was a heritage of conservative philosophy broadened by awareness of new advance. With kind humanity he carried the torch of Robert Jones' [11].

Many believed that Bryan with his kind humanity carried the torch of Robert Jones. Like his son, he also studied at Liverpool and was one of the first four candidates to become master of Orthopaedic surgery in 1926: two years later gaining his fellowship of The Royal College of Surgeons in Edinburgh. Clinically, he devoted a great deal of his work serving crippled children, rickets being a severe problem in those times. In 1948 he became director of Orthopaedic studies, and later Professor, where he was the prime mover behind the remarkable international success of the postgraduate course Orthopaedic Studies, which meant that he travelled and lectured around the world. Curiously enough, I was testimony to this when more than 30 years after his death, I was taken to a traumatologist in Gregorio Marañon Hospital in Madrid who on seeing my surname asked whether I was the son of Professor McFarland. He was not talking about my father but about Bryan who had died more than 30 years earlier.

A close colleague said of him,

> 'McFarland's contributions to the discussions were typical of him, direct, and often pungent, and scorning all pretence and humbug. With McFarland at the head, the postgraduate school flourished.' [11]

These qualities stood him in good stead in the many councils and associations he presided over, including the Liverpool Medical Institution,[5] University Club, Merseyside branch of the BMA and the Liverpool Philomatic Society, as well as founder of the British Editorial board of the *Journal of Bone and Joint Surgery*.

[5] https://www.lmi.org.uk/

He neither went to First World War, being too young, nor the Second World War, being too old. Nevertheless, in the latter he was much needed for Liverpool suffered nearly as much as London with bombing blitzes since it was in those days one of the principal ports in the world. In his inaugural address to the Liverpool Medical Institution in 1956, he spoke of 'Adjustment to Adversity',

> 'No one who has been in practice for many years, even in consultant practice, can fail to be impressed with the incredible variety of human behaviour. The reaction of the human mind and spirit is unpredictable and incalculable, not only by the observer but even by the persons themselves. It is in fact this element of infinite variety that makes mass control of the medical practice by regulation and formula quite impossible. One has but to touch the memory to evoke recollections of incidents and of statements which are so out of the ordinary and so unexpected as to be almost beyond belief. I remember the opening remarks of an old lady of eighty-four, blind and bedridden by an old un-united fracture of the neck of the femur. She was wheeled into the consulting room; there were no preliminaries, no "good morning"; no "how do you do.?"

"Young man," she said, give me your hand, I am blind. I want to say that I don't mind if you kill me by your operation as long as the alternative is that I shall walk' [12]. At the end of this speech he said, 'We must be careful lest by the meretricious temptation of some attractive treatment we are led to obstruct the natural processes of living tissues, and we must be alert to take advantage of the almost infinite capacity of the human body to adjust itself to adversity' [12]. This rings so true now, in twenty-first-century medicine where there is a growing backlash against over-diagnosis, over-treatment and over-medicalization.

Perhaps however he will be remembered for his tenacity and courage; in one of his many after-dinner speeches, The Will to Live, he remarked 'so it is with the will to live: through difficulties surmounted, fear overcome, and pain endured the will is strengthened and the core of endurance is tempered hard'.

In that same speech he said, 'The times are troubled and trying; the present appears treacherous and the future uncertain. But if we put our doubting mind in its place, and if instead we search the hearts within us, we shall find a sense of inevitable success and a feeling of ultimate triumph' [13].

Words whose sentiments certainly ring true now more than ever, perhaps but words that resonate within me, his grandson (Fig. 4).

My maternal grandfather, Andrew McKie Reid, like Bryan McFarland was also President of the Liverpool Medical Institution founded in 1779. He was slightly older than my paternal grandfather and thus was involved in both world wars; his medical training being interrupted in 1914 to enlist and fight in the First World War, where he was involved in the horrors of the battles of the Somme, Messines Ridge and Passchendaele, and received the MC (Military Cross). He was gravely wounded in March 1918, a German soldier, believing him to be lying dead in no man's land, used my grandfather's pistol to shoot the three remaining bullets into his body.

In 1964 (the year I was born) he wrote the following about his experience 46 years earlier,

'I lost consciousness and then came to and felt my breeches filling with blood. I thought the subclavian artery had gone and I managed to roll over, tear open my

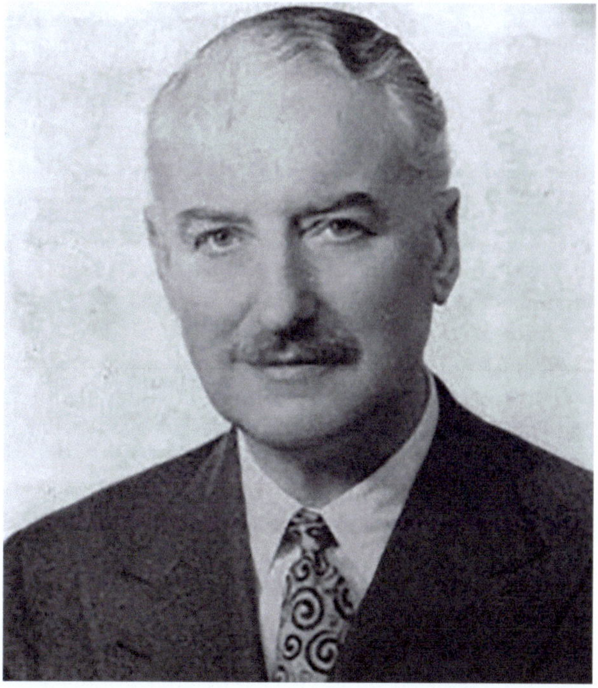

Fig. 4 McFarland family personal collection. Andrew McKie Reid (1893–1973)

trench coat, tunic and shirt with my left hand and saw and felt blood spurting from the cavity round the fold of the right axilla. I plugged the hole with the third finger of my left hand and there it remained for two days. My life, or soul, or spirit, call it what you will, became dissociated from my body, and from a height of five feet I looked at the helpless body.' [14]

Later, in a German war hospital he befriended the surgeon persuading him to save his right arm, and this I am sure played a part in his decision to specialize at the end of the war in eye surgery. This also gave him a peculiar rolling style of fly-fishing. Later in life he used his disabilities cannily. He was deaf in one ear because of his serious wounding at the second Battle of the Somme so his deafness was very useful when it was his turn to pay for a round of drinks. However, he was the first to respond affirmatively when a glass of champagne was being offered. Selective deafness we might call it.

After a year's recovery back in England and finishing his medical studies, he did further postgraduate training in London, Paris and Vienna before returning to Liverpool's St. Paul's Eye Hospital, where he practised and taught both at the department of ophthalmology and the department of tropical medicine. In the Second World War he commanded the First Western General Hospital, seeing service first in Norway and later he was a consultant ophthalmologist in both Africa and India.

He was a distinguished eye surgeon, also responsible for designing the 'recumbent spectacles', which were visual aids for patients suffering from spiral lesions and other diseases who were confined to bed in a supine position for weeks or every month. Those were in the days when patients stayed for prolonged periods hospitalized, and of course, iPhones or iPads had not been invented.

However, he was a true 'Man of the Arts', a collector of modern British Art as well as Chinese antiquities and for many years he chaired the Royal Liverpool Philharmonic Society, once hosting Artur Rubinstein to dinner who, to the delight of the other guests, played and signed the piano. He played an active role in the politics of his city, being on the council for ten years, to such an extent that at his funeral they closed the streets for the funeral cortège, and three thousand attended his funeral at the Liverpool Anglican Cathedral.

In the words of his contemporary and friend, Lord Cohen of Birkenhead,

'His friends will remember him as one who enriched their lives by his devotion to their welfare, by his selfless loyalty to their interests, by his indomitable courage and fearlessness, and by his inflexible integrity. Few have served their country, their city, and their profession with greater devotion and to better purpose.'

Both my grandfathers were on many hospital boards and health board meetings together and the rumour is that if they were both at the same meeting, it might go on for a little longer than expected. The memory of my father and both grandfathers have inspired the idea of this book, since all three, in their distinctive ways, were firm believers that both medicine and surgery were a combination of science and art, and that the relationship between the doctor/surgeon and the patient was the key. A good surgeon needed (and needs) to build a bridge of trust with their patients.

This stance evokes the words written about King James IV,

> 'This noble king James IV was well learned in the Art of Medicine, and also a cunning Chirurgener that none in his realm, that used that craft but would take his Counsel in all their Proceedings.' [15]

Afterword

Late summer of 1994 battling north against the Meltemi, the wind was strong 5-6 Beaufort scale perhaps, the sky a brilliant translucent blue. No clouds to be seen, white, whipping sea-horse waves. The Meltemi is also known as the 'katabalic wind', and suddenly appears coming south from the Bosphorus across the Aegean Sea; it is known as the etesian wind (from the Greek word etesios which means 'annual') and in Turkish it is meltem, meaning sea breeze. We were trying to go straight into it, trying to make progress, sometimes we could go forwards, sometimes backwards, a struggle with nature but the three of us were invigorated by this challenge; the three being my father at the helm, myself and our beautiful boat, Nuada of the Silver Hand, a 32 foot long-keeled Vancouver. The boat's name had been carefully chosen and researched by my father since in Irish mythology Nuada was the first king of the Tuatha De Danann, a supernatural race in Irish mythology. They were often depicted as druids, bards and healers. Nuada is famous for supposedly losing his hand in battle and regaining it after being magically healed by Dian

Cecht, the Irish god of healing who gave him a silver hand and he ruled as king for another 20 years. So, we had an Irish mythological king on our side on the seas of Odysseus, curiously all boats in English are female and Nuada was no exception since we always referred to the boat as ‘her’ (Fig. 5).

Sailing at full throttle into the wind, heading for Patmos, my father turned towards me and with a grin commented, ‘Never forget, these are the glory days’. He was 63 years old, and he, like King Nuada, lived on for another 20 years.

My father ended his interview with these words, later shown at his memorial in December 2013 in Liverpool,

‘It’s often forgotten and crazily overlooked that the sea is larger in area, in capacity, i.e. weight, than the landmass above the sea. There’s more sea and what amazes me is that so much is still being spent on exploring space when we are so ignorant about so much that is going on in the deep part of the sea.

People either hate the sea and fear the sea or they love the sea with a very special feeling and can’t imagine not being able to look out and see the sea, and that’s me’ [2].

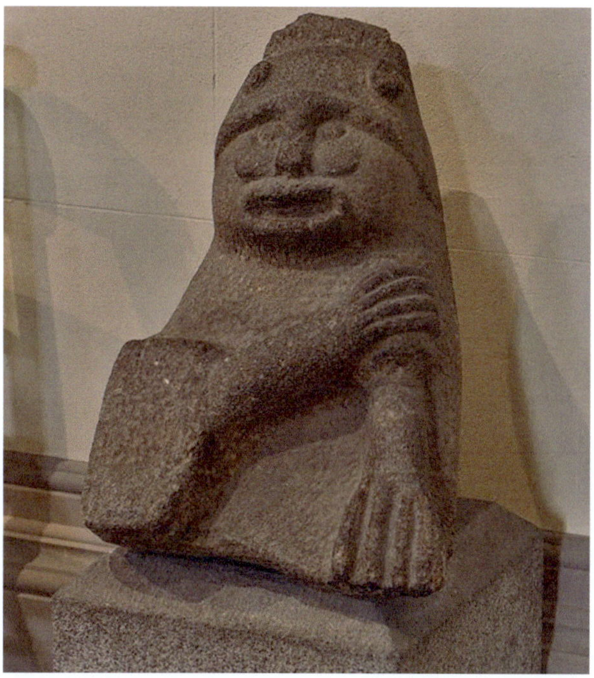

Fig. 5 This sculpture is assumed to be of 1000 B.C. origin and depicting King Nuada who lost his left arm in a battle and got a prosthetic arm which he is holding with his right arm. St. Patrick’s Cathedral of the Church of Ireland, Armagh, County Armagh, Northern Ireland. (https://en.m.wikipedia.org/wiki/File:Armagh_St._Patrick%27s_Cathedral_of_the_Church_of_Ireland_North_Aisle_%E2%80%9CTandragee_Man%E2%80%9C_2019_09_09_(cropped).jpg#filelinks)

Appendices

1. THE SOUL DIVIDED—John McFarland—2010

“A wonderful thing in a wonderful world
Is the healing of wounds” Sir John Bland-Sutton
(events happened during the Mau Mau Rebellion around 1954)

Sing of Africa, the fierce
Amidst jungle and trees, light and shade,
Misty mornings and dark goodnights.
Care for these things, they belong to no-one
but the people who by the river come and go.

The Dawa river ebbs and flows
water and mud the staple source,
Amidst the mud the crocodiles
to the greasy water go,
under thick grass where natives bathe.
A splash, a scream, a blood ripple in the strand
teeth marks score the sand.

Otherwise left alone when villagers from a higher creek
with sticks and stones beat off the muddied bloodied ‘mamba’.
The bone is sheltered by the skin and then the periosteum
clinging like ivy sends its horrors to the brain.
Now wreathed in pus, pus like fire feeds on itself
Grows only to die; it is not itself disease but mirrors death
like plastering snow, sunbaked meringue, the life within her
Flickers three long weeks.

The girl neither lives, nor dies
Awaiting rescue from the skies
But there’s nothing here
only shadows, grassland, swamp, and sand.

“Look! there are the trees”, now gone
The engine, beast of the air, coughs, growls
Beasts of the land moving like oil spilled on yellow plastic
When a door swings into space,
“slipstream” “hold it in” pilot to passenger

Bundled in the back, the girl,
life measured in her fevered pulse,
Beat fails to meet beat.
Above circles vultures of the air, riding the thermals and
surveying the leg and blood congealing in the sand.
Death is fragile.

"Keep the machine running"
"Are you sure about this, Sir?"

But vultures, cleaners of all, know and stay high in the air
The world we fly is not visible,
the plane a tiny thing,
Only the girl and I, and the darkening bush.
No sound beyond the engines roar
And, then the silence of the clouds.
The floor she lay on was like a plastic cage
I heard her moan; I felt her wrist
Can we call one soul an 'other'?
If one fades out, may we expect another

Shadows of darkness cross the sky
I sink morphine into a vein, I cannot take it out again.
She is pulseless on the floor, a "bundle" in my keeping
the pain gone, but in her eyes
No life.

The dead cannot live again, they are gone
A last quick touching of her hand.
The sky darkens in patches, scant blood goes to needed places,
Above the circling vultures, scouts of Zoroaster,
the girl with no leg to speak of.
Casting no shadow in the air, the plane a shadow in the sand
Death now ahead, now trailing,
Through her blood the morphine carried, seeped
and touched the brain which could not touch back.
Spiked with pain, spiked with morphine, she lay a twisted young ghost
I reach to feel the shivering arm, the pulse.
"No insurance for night landing," the pilot whispers;
While many pilots get some small applause
for us, the silence was enough, the kerosene in tubs
The smell of trees above the desert.

On landing, a new beginning,
the girl still breathing.
And on to the hospital,
And the surgeon, grumpy seamster, shiny knife,
blunted fingers, absent wife,
stabbed at the pus to find more pus, and under this, only anatomical
hopelessness, of tendons, nerves and bloody tubes,
Embedded in vats of slimy grey,
"No life here, let's go away."
But pulsing through the slime and squelch

Were vessels carrying blood from one to each,
And, without the leg, to sink the bloody show
The healing process could begin.
God gives but takes away; this from love
Seems strange to me.

2. Kulantapith—John McFarland (the 1980s)

The Bitter Snows, Keylong
The bitter snows of Shingo-La
Whose juice when squeezed
Throws fear upon these Lahaul hills
Send through in torrents death that rides
Far down the slopes we cannot see
But in our hearts, we know the cold that kills.
Here is the Lama seeking his dharma
Muttering prayers for all his souls
Aware of sickness and of terror
That may destroy us now forever.
In days to come we know the moment
When our heart turned in to eat itself
But we shall always hear the screams
Of valleys tearing icy walls apart,
See traces like cobwebs blown
To dust that will lead us only in our dreams.
Yet still the Lama less his dharma,
Mutters prayers for all his souls,
Aware of sickness and of terror
That may destroy us now forever.
The peak ice glistens in the sun,
The rivers trickle where torrents fell
Bridges strengthened, roads are tended
And the sun begins to heal the dread
But the ice knife twisted cut to hurt
That wounded deep, leaves scars not mended.
And though the Lama finds his dharma,
Has said his prayers for all his souls,
He knows his sickness and the terror
That now may destroy us forever.

Jonathan McFarland
Aina McFarland Rojas

Bibliography

1. McFarland JB. Deus Machina, unpublished, written in 1952.
2. Lopez D. Interview with John McFarland. 2009. https://youtu.be/xmhzz3z_P78?si=dmLMt7WKLwJKbz8D
3. Royal College of Surgeons, London. Sir John Temple. March 2014 https://livesonline.rcseng.ac.uk/client/en_GB/lives/search/detailnonmodal/ent:$002f$002fSD_ASSET$002f0$002fSD_ASSET:376972/one?qu=%22rcs%3A+E004789%22&rt=false%7C%7C%7CIDENTIFIER%7C%7C%7CResource+Identifier&h=0
4. McFarland JB. The lengthened shadows of four men. An essay concerning Darwin, Paget, Lister and Thomas, Unpublished talk. 1963. Jackson, Mississippi.
5. McFarland JB. James IV Travelling Report. 1976.
6. McFarland JB. Basic clinical surgery for nurses and medical students. Butterworths. 1973.
7. Peabody FW. The care of the patient. JAMA. 1927;88(12):877–882. https://doi.org/10.1001/jama.1927.02680380001001.
8. Heath I. The patient Earth is sick, but the medical doctors are mainly absent. BJGP LIFE, 30 July 2023. https://bjgplife.com/the-patient-earth-is-sick-but-the-medical-doctors-are-mainly-absent/.
9. Garstin C. Publisher, Frederick A. Stokes Company, 1923. Original from, Oxford University.
10. Taleb NN. 1960- author. The Black Swan: the impact of the highly improbable. New York: Random House. 2007.
11. Journal of Bone and Joint Surgery, pages 196–198. British Number – February 1963, Vol 45-B, No. 1.
12. McFarland B. Adjustment to adversity. Inaugural address, Liverpool Medical Institution, 11th October 1958.
13. McFarland B. The will to live. Presidential address to the Liverpool Philomatic Society, 16th March 1949.
14. McKie Reid A. A personal account of his first world war experiences, 1964. Unpublished.
15. Guthrie D. King James the fourth of Scotland: his influence on medicine and science. Bull Hist Med 1947;21(2):173–192. http://www.jstor.org/stable/44441140/.

Contents

1 Listen to Me: Why Narrative Medicine and Bioethics Matter 1
Susana Magalhães
1.1 The Ethical Node of Health Care and the Role of Narrative Bioethics & Medicine 3
1.2 Narrative Medicine/Ethics: Shifting Perspectives 6
1.3 Final Remarks 8
References 9

2 Conversation with Surgeon 1—Suzy Elneil 11
René Génadry

3 A Personal Reflection on the Core of Medical Practice 23
José Poças
3.1 Introduction 23
3.2 The Mission of the Physician 24
3.3 The Medical Act 25
3.4 Technology in Medical Practice 27
3.5 The Doctor-Patient Relationship 29
3.6 Conclusions 31
Bibliography 33

4 Conversation with Surgeon 2—Manuel Pera 35
Jacek Mostwin

5 Caring for Others Through Relationships: Pedagogical Approaches Inspired by Narrative 47
Ana Filipa Cardoso
5.1 Caring for Others Through Relationships: Pedagogical Approaches Inspired by Narrative 47
5.2 Narrative Medicine 50
5.3 Once Upon a Time 52
5.4 Tell Me More About Yourself 53

5.5 My Story Through an Object . . . 55
5.6 I Am a Person, Not a Number . . . 56
5.7 Assessing People Suffering . . . 57
5.8 Healing by Presence . . . 58
5.9 Being in Other's Hands . . . 58
5.10 Personal Narrative Writing . . . 59
5.11 Our Bodies, Our Selves . . . 59
5.12 Feeling Vulnerable . . . 61
5.13 Empathetic Words . . . 61
References . . . 62

6 Conversation with Surgeon 3—William Reiner . . . 65
Jacek Mostwin

7 Art as Medicine . . . 87
Ana Zão
7.1 Art and the Person-Centered Approach . . . 87
7.2 Art as Medicine: Art Prescription, from Health Promotion to Prevention and Treatment . . . 88
7.2.1 Music as Medicine . . . 88
7.2.2 Other Art-Based Therapies . . . 95
7.2.3 Culture Prescription in an "Artificial Intelligence World" . . 95
7.3 Art and Medical Training . . . 96
7.4 Medicine—The Art of Caring for Others . . . 97
7.5 Conclusion . . . 98
References . . . 99

8 Conversation with Surgeon 4—Christopher Wolfgang . . . 103
Jacek Mostwin

9 To Be or Not to Be . . . 125
Margarida Lobo Antunes
9.1 Education and Future Doctors . . . 125
9.2 Medical Humanities . . . 127
9.3 Narrative Medicine . . . 128
9.4 Literature . . . 129
9.5 Art . . . 132
9.6 The Future . . . 133
References . . . 134

10 Conversation with Surgeon 5—Jeff Wilkinson . . . 135
René Génadry

11 Humanism and Medicine: Quo Vadis 147
Jacek Mostwin
11.1 Medicine Is the Study of the Person 147
11.2 What Is Humanism in Medicine? 148
11.3 What Is a University For? 149
11.4 The Cultures of the Academic World. 150
11.5 Medical Curriculum Evolution 150
11.6 Critical Incidents, Personal Experience and Reflection: Pathways to Learning. 151
11.7 The Natural Philosophy of Medical Students 153
11.8 The Role of the Subjective, Qualitative, and Experiential in Learning. 154
11.9 Experience and Epiphany. 155
11.10 Humanism and Medicine: Quo Vadis?. 158
11.11 Helping Students to Makes Sense of Their Own Experience 158
11.12 The Humanism of Medicine Is in the Medicine 161
11.13 Summary 162
Bibliography 164

12 Conversation with Surgeon 6—John Tarpley. 167
Jacek Mostwin

13 The Word and the Hand. 207
Manuel Pera and Jonathan McFarland
13.1 Introduction 207
13.2 The Word 209
13.3 The Hand (Fig. 13.2) 213
13.4 Touch (Fig. 13.3) 214
13.5 Conclusion 218
13.6 Afterword. 219
References. 220

14 Conversation with Surgeon 7—James Handa 223
René Génadry

15 Shared Decision-Making 235
João M. Silva
15.1 Introduction 235
15.2 Patient–Physician Relationship 237
15.3 What Does Humanism Mean for Us? 239
15.4 Surgery Nowadays 240
15.5 What is the Problem Then? 241
15.6 Shared Decision-Making in Surgery 243
15.7 Conclusion 244
Reference 244

16 Conversation with Surgeon 8—Judith Goh 245
René Génadry

17 Do Surgeons Dream of Robotic Sheep? 255
Paolo Casella
17.1 Surgeon's Hands 255
17.2 What Do Surgeons Think? 256
17.3 Do Surgeons Write? 257
17.4 Do Surgeons Talk? 258
17.5 Do Surgeons Dream? 258
17.6 Do Surgeons Suffer? 259
17.7 Surgeons Are Human 259
17.8 Moscow Rules for Residents 260

18 Conversation with Surgeon 9—Michael Breen 263
René Génadry

19 The Aesthetics of Surgery 271
Pia M. Sorto, Hrvoje Baric, Magnus Tisell, and Antti Huotarinen
19.1 The Beauty of the Physical Dimension and Love of Nature 273
19.2 The Intellectual Beauty of Aesthetic Acts and Reasonable Surgical Decision-Making 276
19.3 The Beauty of the Virtues and of the Absolute Good in Surgery 279
19.4 The Master as the Standard of the Good Taste in Surgery 280
19.5 Surgery Is a Perfect Field for Inquiry into Beauty 281
References 281

20 Conversation with Surgeon 10—Steve Arrowsmith 283
René Génadry
Reference 297

21 Open and Closed Heart Surgery: Reality and Fantasy 299
Mark Mekelburg
21.1 Dr. Pipoca's First Visits in the Operating Block 303
21.2 No Way! Professionals Would Never Do That! 304
21.3 Now That Guy's Got Some Rhythm 305
Reference 308

22 Conversation with Surgeon 11—Ana Pastor 309
Jonathan McFarland

23 Humanism in Surgery 329
Patrick C. Walsh

24 Conversation with Surgeon 12—John Varallo 333
René Génadry

25 Learning from the Human Experience of Patients and Practitioners 343
Jacek Mostwin
25.1 "I Never Understood It Until Now" 343
25.2 Reconstructing Illness from Patient Experience 346
25.3 Lives in Medicine as a Sub-Genre of Life-Writing 349
25.4 The Physician's Voice 356
25.5 Summary 370
Bibliography 372

Epilogue 375

Acknowledgements 377

Biographies of Surgeons 381

Chapter 1
Listen to Me: Why Narrative Medicine and Bioethics Matter

Susana Magalhães

Preamble

Narrative Medicine: dialogical and polyphonic approach to care

> Person-centred care is a question of ethical stance and not merely one of a range of tools in health care. ([17], p. 7)

Defined by Rita Charon as "medicine practised with the narrative competency to recognize, interpret, and be moved to action by the predicament of others" ([4], p. vii), NM has spread from the USA to Europe since 2001, adopting different forms and shapes, but always rooted in the same principles: attention/creativity, representation, and affiliation/reconciliation. Language and Interpretation, which have been central to this interdisciplinary field, are underlined by Brian Hurwitz:

> Narrative Medicine is a practice and an intellectual stance which enables physicians to look beyond the biological mechanisms at the centre of conventional approaches to medical practice, toward domains of thought and ways of telling that focus on language and representation, on the emotions and relationships which illuminate health care practice ([10], 73).

Nowadays two of the challenges we face are how to make the best out of the digital technologies for the benefit of patients, caregivers, and health professionals and how to promote health literacy in the digital world of information (which is not necessarily a world of knowledge). Digital platforms can be user-friendly and provide all these stakeholders access to narrative-enriched healthcare. At the same time, internet pathographies may be a relevant resource for medical providers seeking to develop narrative competence. Studies have been conducted using different categories of illness narratives as objects of analysis and interpretation not only to improve medical practice but also to better understand the social fabric and the

S. Magalhães (✉)
Institute for research and innovation in health (i3S)-University of Porto
University Fernando Pessoa, Porto, Portugal
e-mail: susana.magalhaes@i3s.up.pt

J. McFarland et al. (eds.), *Humanism in Surgery*, New Paradigms in Healthcare,
https://doi.org/10.1007/978-3-031-86018-8_1

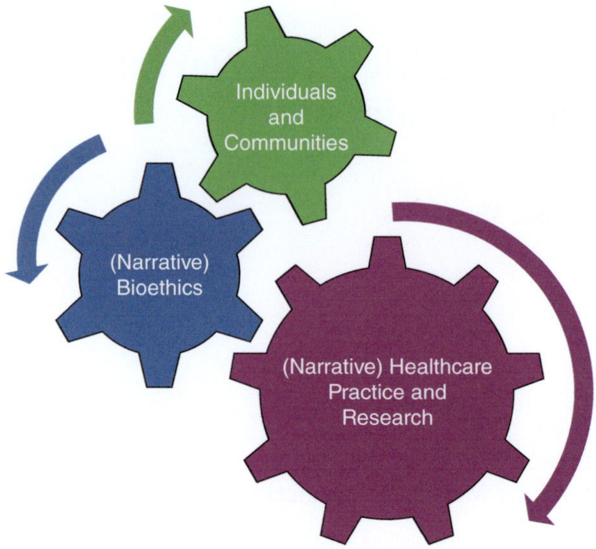

Fig. 1.1 Dialogical and polyphonic approach to healthcare

contradictions of social interaction and self-presentation. According to Marini [12], the studies based on the analysis of "the text written by patients, by healthcare professionals and by relatives provide us with a better understanding of the culture, the values, the needs, the preferences, the personal and professional projects of all the persons involved in healthcare" (Fig. 1.1).

A dialogic and polyphonic approach allows us to open narrative medicine to fields that have not been so much considered throughout NM's (still) short life span: bioethics, health literacy, and scientific research. The narrative categories that are the focus of NM training should be explored not only in healthcare practice, but also in bioethical reflection on healthcare, public health, and biomedical research. Time, Space, Voice, Characters, and Plot are narrative categories that should guide those who interact within these healthcare dimensions. To focus on the person and not only on the patient, on the individual community member, and not only on the profile of the average citizen. Health professionals, researchers, and health literacy experts should have narrative skills that integrate those narrative categories in their reasoning. Making meaning out of conflicting voices is the main aim of a dialogical approach.

The focus of NM is to set up a relational healthcare ecosystem and to provide tools for practice and reflection that can be applied in all the dimensions of healthcare: institutional, communitarian, and individual.

1.1 The Ethical Node of Health Care and the Role of Narrative Bioethics & Medicine

Together with the ethical question "what should I do?" NM requires us to think about the journey that has led us to a particular problem. Narratives make us aware of our finitude; allow us to imagine ourselves in the future and to design possible futures. According to Weiss and Swede [18], "narrative reciprocity implies that the care situation is an interaction between equal participants who collaboratively construct meaning rather than one where the expert practitioner dictates meaning to a patient". This is contrary to the common bioethical view on the role of the ethicist "as a disinterested expert providing counsel rather than a community member who is intractably involved and invested and has particular interests. More important, bioethics usually insists on separating theory from practice, missing the point that theory finds its meaning only in the context of the inquiry." ([13], 27). NM provides tools and concepts to address the narrativity of ethical issues within healthcare, while allowing patients, caregivers, and health professionals to see themselves in the mirror, recognizing their own vulnerabilities.

The approach applied within narrative medicine & narrative bioethics is based on the concept of thinking about and thinking with ethics:

- To think about ethics is to reflect on ethical questions, on different approaches to ethical problems, on different ways of responding to the concerns, which we face in our personal and professional contexts.
- Thinking with ethics happens whenever the reflections we make in a certain time and place perpetuate and accompany us, like characters of movies/novels that revisit us and are part of our interiority (Fig. 1.2).

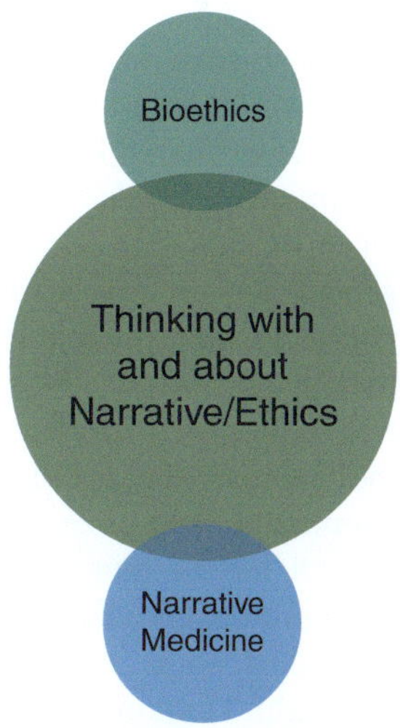

Fig. 1.2 Relationship between narratives and ethics

Using the lens of this approach to reflect upon values such as Dignity, Autonomy, and Vulnerability sets up the bridge with the depth of lived experience, giving meanings that would otherwise be too much abstract for clinical ethical reflection:

> Suffering. I know a lot about the suffering of parents, because I have felt it and because I can guess it in other parents, based on my experience and imperfect knowledge of the human species. However, I do not know if I can talk about doctors' suffering with the suffering of others, what that suffering does to them, if they tell a story or if they come home having left their suffering in a locker, along with a gown and a stethoscope. I think a lot about the two doctors who were in Madalena's room the minute she died. They left the room discreetly, to give the parents a space of intimacy. Where did they go after leaving a room where a seven-year-old child had died? What did they say to each other? What did they say to their husbands/children when they were asked, "So how was your day?"
>
> I don't know, but I think a lot about it.
>
> Is there a crossing for health professionals? (João de Bragança, President of Acreditar and Former President of the Childhood Cancer International Organisation)

The testimony provided by João de Bragança points out the importance of paying attention to the way patients and their families "read" their physicians and how they need health professionals to remain persons. The doubt signaled above—"Where did they go after leaving the room where a seven-year-old child had just died?"—echoes the position of humility that should be required by the health team. A position of cultural and narrative humility, based on the development of self-awareness:

> Narrative humility acknowledges that our patients' stories are not objects that we can comprehend or master, but rather dynamic entities that we can approach and engage with, while simultaneously remaining open to their ambiguity and contradiction, and engaging in constant self-evaluation and self-critique about issues such as our own role in the story, our expectations of the story, our responsibilities to the story, and our identifications with the story—how the story attracts or repels us because it reminds us of any number of personal stories. ([6], 981)

This is particularly relevant concerning the use of AI in biomedical research and healthcare: humility is the cornerstone of ethics by design since it is precisely because we do not know what the future holds that we need to reflect ethically from the moment we plan and design an AI system until it is implemented and beyond. Uncertainty looms ahead regarding the benefits and risks posed by AI in our lives in general and in healthcare in particular. The European AI Act points out potential risks regarding the manipulation of human beings, with specific emphasis on vulnerable groups; the discrimination driven by biased algorithms and the generalization of biometric identification systems that can eventually lead to remote control of individuals and populations. The framework of principles proposed by the European Community addresses these risks and has a substantial echo in the scientific world: respect for the human agency (keeping humans in the loop), that is, respect for autonomy, dignity, and freedom; the right to privacy and data protection; fairness; individual, social and environmental well-being; transparency; accountability and oversight. Thinking with and about ethics requires the normative framework of principles and values pointed out by the European Community, but it also demands *listening to the narratives of all the stakeholders*, who live in these times of uncertainties masked by the certainty provided by some kind of storytellers. Therefore, we are facing a quite challenging time: reflecting ethically upon AI is worthwhile only if we seize the opportunity to reflect upon the society that is feeding the AI systems. However, this does not seem to be a time prone to ethical reflection, due to the current cultural context: we are immersed in information that tends to discipline our communities, to close the entrance to other worldviews, to provide recipes for healthy, successful, and productive individuals, within an anesthetized/palliative society [8].

Regarding the use of AI in healthcare, the pace of technological advances is much faster than the rhythm needed for stepping back and looking into the mirror. Trust is the basis of physician/patient relationship and AI can deconstruct it in case it is used as a black box. Even though explainable AI is the only acceptable form in all the European guidelines, it can easily get lost in the winding path we are walking:

> AI models simply learn correlations in data, not the causal relationships involved. Causal models are needed to disentangle correlation from causation. For example, if a study indicates that levels of vitamin D in a population correlate with depression, that does not mean one caused the other, or they are both simply symptoms of an (as yet unknown) underlying problem» ([15], p. 110).

Assuming AI as a tool supervised by human agency is crucial with a special focus on promoting empathy and compassion side by side with non-empathic technology. Programming AI to be nonbiased, non-discriminatory, fair, and protective of human rights and personal data requires reflecting upon the reality that is feeding the algorithms: metrics, evidence-based medicine, technology mediation in healthcare, healthcare curricula with humanities as appendixes that try to convey the meaning of empathy to a student while presenting role models that are contrary to empathic relations. As Offri points out,

> No matter how efficient medicine becomes, no matter how computerized, automated, algorithmed, wireless, evidence based or 'QA'ed'it becomes, medicine will always boil down to one caregiver with one patient, in one room, with one story. Effective healthcare, therefore, requires narrative competence (…). ([16], p. 1006)

The humility required for ethical reflection on AI should be the basis of medical education regarding a doctor-patient relationship, assuming that in some cases empathy may not be possible. The gap between health professionals and patients regarding the social, literacy, and medical context may be so wide that empathic attitudes might get hampered. Moreover, the whole ethical reflection taking place around and on AI should be framed within the historical background of ethical thinking in healthcare, making visible the (sometimes) invisible framework of human values underlying the healthcare ecosystem.

Narrative competence is required not only to set up meaningful relationships with others, but also to be self-aware, to know one's own strengths and weaknesses, as well as one's own biases and perceptions, which "can lead to attitudes that are tone deaf and decisions that are discordant with patients' perceptions, values, and goals. Distorted compassion—that is compassion based on tainted or inaccurate perceptions of another person's suffering—can lead to ostensibly well-intended advice, actions, or inactions that may be completely at odds with what the patient really wants. Rather than feeling that they have been heard, distorted compassion can result in patients feeling devalued, misunderstood, and further demoralized at the very hands of those who are meant to help." ([5], p. 855)

Likewise, revisiting the concept of Vulnerability as layers and not as a label generally applied to the average citizen, and perceiving the depth of it, will certainly influence the way scientists and healthcare professionals relate to different vulnerable persons (from a cultural and narrative humility position). Being aware of the different types of vulnerability—medical, cognitive, deferential, allocational, and infrastructural [11]—together with healthcare practices that keep the personhood of patients and professionals can actually make a difference in avoiding the trap of false information and imprudent ethical decisions:

- Reflective practice among healthcare team members can provide safe spaces for revisiting terms and concepts that need to be clear to all, so that the message conveyed to patients is not contradictory and can actually add up to health literacy. Terms and concepts such as advanced health care directive and living will, end of life, terminally ill, futile treatments/interventions, therapeutic obstinacy, death, health, and normalcy can be revisited by healthcare team members, using reflective writing and reflective sharing tools provided by NM to outline guidance on the meaning of the words used in their daily practice.
- Being aware that our communities are affected by chronic diseases and multiple comorbidities, it is clear that self-management of the health condition already plays an important role. Not only are communities required to share resources that address their own members' needs, but the healthcare system and decision makers are also challenged to design interactive pathways based on sound communication, integration, and collaboration.

1.2 Narrative Medicine/Ethics: Shifting Perspectives

> Oral historian Alessandro Portelli has written extensively about mutuality in the relationship between field researcher and subject, but his comments can be easily applied to the clinical relationship. He writes, "an interview is an exchange between two subjects: literally a mutual sighting. One party cannot really see the other unless the other can see him or her in turn. The two interacting subjects cannot act together unless some kind of mutuality can be established. Thus, the [clinician] has an objective stake in equality." In other words, by entering into a stance of narrative humility, the physician is fostering a state in which, as Broyard has observed, even as the physician examines the patient, the patient is able to examine the physician. ([6], p. 981)

NM is three dimensional, including training, practice, and research. In these three areas, narrative is the key point, being both a tool and the content of the interactions taking place. Narrative-based training, narrative-based practice, and narrative-based research use transversal methods, namely closed reading, reflective writing, sharing to care, and caring to share. To these strategies, we can add two more proposed by Nash et al.[14] as the basis for a co-curricular medical storytelling program: co-construction and compelling performance of stories. Close reading and collaborative creative writing, followed by the performance of the story, raises awareness of narrative reciprocity that characterizes all care settings: equal participants interact and collaboratively construct meaning ([18], p. 4).

Writing is not only a way to represent reality, but it is also a tool that accrues knowledge to previous representations and allows for uncertainty to be expressed, unveiling aspects of the patient's journey that are not possible to grasp in the conventional electronic medical record:

> I came to understand that I had accrued deep knowledge about my patients that remained unavailable to me— and, by extension, to them— until I wrote it down, whether as a representation of so-called fact or as fiction. I often show patients what I've written about them, mostly to check my understanding of what they have told me. I ask them, in effect, 'Did I get it right?' The dividends of such simple doctorly writing are many. Patients have evidence showing that I'm trying hard to listen. More powerfully, my writing, I believe, helps my patients to feel heard. After reading what I've written, a patient might say, "We left something out", and then tell of clinically important matters that otherwise would have taken years to disclose. ([3], p. 404)

Based on this perspective, Charon implemented a new tool, the so-called parallel chart, as a narrative-based medical record where there is space for health practitioners to register how their interactions with patients affect or resonate with them, exposing unique dimensions of care. This tool is used not only in training sessions in narrative medicine (to promote reflective skills and to underline the role of the subjective dimension in healthcare), but also in the daily routine of healthcare teams. Reflective practice, using writing prompts, can be implemented in their meetings, shifting the focus from electronic medical records and clinical decision-making to narrative parallel charts and ethical deliberation. The writing prompts in training sessions are often used after close reading activities that require attention to all the narrative categories of the text, highlighting the ethical relationship between the reader and the text as the Other.

"The patient who died [to me]"; "The day I met error"; "Vulnerabilites in the face of difficult news"; "Being in the waiting room"; "On my way to hospital" are some of the writing prompts that can be worked out in narrative medicine training programs and at scientific and academic events, opening up safe spaces for sharing perspectives on issues that are usually left out of the clinical setting.

Intensive care and emergency rooms are not expected to be places of (self)-reflection due to the need to act promptly. Constant readiness to respond to the needs of those suffering in such hard contexts demands times of reflection on how one is acting and reasoning, and above all, on how one is being. In hospitals, patients experience a certain type of alienation from the time-constrained world of work, of commuting, and of opening and closing schedules. It is a similar experience to imprisonment, with the same type of depersonalization, defamiliarization, and Unheimlichkeit, thus demanding particular attention to all the dimensions that can improve the quality of this experience in the hospital, at discharge, and in the community. Listening to patients' perspectives on the impact of light, lack of privacy, noise, prescriptive environment, and lack of connection to the community is of utmost importance to implement person-centered care. The narratives of caregivers and health professionals also contribute to getting the gist of the text. The challenge lies in integrating these reading and listening attitudes and practices into a professional routine. The answer may be found in the integration of parallel charts in the conventional medical record, while providing patients with the opportunity to register their questions, suggestions, uncertainties and perspectives either in writing or by visual or recording mediums. Both parallel charts and patients' experience (digital) notebooks could provide narrative input for doctor and other health professionals/patients encounters, promoting practice-based evidence and practice-based bioethical deliberation.

The ethical stance mentioned at the beginning of this chapter would benefit from medical education that adopts NM in a transversal way. Ensuring this integration requires planning and ongoing evaluation. Remein CDiF et al. conducted a systematic review of the literature published in 2020 with the aim to address the question "how effective is the implementation and evaluation of NM programs in academic medicine and health sciences?" The conclusions were highly positive:

> Our findings demonstrate that NM has shown potential for enhancing communication and team-building skills, encouraging perspective-taking and reflection, promoting empathic behaviour, detecting/mitigating burnout, cultivating narrative competence, augmenting pedagogical and clinical skills, and fostering ethical inquiry. Based on our analysis and interpretation of the programmes reviewed, we recommend considering the inclusion of narrative-based education in curricula for medical/health sciences students, trainees and faculty. ([7], p. 10)

Narrative Medicine tools and concepts can therefore be applied in community at large to build bridges among biomedical scientists, health professionals, caregivers, arts and humanities researchers, journalists, patients' associations, and individual patients. Talking about the meaning of illness experience, scientific evidence-based knowledge on disease, and social constructs of illness can promote literacy, reducing the spread of false information and allowing decision-makers to actually address people's perspectives and their needs. Bearing in mind all the benefits of NM mentioned above, we believe it is high time we promoted this field in training, practice, and research.

1.3 Final Remarks

In a nutshell, NM gives depth to the healthcare ecosystem and deconstructs the threats raised by prejudices and stereotypes that can easily spread in the palliative society of our times. Instead of a one-size-fits-all all approach, narrative categories like voice, character, time, space, and plot remind us that evidence should also be practiced and individual-based. Only then can care delivery, design and management be actually improved.

The main resistance to NM implementation is rooted in the current mindset, focused on metrics and quantitative data, burdened with technology and checklists. Narrative and medical humanities are relationship-based, driven by the scent of time [9]:

> The current time crisis is connected with the absolutization of the vita active. It leads to a work imperative which reduces people to beasts of burden (animal laborans). Everyday hyperactivity depletes people's lives of all ability to linger and be contemplative. This renders a fulfilling experience of time impossible. Revitalization of the vita contemplativa and relearning of the art of lingering are essential to overcoming the current time crisis. (p.2)

Bearing in mind the acceleration induced by artificial intelligence, current and future healthcare professionals need to improve their relationship literacy, so that decision-makers, patients, and caregivers can see why relationship-based care really matters: a person taking care of another person requires the preservation of personhood [2] and personhood is rooted in time, narrative and alterity. NM provides unique resources to face our and the next generations' brave new world.

In this reflective, argumentative, and critical analysis, based on assumptions, concepts, and principles of NM, we have pointed out the central role of communication, relationship, trust, and context in healthcare. All stakeholders are involved in this narrative approach—patients, relatives/caregivers, and healthcare teams. It presents the same kind of challenge that an evidence-based approach does knowing how and when to stop. To preserve the integrity and the humanity of patients and healthcare professionals, we need to listen to each other's narrative, knowing that telling our story is essential to give a future to our memory:

> These are the last things, she wrote. One by one they disappear and never come back. I can tell you of the ones I have seen, of the ones that are no more, but I doubt there will be time. It is all happening too fast now, and I cannot keep up…The government doesn't like it when people make up stories. It's bad for morale. You see what you are against here. It's not just that things vanish –but once they vanish, the memory of them vanishes as well. [1]

Acknowledgements The work developed by the researcher is funded by FCT: CEECINST/00091/2018/CP1500/CT000.. 10.54499/CEECINST/00091/2018/CP1500/CT0008.

Conflicts of Interest The authors declare no conflict of interest.

References

1. Auster P. In the country of last things. Faber and Faber; 1987.
2. Casal T. Between patients and doctors: it takes a person. In: Bray P, Casal T, editors. Beyond diagnosis: relating the person to the patient—the patient to the person. Inter-Disciplinary Press; 2014. p. 83–110.
3. Charon R. Narrative and medicine. N Engl J Med. 2004;350(9):862–4. https://doi.org/10.1056/nejmp038249.
4. Charon R. Narrative medicine: honoring the stories of illness. Oxford University Press; 2006.
5. Chochinov HM. The platinum rule: a new standard for patient-centered care. J Palliat Med. 2022;25(6)

6. DasGupta S. Narrative humility. Lancet. 2008;371(9617):980–1.
7. Remein CDF, et al. Content and outcomes of narrative medicine programmes: a systematic review of the literature through 2019. BMJ Open. 2020;10(1) https://doi.org/10.1136/bmjopen-2019-031568.
8. Han, B.C. 2021. The Palliative Society: Pain today. John Wiley and Sons.
9. Han BC. The scent of time: a philosophical essay on the art of lingering. Polity. 2017;
10. Hurtwit B. Narrative (in) medicine. In: Spinozzi P, Hurtwitz B, editors. Discourses and narrations in the biosciences. Vandenhoeck & Ruprecht Unipress; 2011. p. 73–87.
11. Kipnis K. Vulnerability in research subjects: a bioethical taxonomy. National Bioethics Advisory Commission [NBAC]. In: Ethical and policy issues in research involving human participants, Commissioned papers, vol. II. National Bioethics Advisory Commission [NBAC]; 2001. p. 1–13.
12. Marini MG. Interview to Maria Giulia Marini, La Repubblica, June 12, 2012. https://www.medicinanarrativa.eu/narrative-medicine.
13. McGee G. Pragmatic method and bioethics. In: McGee G, editor. Pragmatic bioethics. Cambridge: The MIT Press; 2003.
14. Nash W, Erondu M, Childress A. Expanding Narrative Medicine through the Collaborative Construction and Compelling Performance of Stories. J Med Humanit. 2023;44:207–25. https://doi.org/10.1007/s10912-022-09779-6.
15. OECD. Artificial intelligence in science: challenges, opportunities and the future of research. Paris: OECD Publishing; 2023. https://doi.org/10.1787/a8d820bd-en.
16. Ofri D. The passion and the peril: storytelling in medicine. Acad Med. 2015;90:1005–6.
17. Öhlén J, et al. Person-centred care dialectics—inquired in the context of palliative care. Nurs Philos. 2017;18(4) https://doi.org/10.1111/nup.12177.
18. Weiss T, Swede MJ. Transforming preprofessional health education through relationship-centered care and narrative medicine. Teach Learn Med. 2019;31(2):222–33. https://doi.org/10.1080/10401334.2016.1159566.

Chapter 2
Conversation with Surgeon 1—Suzy Elneil

René Génadry

Conversation with Pr. Sohier (Suzy) Elneil (SE).
Recorded online on May 3rd, 2024, by René Génadry (RG).

Abbreviations that follow:

SE: Sohier (Suzy) Elneil
RG: René Génadry

RG: Hello Suzy, I just wanted to benefit from your experience and your insights as regards the issue of educating the next generation of physicians to become more humanistic.

SE: At the outset, I would say that one of my anxieties over the last few years, and I use this terminology for a long time, has been the lack of humanity. Those people have kind of forgotten the Hippocratic Oath, particularly the modern version from 1964 that states very clearly that Medicine is not about the science aspect of it, it is about bringing the art to it and give equal weight to other priorities which are not parameters people think matter, such as kindness and empathy. And I think one of the problems that has happened in the last few years, well probably the last three decades, medical education has become increasingly technical, and it has become all about ticking a box to say you're confident in doing the technical procedure whatever that technical procedure may be. There's also a box for ticking whether you're a good communicator or not, but it isn't judged on your ability to work with people or deal with people, it is just on your ability to communicate well directly with colleagues and management. It has nothing to do with the patient, so I think we've lost our way hugely. It is a battleground that's very difficult to fix, because it is not given any priority, and if anything, it's seen as a sign of weakness if you are

R. Génadry (✉)
Carver College of Medicine, University of Iowa, Iowa City, IA, USA

J. McFarland et al. (eds.), *Humanism in Surgery*, New Paradigms in Healthcare,
https://doi.org/10.1007/978-3-031-86018-8_2

thinking that things should be about kindness, empathy, generosity, time, patience, and yet those have always been the basis of medicine. And if you look back to the times of the great philosophers, you know go back to Socrates and so on, they all talk about this problem which preexisted us many centuries ago. There is a famous quote from Socrates where he talks about the physicians of Hellas, in other words the physicians of Athens in Greece, and how they failed to recognize their role in the humanitarian aspect of caring. So, it's not a new problem, it's a revisited problem, and it's one that as physicians, we have to really grow and think about, and we should give weight to: but to give it weight, it has to be recognized, and for it to be recognized, it has to be valued, and from what I see, the value isn't there!

RG: Well Suzy, you have summarized the whole problem very nicely. I'm sure you must have been thinking about it for a long time, and before getting to see what you would perceive as solutions to the problem, and knowing how much involved, engaged, empathetic and committed you are, I wonder if you could tell me a bit about your journey to that point.

SE: OK I think the way I would describe it, it started basically with watching my parents and what they were doing for humanity. My father was a doctor and a professor, he was a medic, but he specialized in the basic sciences and was the director of emergency relief operations, occupying one of the deputy director general roles at WHO and he did a lot of his work when he was appointed to the region. He chose to be appointed to the region of Africa although we're from Sudan and he could have been appointed in the Middle East regions, he chose Africa because he felt that's where he could do his best work. What was interesting is that dad was in the process of building up institutions, like better medical schools for doctors, but he was also building public health schools, nursing schools, middle level healthcare management schools which were providing healthcare teaching and tools to nurses, midwives, and others. In the process of doing that, this is now we're talking about the 70s, we were based in Dar as Salam, Tanzania, my mother was involved with the freedom fighters and the liberators of eastern and southern Africa: she spent a lot of time raising funds, promoting the lives of, supporting the lives of women and children, ensuring legal access to healthcare, and so on. That's where it started. So I grew up watching these two people giving and giving and giving… when I went to medical school that was my natural empathy drive because I saw that with them it was all about giving the best and I realized that if I was going to do medicine that's what I had to do: I had to give my best, I had to listen and I felt that going to medical school was important; so I learned the tools of the trade but being a doctor wasn't just about the tools, it was about the humanity of the trade, and the humanity came from my parents so I remember that one of the things that happened sort of set me on this path: I had a 6 months hiatus between two particular jobs in Cambridge in the UK, and I had about 3 months when I had some free time, so my father's natural advice was: well you can do something good with that, and that was when I went to the Addis Ababa Fistula hospital. I told them I was being self-funded and wanted just to help and not necessarily to learn surgery. All I wanted to do was just help. I was just going there to help anywhere I could. I said I'm here to do anything, I will mop floors, I will cap pills, I'll do anything; but Catherine Hamlin decided that that wasn't what I was going to be there for, and she insisted that I had to learn how to do the surgery. Now when you've looked after women who are right at the end of human existence, they are at the point they want to give up, they want to leave, and these are young women not always very young women but young enough you realize that the only way you could gain their trust is for you to sit with them, be with them, understand them, and that's where my listening really developed: I used to see my parents doing it, so I took it forward myself, and what I learned was to always say to people and I've done that in all the training I've done with my students and the people I've worked with which is focused hugely on training people by teaching them to listen to the person who has the problem, it is not about you giving out what you want people to think or see, but about what the person who has the problem; listen to see how you can use your tools of trade to help out and help that person. So, that's where it comes from Rene, and it comes from that place and that has never left me, that has been throughout my life, and I feel that if I lose that, I lose the ability to be a good doctor.

RG: So basically, the example of your parents was critical. Was there anything during your education that was formal in bringing out that which was innate in you obviously?

SE: No because our educational process was very much dependent on who trained and taught you: if I saw those who trained and taught me following that line, I wanted to be like those individuals much more and I aligned myself much more with those people; whereas I often saw bad behavior as well, and I remember distinctly saying: I don't wish to ever be like that; but I saw good people, the vast majority of our very senior mentors were good people, they did do it this way, they did spend time, they did think it was important to sit with your patient, with the family, with the team. They built that trust, not just in their personal interaction with an individual that needed your help, but the entire team structure and support for all that; so, I learned that from there, but there was nothing formal in the curriculums, nothing formal in our training process: this was literally by osmosis, you imbibed it from the environment you're in and the people you are surrounded by.

RG: So, do you think that a humanistic attitude is teachable?

SE: It's a very good question because I think we have gotten in this era of electronic technology of all sorts and you know people will often quote things like social media and so on, but in my mind when you teach things you kind of need a structure, but also I found that the tendencies most people learning things nowadays do tend to want a kind of tick box to some extent: in other words, do you know what compassion means and they can define it, doesn't mean they do it, they don't, and if they do it once they might not do it 10 times. So, my anxiety with teaching it is that I think it must be taught partially by example. You can be given the tools and be told you do need to understand that your work involves compassion, kindness and empathy but unless you see it in action and in working, I don't think they totally understand its relevance to them.

RG: Moving forward Suzy, do you see any solution or any possibility of solution besides good example, good environment and good role modeling?

SE: When I'm talking about that, that's quite a time intensive one-on-one basis and that's the difficulty of it. I think it needs to be normalized. It needs to be included in everything and normalized, in other words you can't move on in a job unless you know the people see you as that person, see you as a person who's done a good job on that front, who's been caring, who's been kind, who's been helpful etc. Because at the moment, what happens is: are you the person with the highest marks in something who gets through that process rather than the best person with the best ability and the kindness and so on? My dilemma is that the value component isn't seen, and the value component isn't applauded: so, if somebody is empathetic, kind, compassionate, etcetera and is humanitarian in their approach of caring people, you can teach the process in my view. For instance, when I develop pathways of care, I always start with the service user, the patient; the patient using that pathway needs to be integrated into developing that process, and that means listening and being in that environment. In this sort of arena, we almost need to do the same thing, we need to sit people down and show that there is no shame in being kind, compassionate, caring essentially in fact it's an asset; but to make it normalized and to make it acceptable and to applaud it, it needs to be put in a position where it matters. Right now, my opinion Rene, I don't think it matters to many people.

RG: So how can one make it matter? is it a matter of evaluation as part of the graduation process, or is it evaluable otherwise?

SE: That's a tough thing because these are human characteristics. They're very difficult to teach, they're easy to evaluate that's not difficult, but they're difficult to teach and embed and maintain. But the only way we can improve on the situation as we have it is to somehow teach it formally and informally. And perhaps just like many years ago you recall Rene, in medical schools we never had a communications module, did we? And now everybody has a communications module where they must learn how good communication works, the same with so many other sorts of what I call soft skills which you would have anticipated most people would have but they don't. I think that would be a start, but I think it also needs to be embedded entrenched in everything that we do at all levels. Perhaps even something like the WHO checklist should it be included at the end and at the beginning of what kind of thing is going to be done today: how did you demonstrate this, and then at the end how do you feel we as a team when you do your debriefing, do you think we were kind to each other, were we empathetic, were we supportive of each other? Those soft things need to be asked, maybe perhaps at the beginning people will feel uncomfortable, but eventually it will become part of you because you'll be thinking about it. You think gosh we're going to get to the team debriefing after every case, and everyone's going to be asked were we kind to each other? Were we empathetic? Were we compassionate? I think that would help change behavior because you are being watched all the time.

RG: Yeah, so do you think it's the intentionality that would be critical? As I recall most of these changes that have occurred over time have been pushed and promoted by institutional concerns about the relationship between the physician-technician and the patient as a client receiving care, and it is from there that those that have a humanitarian incline have promoted it internationally, but otherwise in a lot of institutions, I get the feeling that the intention is not necessarily a humanistic approach as much as a defensive approach.

SE: I would agree. I would agree that institutions are more about protecting their brand and they are protecting their income and protecting what they think the people need to see or want to see; even the fact that we have taken the name patient out of it and made them "clients" or service users, etcetera: it dehumanizes the person in front of you. Then it is the number rather than a person, and there's no interest in them as such or their family etcetera, it's just "an appendix that needs to be removed." It isn't Mrs. X who is the mother of three, who has appendicitis and needs to have her operation today because she is in a lot of pain. There is a lack of understanding. Interestingly in medical school, you are trained when you speak about a case: this is Mrs. so and so who has such and such; but somehow, from medical school to where you are delivering the care, it has disappeared en route. That needs to all be brought back. But I agree, in my view institutions have made us into a sort of little tick box technocrats for "doing the right thing." I'll give you an example, my sort of favorite is the so-called "learn, not blame culture" you know everything is about: we want to learn from our mistake, we don't want to blame anybody, and yet the whole process is blaming… The learning might be there, but it's done as an afterthought; the first thing is how it all went wrong, why it went wrong, who made it wrong, and then they say: in the future, all registrars must do this, all consultants have to do that. The learning bit is the last bit, the first bit which they spend a lot of time on is the blaming bit. So, there is no learning culture really, and everything is about blame first. So, if you don't take that so-called system of governance away, you can't build compassion to the process. There is no compassion in the process.

RG: You've had a lot of experience with that with the mesh business.

SE: Ohh huge amounts, huge yeah huge! so of course when I spoke about it, and I actually came at it from the point of view of the patient saying look they are right, there is a problem, and we are the ones who should look for a solution: my colleagues saw it as an assault on them. So, their answer wasn't ohh my gosh we have a problem let's investigate and find a solution, their problem became get rid of El Neil and by getting rid of El Neil, that's the solution. Because then the patients have no one they can talk to. It's still ongoing to be honest Rene, because a lot of these colleagues are funded by various agencies and groups whose purpose is to try and bring mesh back so in the UK as you're aware the UK has put a halt on all mesh insertions for continence and prolapse through the last four almost five years, but there are still people who would like to bring it back (in its current form).

RG: That's why I kept getting back to the intention and that's why you have a wonderful way of presenting it, because in whatever talk you do about it, you keep the patient at the center of the controversy whatever it is…

SE: I was just saying that is how I feel, and that's probably why you will find me in the arena of where I can do humanitarian medicine, where I can actually practice it. In a way, that's how I can give back because I always felt that if you're pushed out of an arena because you're trying to do the right thing, you need to restore your faith in other arenas as you need to work as much as you can to reinforce that approach to care.

RG: You need to fight back, you need to maintain because you can let these situations deter you.

SE: Exactly it's about truth and justice and you must keep fighting.

RG: Suzy, let me get you back a little bit just to get your take on that: would you think that humanities introduced in pre-Med or whatever level before medical school would have an impact on creating that kindness, compassion and empathy toward the patient?

SE: Yeah, I think if it wasn't so much about the purity of the science should I say, well the big scientific groups you know natural Physiology etcetera where there's a dissociation from yourself to the human being who's providing you with that information. In other words, if you go to the lab and you are doing your assessments and now of course everything is technology based you don't even have that contact with the person who's given themselves up for this medical science: so those aspects of that disconnect, that that person doesn't matter etcetera, but I don't think it's meant, it's just that people don't see that person as human, they're not part of them as it were: so bringing in the Humanities I often think that things like philosophy, understanding the history of where we came to, how we are created, and where we are now is quite important for us as medics. So, we shouldn't be about who's got the highest mark in something, we should really be talking how did you get here, why did we get here, what are we going to do about it and what should we do to improve Women's Health for instance in my case, and in others it will be how much will we do to improve humanity. So yes, I think there is a role for it Rene. I think it should be pervasive I think it should be pre-med, it should be med, and it should be post-med. it should be part of your entire training and perhaps even organizations and professional societies should have a section on it because that will then embed it more and make it better.

RG: That's what really brought the idea of trying to have these conversations with people that have been involved in humanitarian work, because most of the push has come essentially from anthropologists and writers but very few physicians have been as active as you have in trying to promote the humanity in medicine. I hope at least the readership or whoever gets the information will make use of it to try to alter the medical curriculum or pre-Med or post-Med as you said to try to change a little bit the perspective of what it is to be a physician, not just a technician.

SE: And that's a very important word physician, because I always say to my trainees, you're a physician first, a surgeon second. Even that separation is key: surgeons have a worse disconnect I feel than physicians. Physicians can be involved because if you look at a physician taking a history of school style they are very much into the family: what happened to your father, your mother, your siblings etc., surgeons tend to not be interested unless they're dealing say with cancer, and they will say did your father, mother or somebody have cancer and that's the extent of the association.

RG: Is that differentiation between physician and surgeon as significant as it has been developing in the UK?

SE: I think there is yeah, I've noticed that the surgeons are increasingly more distant, they are increasingly more aligned with technical ability, technical skill and technical know-how and that's how they're actually treated by management. It's how many cases of X can you do, what on average does it take to do a case of X, so if I give you 12-h theater session you should be able to do six of these or five of these or four of these whatever it is. So, the technicality is the key, the ability is the key, not the interest on the quality of the delivery to that patient or their needs.

RG: With the common use of physician assistants and the introduction of robotics I think the surgeons are losing "touch" with the patient, aren't they?

SE: Totally, totally! so I have noticed the same patients, the same doctors who were ballistically crazy about laparoscopic surgery, or in my case also the mesh surgery, felt very left out when mesh was withdrawn: they didn't know what to do with themselves. So, they've now all suddenly found robotics, and it made me question exactly what you're saying: why it is so easy to turn to robotics because robotics you could be anywhere in the world doing the operation frankly because somebody else could put your scopes and instruments there, you could be sitting at home doing it if you wished. It's not that difficult as it were and I noticed people laugh about it they'll say you know "boys and their toys" but I don't think it is funny, because I think the patients are being sold a method of doing surgery because everybody's trying to tell them it's better for you but realistically, it isn't necessarily better for you. The jury is still out, and we need the evidence. So, there's that aspect of it and as you correctly say the surgeons and I and as I'm speaking to you, I can envisage our surgeon's coffee room on a typical Wednesday when I'm operating, I could see the disconnect not just between the surgeons and their patients but the surgeons and each other: there's no communication.

RG: That's true. Well Suzy, when you mentor someone who is interested in getting into a humanitarian career, what do you recommend, what do you suggest, how do you make them approach it?

SE: The first thing is to make it very clear to them this is not an easy "I wish to do this because I think I'm a good person etcetera" approach, because there are some people who think it's just about being a nice and good person. There's no point going anywhere if you cannot be prepared to have a dialogue, and by that, I mean you take your skills and share but you equally learn from that environment and bring back. It's all about being together in a dialogue and you have to respect who you're going to and respect how you bring it back, so that's the first thing. The second thing I always say to them, because it depends on the level they're at, the people working in that environment they know what they are doing, they sometimes need an extra pair of hands, they need somebody to be with them for whatever reason that means when you go out there your first job is to learn, nothing else. They say to you, you need to mop the floor, you mop the floor if that's helpful, and that's just as well: so that's how I do it. I say you're not going there as a fabulous person who you think the world should be at your feet, you're going there to learn, to develop yourself but to help develop others in any way you can with any skills you have, and also to simply listen and come back and rethink what you want to do because I don't think all this work is always suitable for everybody. I think some people are misguided in what they try to do in those environments. I do start off with that, so the first trip is about learning, listening, speaking and sharing: it's all about sharing. After that, you need to be committed. You cannot just go when it suits you and not realize that everybody else have their own schedule. so, you need to be committed, and you need to work with them and decide together how you're going to make this work. Nowadays with all the improvement in technology you can stay in touch even more so than you could do 15–20 years ago, so no excuse. And then also what their needs are, work with them to find a sustainable way and I don't mean green economy here I'm talking about sustainable way to ensure equipment can be sent to them on a regular basis, or teams can be supported on a regular basis etcetera. If you ask me to write it down 1234 I probably wouldn't be good at it, because you base it on the needs of the place you're going, so every place is unique, every group of people you're working with is unique, so you need to go really with an open arm policy to go and learn from that environment and learn what they need. It's not about what you want to give, it's about what the need is, and how you can share the knowledge to deliver on that need.

RG: So, with open heart, open mind, and a lot of humility.

SE: A lot of humility!

RG: What advice would you give a potential candidate for dealing with the patient, how do you tell them to approach the patient in a different environment?

SE: So, I think one of the first things is sitting with the team that are there first of all. This is about learning again, often the place you go to they're extremely good at providing support and they are a welcoming environment: you need to be ready for all sorts of things you know: sometimes it's a 7:00 start, so a lot of doctors in different countries don't always have that start so in the UK it's unusual to start at 7 although it's more common to start at 7:30 or 8:00 but it is those simple things like adjusting yourself to the routine of that place, go with the team in and learn from them, and then when you start to do your own one-on-one, the important thing it's a bit like, I don't mean to sound patronizing, but you must gain the trust of the person sitting in front of you; and anyway you can do that is to be kind, compassionate and listen to them and work with them and you take it at their pace not at your pace, that's very important, and once you do that, people will see it in you, and the trust will come because you're not pushing them but asking them how they like to be helped.

RG: Suzy I'm very impressed by all that you do and your journey but what did you do after medical school? You said you went to the fistula hospital and then how did you carry whatever you've learned there to the future?

SE: At that stage I had just literally graduated medical school and finished my house officer jobs, so I came back to England and the plan was to train: now I was trying to be a surgeon and not a gynecologist. But again, on the advice my father and my parents really, they said to me, look, women need women to do more of their care and surgery. I remember saying to my dad I wanted to do surgery he says, well you can do that from within the realms of obstetrics and gynecology, but if I do anything on women the most important thing is you have to understand how women work, you need to understand childbirth, you need to understand periods. You need to understand everything and anyway you could do that is to do obstetrics and gynecology. So, I came back to the UK with a view to start my training. But before I could actually do a cesarean or an abdominal procedure, I was already repairing fistulas, so I did it sort of back to front and because I could see the damage and Catherine Hamlin (Addis Ababa Fistula Hospital) had insisted, Reginald Hamlin was still alive bless his soul as well, and so Catherine had decided I was going to do fistulas no matter what. So, I started on that front and by the time I came to the United Kingdom, I went straight to Cambridge to start my postgraduate training. I was already ahead of all my classmates as it were because I could do things none of them could, but some of them could do cesareans I didn't know how, but it doesn't take you long to learn especially if you know that environment; and most of us are slightly workaholic in that sense, so that's how I first did it. In the midst of doing all of that, I came to the realization that despite fixing the fistula in women, and even though they didn't have incontinence because of the fistula, they still had other forms of incontinence and infertility: they had overactive bladders, they had stress incontinence and so on. So, I came back again and decided to do a PhD in bladder mechanisms: now that's in the late 90s early 2000s everybody's focus was on the bladder muscle, and I just inherently knew it wasn't the muscle that was the problem, I just felt it was the nerve that was the problem and there wasn't much research on nerves and their impact. so, I did my work on that, got in my PhD from there, and then I was looking at what therapeutic options were available to make nerves function better in such conditions, and that's where we developed for my work on neuromodulation and both electrical and chemo neuromodulation and then develop that sort of skill. So, I became aware that I had to not just be a good surgeon in restoring anatomy, I had to be good at restoring function, I had to understand where I could apply my various techniques and technologies. I saw myself as a person who had an armamentarium of approaches and I could individualize that approach to every patient specifically, and that includes everything from physiotherapy, nutrition you know it wasn't just surgery it was what goes with the rehabilitation of the whole patient and looking at them from top to toe, working out what was leading to what, and how to get it better and not just getting my area better but the rest of it better. There's no point me doing all this work on an overactive bladder from diabetes that is out of control.

RG: While you were doing all this work in developing your skills, your research and so on, were you approached by people who were interested in doing similar endeavors or did you have to try to convince people that it's something that they should get involved?

SE: I think it was more convincing at the beginning, I realized it's a slightly lonely road because I remember distinctly being asked by my professor in Cambridge, what was my interest in "wet women" and that kind of told you everything… it made you realize that people don't value or don't get it: he was a fertility expert, and he thought everything had to do with fertility. Fertility is only one part of a woman; the rest of her life needs to be lived as well so that was my approach. It wasn't easy to get that interest and I remember when I did myself specialization training which involved urology, gynecology, colorectal, oncology, neurology the whole lot, it was just a specialty that wasn't really that important: people felt it's not that critical and I remember a colleague who was supposed to be my trainer saying to me that he was going to give me a "poisoned chalice," that I was to be part of the neurology hospital because that's where part of my job is at the National Hospital for neurology and neurosurgery. I actually couldn't understand how he thought it was a chalice because I saw it as a huge opportunity to understand the nerve dysfunction in patients with pelvic floor dysfunction; and a lot of my work went on to do that. So, coming back to what you're saying I did get approached: it was interesting as you did more and more you got a lot of approach from companies, from colleagues with similar interests around Europe and the US, and a lot of collaborative work which was very helpful when looking for trying to encourage and build the team. It was a real struggle to find funding, to find support and so on because it wasn't seen as a needful issue. If I was doing cancer, if I was looking after women in their pregnancies and babies, there was money in that, and that was the only two areas. This area among the benign specialties is also the poorest of the poor in a sense that a lot of focus goes on other aspects of the benign specialties. So, it took a little while, you then get a name, and you know people would start to come and want to work with you but what I realized and I'm sure you've got this as well, really a lot of people want to work but they'd rather you did the work. That's the same picture of the world I'm sure: there are very few people who sat down and actually wrote with a lot more people wanted to just be part of the party should I say.

RG: This is wonderful Suzy I really appreciate all your insights. if I were to ask you, who are you? how would you describe yourself.

SE: I am not very good at describing myself. I'll give you an example of what I mean: I got a message from one of the hospitals I work in, and they said to me we've just looked up your bio on our website and it doesn't do you any favors. We know the fantastic work you do, why on earth isn't it all over this bio? And I thought well that's sort of typical of me. I'd like to be thought of as first of all a person of humanity, very caring person. That would be it, that would be my main things but that whatever I try to do, I honestly do try to do my best to make it better. That's the way I would put it; sometimes that's much harder to do than at other times, because sometimes you're going across the beliefs of others who don't see that, they see something else and it always surprises me when people see when you think you're trying to do good and people see you as not doing good for whatever reason, so I feel that, even in that circumstance, I must maintain my humanity first and I must look to them and think maybe one day they will see it as well.

RG: They feel obviously threatened but instead of learning from you they try to ignore the process.

SE: I think you're right. I do win a lot of awards, and I do get lots of accolades and so on, but you don't celebrate them because I feel it is something we should all be doing. So, I don't see why I should be rewarded or awarded for it because that should be the norm, that's how it should be.

RG: You're not doing it for the glory, you're doing it because it's the right thing to do; so why be rewarded for doing what you're supposed to do.

SE: Exactly and even as you're speaking to me Rene, I'm cringing thinking, ohh gosh that sounds so self-serving about me but you're absolutely right.

RG: It's not self-serving, it's the truth and it comes from your commitment, your engagement and your enthusiasm in what you're doing.

SE: You're right if you mean something and you mean it truthfully, it's very hard to fake it.

RG: Absolutely. Well thank you so much Suzy.

Chapter 3
A Personal Reflection on the Core of Medical Practice

José Poças

> An empirical science deprived of reflection as well as a purely speculative philosophy is insufficient. Consciousness without science and science without consciousness is radically mutilated and mutilating (Edgar Morin, French philosopher and sociologist, 1921–)

3.1 Introduction

> No one is equal to anyone. Every human being is a unique stranger (Carlos Drummond de Andrade, Brazilian poet, 1902–1987)

We live in a time when the virtues of science are idolised almost as if it were a new religion. Science is believed to be based exclusively on technology, and technology is based only on mathematics. We theorise that all humankind's enigmas and problems can be expressed through numbers and equations, and the qualification of something can boil down to its mere quantification. Therefore, distinguishing the virtual from reality is increasingly more difficult. More and more, people tend to go through life alone, surrounded by many other humans who share the same loneliness. The hyper-information of contemporary society often makes it difficult for anyone to have an informed opinion and make a conscious and autonomous decision. Fruitful introspections and dialogue are increasingly rare. In a society where everyone runs, often by inertia, uncritically mimicking what they see in others or at the behest of some sinister 'Big Brother' because they are no longer able to stop, to appreciate silence, stillness, be enchanted by the simplest things or sympathise with the fragility of Man. For the remaining minority, time has become a secret luxury

J. Poças (✉)
Internal Medicine, Infectious Disease and Travel Medicine Specialist, Consulped Clinic, Setúbal, Portugal
e-mail: josemdpocas@netcabo.pt

J. McFarland et al. (eds.), *Humanism in Surgery*, New Paradigms in Healthcare,
https://doi.org/10.1007/978-3-031-86018-8_3

that cannot be dispensed to maintain the indispensable emotional and psychological balance and thus face daily life better. Life, at present, has all of this and, therefore, there are clear and substantive implications for the practice of clinical medicine.

As far as medicine is concerned and regarding the exercise of clinical activity, which I consider to be its core, present times are characterised by the progressive devaluation of clinical semiology and anamnesis as a structuring element of the medical act, by the artificial refuge in solutions that predominantly refer to the use of technological means, by the unconscious escape from scenarios in which the suffering of others—as well as one's own—by the subconscious denial of the inevitable finitude of life, as well as the conscious, unconditional, and sometimes even unbridled search for pleasure, infallibility, and fame at any price. Unfortunately, the practice of medicine is increasingly submerged in a complex, inoperative, and absurd bureaucracy, implemented with the official seal of a hierarchy that has led the policy of this complicated sector, with the unacknowledged and apparent purpose of making the time spent by its professionals profitable when what is essentially intended is to have obsessive control over all countable indices; even though, in reality, this is not even adequately achieved, in many circumstances, due to the blatant inoperability of the computerised means made available!

It is a scenario where the excessive and indiscriminate overvaluation of the results of auxiliary diagnosis means prevails, not rarely as a means of promoting them, as if it were a mere business, to the detriment of humanisation in the attitudes and empathy in the decisions between those who are supposed to be the 'only' and 'true' interlocutors in this particular relationship: the Doctor and the Patient.

3.2 The Mission of the Physician

> The thought of death deceives us; for it causes us to neglect to live (Luc de Clapiers Vauvenargues, French philosopher and writer, 1715–1747)

There is a notorious and growing gap within the community of medical graduates: those who are physicians and those who, by not being so and working in the execution of additional diagnostic tests or techniques or the planning and analysis of the determinants in health or Politics, never lose sight of the notion that their work is equally fundamental to compose, with the necessary adequacy and intelligibility, the indispensable puzzle to arrive at a correct diagnosis (clinical, psychological, and social). So, for the best possible treatment of the patient (and the citizens), and when seeing an image of a fragment of the body of an anonymous human being (on the computer or under the microscope), when handling any of its biological products, when performing an instrumental procedure, more or less invasive, when writing or analysing reports, or when legislating on the regulation of this complicated sector, never forget that all actions have repercussions, directly and indirectly, on someone who is suffering and needs their decisive contribution… and the others! Those who only see figures and financial returns, often for their profit and of speculative origin, look at the patient as a mere means of survival. Or equally reprehensible, those who only care about their fame and appearing in columns at the expense of disproportionate propaganda of their successes. Those who sit comfortably at a desk across multiple departments (governmental or private), exercising their power in a detached, despotic manner, constantly using linguistic euphemisms to hide their repugnant hypocrisy and their profound indifference to those who suffer and to whom the first and last mission is to alleviate physical and psychological pain, contributing decisively to restoring possible autonomy (those of the first group).

Being a physician and practicing medicine is not to have a profession like any other. Health and disease, life and death, suffering and physical and emotional well-being, are anything but irrelevant and what we should cherish the most. Because our more precious collective civilisational heritage is the uncompromising defence of these principles, since we are invested in the honourable and timeless role of being our patients' most interested and competent advocates. With competence, empathy, compassion, humanism, and common sense, we should try everything to avoid or minimise the patient's suffering because making them suffer without a reason will never be part of our mission. This job will be all the more successful if a physician knows how to be more than 'just' a doctor, adapting to each particular case and transforming this point of view into something special that becomes an integral and inextricable part of his being. We should always bear in mind that clinical activity lives from its context. Feelings and antagonistic realities such as successes and defeats, hopes and frustrations, suffering and joy necessarily abound because man's journey on Earth is composed of a mixture of life, health, sickness and death, pleasure and suffering, and in all of these stages, a doctor may be called upon to intervene and help.

Given what has been said, if anyone thinks the mission of a physician is only the proper diagnosis and treatment of the diseases, he his entirely mistaken. I could not agree more if we add the vital respect for the norms of medical ethics and deontology, but I still find it largely insufficient. By adding empathy, compassion, and concern for the psychological and social conditions of the patient and their family and professional environment, we will be much closer to the ideal. However, even then, it will be insufficient. Isn't renouncing to agree with the patent exiguity of the minimum conditions for treating patients with adequate dignity and humanisation the last mission a doctor can resist investing in, when everyone collapses in front of him? Because to do so, when dealing with the problem of health and disease, particularly in the context of a real catastrophe, is really to be a doctor. Furthermore, either we are that way, or our mission is inescapably lacking and incomplete.

3.3 The Medical Act

> We are completely immersed in this world belonging to our sufferings, our happiness, and our loves. Not to feel is to avoid suffering, but also rejoicing. The more qualified we are for happiness, the more qualified we are for unhappiness. (Edgar Morin, French philosopher and sociologist, 1921–)

Figuratively speaking, the medical act is a meeting between two persons of sound body and mind, resulting in the correct diagnosis and effective treatment of the patient's disease, even when palliation is the only option.

The Hippocratic Oath, so often repeated, only because it seems wrong not to do so, 'to cure sometimes, to relieve often, and to comfort always' is what best defines the physician's mission. A timeless imperative of professional conscience, it also contains something of such transcendent importance that it can only be accomplished, step by step, in a path of solidarity and unreserved partnership, in which the idiosyncrasies of both physician and patient enhance in favour of spiritual communion, imbued with solidarity, compassion, trust, and empathy. This allows, where applicable, an acceptance, with the least possible suffering, of disability, when not, of death itself, however, without ever removing the last spark of hope. It is necessary to recognise that the indispensable dialogue continues beyond simple words, and a therapeutic result is not restricted to the adequate use of drugs or surgical instruments. Therefore, the actual dimension of this unforgettable act, from beginning to end, should only bear these two committed protagonists: The Patient and the Doctor.

I often whisper to myself, 'How do I do it?' when addressing unique issues, for example, impending death, with patients or their relatives. I always conclude that one should never try to anticipate the natural development of events, show as much calm and availability as possible, make others feel our presence in a supportive and professional way, not rationalise or overdramatise our speech, and know how to use body language appropriately and spontaneously. To know how to listen attentively to the family members' venting, look each other in the eye, not be afraid to get emotional and provide a space for others to do so naturally, are ways of transmitting the necessary messages of serenity and complicity that allow us to mitigate the suffering of others.

It is also relevant to mention, besides the physician never abandoning a patient, even if the pathology has no cure or specific pharmacological or surgical treatment available, he must always know how to comfort, give hope, and help to accept and understand the nature of the disease and, if necessary, death itself. Whenever, when I have this kind of conversation with patients with a reserved prognosis because they suffer from evolutive diseases that spare consciousness and lucidity, I always end up concluding that we have to do it without any reservation or previously established clichés, letting the speech flow spontaneously with a serene tone and in an environment as calm as possible.

It is crucial not to stray from the point, not treating the patient as if they were an 'ignoramus' or a 'poor thing'. Knowing how to convey the truth, which means to know his personality and making yourself known as a person, is fundamental, as is having the courage to openly acknowledge what you do not know and be willing to ask for advice from more knowledgeable and experienced colleagues. Respecting their wills and values and being firm and cautious in dismantling the web of ideas devoid of any scientific basis, without ever withdrawing the last shred of hope, completes the list of requirements. This is learnt through experience, dialogue with our mentors and patients, their families, and friends, as well as vital constant reflection on our professional practice and its fundamentals—writing, reading, analysing, and discussing. True medicine is precisely this—everything that the venerable tradition going back to Hippocrates has handed down to us over the centuries and nothing else.

Knowing how to support those accompanying the last moments of someone's life, showing gestures as simple as looking into the other's eyes with tenderness, gently holding hands, and silently listening to their loved one's breathing is, in fact, the most humanising way for a person to say goodbye to this world, being the most human of all available treatments. As long as the gesture is spontaneous, it can be immediately felt by the patient as a form of warm bodily, tactile, and auditory language that carries a message of professional competence, availability, solidarity, and relational affection. It can trigger a subliminal expression that must be correctly interpreted and contextualised by the physician, materialised in the exteriorisation of a whole important set of feelings often reflected fleetingly, although quite significantly, in the patient's face.

Suffering is a part of human life. The search to avoid it is one of the physicians' inalienably noblest missions, as much as speaking the language of truth and knowing how to transmit the prognosis inherent to the formulated diagnosis properly. However bad it may be, it is necessary to find the means, the time, and the place best suited to the specific circumstance and with respect for the patient's autonomy and personality in an atmosphere with indispensable affectionate complicity. This is one of the pillars upon which the ethics of interpersonal relationships must be based, especially in the context of the physician's relationship with the patient and even more so in the context of diseases with a reserved vital or functional prognosis.

3.4 Technology in Medical Practice

> We cannot stop in time… for the first time, an invisible and unknown being has paralysed the entire civilisation of technique. Until yesterday, we could consider ourselves omnipotent amid the rubble, the first and only ones also in our primacy of destruction. We had forgotten that to exist is to breathe (Donatella Di Cesare, Italian thinker and essayist, 1956–)

Technological development will always continue to improve. It has brought and continues to bring new and substantial benefits to humanity. So, it is not desirable, nor possible, to claim that it should be merely suspended, just as it is also undesirable to deny the clear evidence of its recognised virtues, which imposes the recognition that the resulting scientific advances have brought about a notable increase in survival and quality of life for patients and populations.

However, it is equally valid that clinical activity is increasingly being (unduly) subordinated to the blind and crushing advances of technology and the absurd demands of the bureaucracy imposed by the most diverse institutional hierarchies. As referred before, semiology and anamnesis have progressively been devalued and no longer occupy their rightful top position. In fact, they are the first indispensable pieces to guide the judicious requisition of auxiliary means of diagnosis and to the formulation of a prior assertive differential diagnosis. However, they are nowadays unfortunately neglected as a privileged way of emotional closeness between doctor and patient.

Acknowledging that using technological means, in the context of the medical act and the doctor-patient relationship, should come first and foremost in the course of a path mapped out by these two persons and with the necessary logic and coherence, but never at the beginning or end of it, or even as the result of a solitary decision removed from the respect due to the expressed and informed will of the patient, even if well-intentioned.

For example, remote work and telemedicine are not to be thought of as anything more than a possible, albeit merely transitory, means in particular contexts, such as that of the pandemic or when accessibility is an insurmountable obstacle or one that is notoriously difficult to overcome because they will never be able to resolve, in the long run, most of the dysfunctionalities concerning the mission of health-related professions that provide direct clinical care, since human contact is something irreplaceable because it is only through this that the medical act performs with all its full humanisation.

In the doctor-patient or mentor-student relationship, replacing face-to-face consultations with a computer or a telephone conversation and a live class with a computer might be the most acceptable transitional measure as an alternative to its endless postponement. Alas, that it is, and will never be the same, must be pedagogically recognised. Just like in the relationship between two lovers or friends, the touch, the variations in physiognomy and tone, the spontaneous smiles and cries, in short, the availability of healthy face-to-face interaction, transmits semiotic and affective signs that duly contextualised allow each of the actors to leave, saying that it was worthwhile, that it was for this that they went there, or that time was well spent.

I believe that 'voluntary' limits should be set to scientific and technological development so that they do not give us the intoxicating prospect of becoming immortal or turning us into mere bionic beings. Because that would make Man a predator of his fellow Man, as well of himself and all Humanity. Because that would be equivalent to becoming equal to divinities and therefore ceasing to be fully-fledged Human Beings. Because that would mean pretending to materialise the spirit in total opposition to its essence. Because that would represent something that would contradict the timeless logic of the universe, in which everything is constantly recycled and transformed. Because life must originate from another life and never be an obstacle to continue so ad eternum. Because nature's resources are finite, we cannot lose this vital notion of survival and healthy coexistence. Thus, we must contribute that those to come will also have the conditions to carry out their projects with the same freedom and responsibility, as well as with identical social rules and imbued with identical values of previous generations. We have to accept that the iron molecule of haemoglobin that is in the blood of any one of us, nobody knows where it came from or where it will go after we die, but that it should continue eternally to circulate in the same way throughout the cosmos, just as it did before. This is an absolute condition for maintaining the existence of our collective home, called Earth, which we have no right to mortgage for excessive ambitions and empty of any real sense of civilisation.

Thus, we can consider that technology should be used as a mean, but not as an end in itself, since, as the venerable colleague Mário Moura says in a certain text full of provocative interpellations, 'eye to eye' and 'skin to skin', (to which I would add 'mind to mind') is something simultaneously so simple, so intuitive, and so transcendent, that it is capable of carrying an irreplaceable intrinsic therapeutic and civilisational value, whether from a strictly medical or psychological point of view or an anthropological and even philosophical one. Something that the cold contact between man and machine can never provide.

3.5 The Doctor-Patient Relationship

> No human life, not even the life of the hermit in nature's wilderness, is possible without a world which directly or indirectly testifies to the presence of other human beings (Hannah Arendt, German American philosopher, 1906–1975)

The doctor-patient relationship is that special *meeting* between two people, where respect for the right to confidentiality and free choice, without prejudice to others, must never be absent, just as the timeless values of professional ethics and deontology can never be alienated. Attitudes are best born from the genuine feeling of solidarity and compassion of the doctor involved, where physical and affective closeness between the doctor and the patient is determinant because indifference and distance between these characters should never be part of the essence of the medical act.

One of the practitioner's noblest attributes is to decode, through clinical observation, the moods of their patients. In their facial expressions. In their eyes. In their gestures. In their voice. Taking a humanised and individualised clinical approach by reading between the lines of the patient's speech, in the sense that the patient will accept the decisions as they feel well-founded. This allows for the necessary internalisation after they have had the opportunity to express their fears, their doubts clarified, and their idiosyncrasies and wishes respected. If deciding and acting is an intrinsic part of the essence of the medical act, we must also bear in mind that, however much medical science we may know or clinical experience we may have, its consequences are unpredictable. We must strive to find the right balance between our convictions and intentions and the will that emanates from the values of the patient and/or their family, however unexpected the events may be.

This relationship implies being available to know how to overcome, if appropriate, the traditional conventionalisms imposed by society, from the time, place, or fees, to the use of the typical instruments, exchanging the stethoscope and the sphygmomanometer for the use of the word, the look and the gesture, promoting the creation of an environment in which the exchange of emotions is much greater than the faultless compliance with the dosage of any medicine. It will be, therefore, caring for our fellow man, where elements such as music, for example, can work true 'miracles'. This is inferred from what Plato, the great philosopher of ancient Greece, wanted to express when he said, '[music] gives soul to the universe, wings to the mind, flight to the imagination, and charm and gaiety to life and everything'.

As I am trying to demonstrate, being a doctor is knowing how to go beyond the strict role of a mere 'physician'. In a broader sense, it may even mean not having the mission to prescribe additional diagnostic tests or pharmacological therapy. It can be materialised 'only' in an encounter capable, more than anything, to provide the possible pleasure in each circumstance to someone concrete, to whom we help, understandably full of uncertainty about his future, that find the way to free himself from the interminable labyrinth that the incessant search for knowing how to answer the questions relative to the causes of the cataclysm that has suddenly and inexplicably fallen upon him. Why me? Why now? Why this one and not another disease with a not-so-inexorable path to almost complete dependence? Why is this disease still untreatable? Why does this pathology spare the mind but leave the body completely inert?

Every time I left Fernando's house (a pre-terminal ALS patient I regularly followed for several months), I wondered what the real impact of my visits would have to him. Perhaps the comfort provided by friendship and empathy, the only possible 'medicine' in these circumstances, would be much more effective than the remote possibility of having had access to any pharmacological innovation, the usefulness of which, at that exact moment, would have been highly doubtful, as he lucidly recognised, given that the reversibility of the clinical picture would not be within reach of any reasonably expected scientific advance. Moreover, the true purpose of medical art was fulfilled, even in an unconventional way: that of making the patient accept, with the most extraordinary possible tranquillity, the prognosis of his illness, without ever resorting to the trick of shirking this responsibility by giving false hopes.

However, as I experienced during the pandemic, there are circumstances in which words are of little help. What they express needs to include the effective translation of the reality internalised by the emotions we share with the patients. Pertinent information and, at the same time, knowing how to convey hope is one of the doctor's noblest missions, even in clinical situations of recognised poor prognosis, above all in the case of major natural catastrophes. Besides having to try to respect (if possible) everything that is required in the most common clinical situations, it has the particularity of taking place among people who are subject to overwhelming emotional stress, in which the feeling of vulnerability of the Human Being is terrifying, the lack of resources is extremely limiting, the time available for each medical act is extremely short, the pressure of the circumstances and surroundings is overwhelming, interpersonal, verbal communication is difficult or even almost impossible, in short, the prevailing feeling will often be that the end of life, and perhaps of the world itself, may be imminent.

Although all this may undoubtedly be a reality at any given moment, it does not imply that the spark of humanism and goodness, capable of transforming that moment into an unforgettable one for both protagonists, is missing. There are times when what in other circumstances might have been trivial and devoid of any noteworthy meaning can become something so precious that no words can describe it.

Only the heart can understand, and the participants' memory makes the correct registration. Forever.

In other words, as long as Man is the Being that we know today, with the ability to feel emotion, to feel compassion, to feel indignation, to carry a remarkable set of civilisational values accumulated over countless generations, to be able to make choices and ethical judgments based on them and to possess body and spirit, he should always be treated by someone with identical attributes. When one of these days, in a more or less distant future, comes to be a bionic Being composed of a set of electronic circuits and pieces of disposable inert material, it will then make all the sense that it is treated as a mere 'robot' and not as someone originated and created with love by fellow beings; perishable, fallible, endowed with emotional intelligence, and a rough amalgam of hair, skin, muscles, bones, nerves, blood and soul made, because that is the biological magma sprinkled with feelings where the beautiful and imperfect structure of the Human condition is based.

3.6 Conclusions

> In the depths of love there is the desire for eternity (Friar Bento Domingues, Portuguese theologian, 1934–)

The 'idolised' quality of life does not necessarily translate into a long one. Functional aspects and the capacity for self-sufficiency are fundamental for each person to feel true happiness. Not to be in pain. To have a restful sleep. To take pleasure in relating to others, be it family or at work, when eating, when drinking, when smelling a perfume, a delicacy, or your lover. When contemplating your partner, children, parents, grandchildren, siblings, colleagues, neighbours, landscapes, poems, or canvas. On holiday or in the hustle and bustle of daily life. When hearing the first cry of your first child, the moan of sexual pleasure from one's partner, or a favourite tune. When feeling the energetic handshake of a long-standing friend or the caress of someone with significant emotional ties to us. All this is fundamental to the fulfilment of each of us, although each one is free to have their natural preferences in how, when and with whom. Or with no one else!

To safeguard an eminently humanistic posture in the medical practice it is necessary to invest in the training of new students and interns in Humanities (Ethics, Philosophy, Sociology, Anthropology, History, Literature, Painting, Music, Theatre and Cinema), together with the study of the medical field itself, instead of always deifying the omnipotent, omniscient and omnipresent capacities of cold technology, which seems to make everything credible in the eyes of men and represents the infallible answer to all their doubts and problems—addressing that there are not just one, but two equally valid meanings for 'Personalised Medicine'. The traditional version that should never be abandoned, according to which its exercise should always assume respect for ethics and the set of characteristics (psychological, philosophical, anthropological, sociological and religious) of each individual in pursuit of the principle that says 'an identical disease in a different person is a distinct disease', and, the most recent, but equally valid and promising, in which what is valued above all is the singularity of the genetic heritage of each being, and, in this way, one can better understand why a particular physiological phenomenon, in different patients, produces different effects, or why, for the same disease, different people react differently to the same pharmacological treatment.

To obtain the maximum benefit for the patient, it is necessary to improve knowledge in clinical semiology to make better use of technological means and not by its mindless generalisation as if it were a panacea or an obsession taken to the extreme. We should be concerned with promoting the return of a particular tradition of respect for hierarchy based on professional experience, solid scientific knowledge, the capacity for intergenerational transmission of knowledge and the establishment of empathetic inter-human relations, and mutual trust and respect, solidly based both on professional ethics and deontology, and also on the venerable collection of values inherited from our timeless mentors, instead of, counterproductively, relegating it to second place before the whirlwind of required assistance goals, calculated according to mere quantitative indices, but increasingly separated from the fundamental needs felt by both professionals and the patients themselves, and also because this is very important for the training of new generations of doctors and the practice of humanised, holistic, personalised and quality medicine.

For these reasons stated above, the medical practice of this unforgettable craft and its teaching must be founded to avoid being overwhelmed by anguishing and lacerating doubts accompanying us in our professional life. In reality, we have not been formatted to peacefully accept the error, even if inherent to all professional activity and involuntary, and of not having managed to avoid the unexpected death of our patient or to arrive at the exact diagnosis in time. As much as we do not want it to be, this is like an accusation before the court of our mind and soul. We assume it, subconsciously, as a defeat that is difficult to accept naturally. Where did I fail? Where I was not assertive enough in the timing of the clinical process? What alternative therapy should I have prescribed? What diagnoses have I not thought of?

My opinion regarding the eternal and never conclusive debate about the nature of medicine in which it is discussed if it is an Art or a Science is that it could, and should, be both! It is an 'Art' that aspires to use scientific methodology and adopts the so-called basic sciences to construct its principles and values without being a pure science itself, nor even claiming or having to restrict itself to this condition. Therefore, it is Art in the way of the relationship between the Doctor and his patient. It remains Art in the appreciation and context of the subjectivities of anamnesis and emotions in the clinical decision. It is also Art in the intellectual and aesthetic conception of the architecture of differential diagnosis. In everything else, it is Science.

We must assume without subterfuge that to diagnose, treat, cure, care for, accompany, or share in solidarity the joy, anguish, and suffering of others is to understand the essence of Man and Humanity, dictates to which no one should remain indifferent, especially not a doctor, nor a good governor, being unaware of the singular core of human nature or being indifferent to the consequences of suffering and disability. Understanding someone's illness goes far beyond diagnosing and treating it with competence and professionalism. It must also aim to seek knowledge of the multidimensionality of the person suffering from it. Medicine should always be practiced from Man for Man, or it will never be able to use this millenary epithet.

In an admittedly provocative conclusion, the physician should never contribute, within the scope of their correctly understood mission, directly or indirectly, implicitly or explicitly, to any member of our species taking possession of what should remain the exclusive and distinctive property of divinities that is, access to eternity, as I think is symbolically underpinned by the 'almost touching of the fingers between God and Man' in the timeless painting by the brilliant Michelangelo, called The Creation of Adam, on the ceiling of the Sistine Chapel. Death is the last chapter of life and an indissoluble part of it, and also an indispensable condition for the dignity and maintenance of our collective existence in this 'house called planet Earth' that we inhabit and must continue to healthily inhabit so that future generations may feel the pleasure of living there, a condition to which all Human Beings legitimately aspire to.

In short, not everything that is technically and scientifically possible to implement is ethically licit since the eventual implementation of that hypothetical scenario would be like a new Holocaust, in which the victims would not now, as in the past, be only the believers of a particular religious faith or ethnic group, but rather all of Humanity. Signalling the end of medicine, the Medical Act, and the Doctor-Patient relationship as I think it should be understood.

Bibliography

Books

1. Poças J. Ode or requiem: allegory about the nature of the medical act, about some real clinical histories. 1st ed. Lisbon: ByTheBook; 2015.
2. Poças J. Reflections in times of a pandemic: stories of life, pleasure, suffering, and death. 1st ed. Lisbon: ByTheBook; 2021.
3. Poças J. A global perspective from a few fragments in the doctor-patient relationship: a contribution by the Portuguese medical association. Lisbon: ByTheBook; 2019a. p. 221–55.
4. Poças J. A possible summary: editor's text in the doctor-patient relationship: a contribution by the Portuguese medical association. Lisbon: ByTheBook; 2019b. p. 748–55.

Internet

5. Poças, J. Razão de ser. 2020. https://www.josepocas.com/razao-de-ser/
6. A specialist in Internal Medicine, former President of the National Medical Committee of Setubal, former Director of Urgency Department, former President of the Infection Control Committee, former President of the Pharmacy and Therapeutics Committee, former President of the Antibiotic Committee, former member of the Medical Directory and also Head of The Pandemic COVID-19 Committee of the same Hospital, as well as Patient Provider of the Friend's League of St. Bernardo's Hospital (LAHSB) and President of the Consultive Committee of the Community Support League for the Study of Infectious Diseases (LACPEDI). Since January 2024 only practice ambulatory internal medicine in a private clinic in Setúbal. As a writer, published four books and was editor of another three.

Chapter 4
Conversation with Surgeon 2—Manuel Pera

Jacek Mostwin

Interview Dr. Manuel Pera March 8, 2024, by Zoom at his office in Barcelona, Spain
Abbreviations that follow:

JM: Jacek Mostwin
MP: Manuel Pera
March 5, 2024

JM: This is a conversation that recalls one we've had many times. But perhaps we'll go a little further today. You know this is for the book on humanism and surgery and I know that you and Jonathan are working on a specific chapter for the book, which I think sounds very interesting about the word and touch.

MP: That's right,

JM: I think I understand exactly what you're getting at. Sometimes it's hard to know exactly how to phrase this word 'touch', but I think you've got it just right. So, this is part of our conversation with surgeons about humanism and surgery, by which I mean the human side of medicine, the human side of surgery. I know that this is something that matters to you, so this is an opportunity for you to get your words down on paper, perhaps prompted by a few things that I say. Maybe you could tell me a little bit about yourself, where you grew up, what your home was like and how it all started for you?

MP: I was born in the South of Spain. My grandfather was originally a general practitioner in a small village in Extremadura, an area close to the border with Portugal. His brother, Cristobal was also a doctor, a surgeon, in Seville at that time. He became a very prestigious surgeon in Seville when my father was very young, just 2 years old. So my grandfather moved to Seville, a bigger

J. Mostwin (✉)
Department of Urology, Johns Hopkins Medical Institutions, Baltimore, MD, USA

J. McFarland et al. (eds.), *Humanism in Surgery*, New Paradigms in Healthcare,
https://doi.org/10.1007/978-3-031-86018-8_4

city, to provide a better education for my father and his sister. During my childhood I always had the experience of talking to my grandfather about medicine, his practice in that small village, doing everything from obstetrics and every kind of procedure. My first memories…I always remember that on Sunday my father used to take me and my brother, now living in United States, to the hospital. We would drive to the hospital and wait for him while he was seeing his patients who were at the University Hospital. So I have those memories. After that we used to go with my mother to a beautiful park in Seville to go for a walk. So those were my first memories.

I always understood at that time the commitment of my father to his patients. Even on Sunday he used to go to see them. My grandfather built a beautiful small house on the coast near Portugal and during the summer I used to share the bedroom with my grandfather and and he would tell me about his practice. I remember when I started medicine, as a present he gave me a book, my first book for my medical studies about the importance of physical examination and how to approach the patient. Those were my first steps, and those experiences were very important for me.

After that, we moved to Barcelona when my father was 38 years old. He was appointed Professor of Surgery in Barcelona. We were seven at home and for my mother it was not easy. My father, my mother, the whole family. My father was very busy in the hospital and my mother, always my mother, who passed away a year and a half ago, she always took care of us. We knew everyone there in Seville so when we moved to Barcelona it was a challenge. And well, I did my studies here in Barcelona. I always thought that medicine was my future career and and I was fortunate to get a good mark in order to start my medical studies at the the School of Medicine at the University of Barcelona. I was not sure about whether surgery would be my my career, my profession, but well, at that time I enjoyed basic [science] chemistry, biology, and pathology. But, at that time at the School of Medicine in Barcelona they opened a position called *internal alumni* (similar to an internship) at the Department of Surgery. You had to pass an exam if you wanted to apply for the position. So, it allowed you to be on call with the seniors and residents and also to spend some time on the hospital wards. I applied and got the position. It allowed me to be closer to surgical practice, and it reinforced my idea that surgery would be my choice as a future career.

Well, in Spain after finishing medical studies, we had to pass a national exam, and everything depended on the score you got. You could choose the specialty and also the hospital. So, I was also fortunate to start my residency at the Hospital Clinic, the University Hospital in Barcelona. Also, it was a quite interesting experience because it was not easy because at that time my father was the head of the department. It was not easy being the son of the head of the department and being in the same department. I always remember the words of my father. He told me that you must stand up for yourself: you must do that. In the end, in the future, people should recognise your achievement by what you have done, not by being the 'son of', And I tried, but it was not easy. And sometimes, well…I had some problems, but I think it made me be more resilient, I could say. And I always tried to demonstrate that I could do things by myself. And this is why during my residency, I worked very hard, and I was able to do well.

I can say that during my career, I've had several persons that have been very, very important in my career (good mentors) who have helped me a lot. For instance, one of them was Antonio Cardesa, Professor of Pathology, who had moved from Valladolid, a small town in the north of Castilla-Leon, to Barcelona. He had very good training in Germany, and also in Nebraska at the Eppley Institute. He was an expert in carcinogenesis, and he was very influential in facilitating my move to Hannover, where I completed part of my doctoral.

Another example is Mr. Adrian Marston, a general and vascular surgeon at the Middlesex Hospital in London. I was able to spend two summers there. The general surgeons also had some practice in vascular surgery, but he was mostly a vascular surgeon with a special interest in intestinal ischaemia.

For me, it was an incredible experience seeing how he would do his rounds, how respectful he was with his patients, and this ritual was at that time for me very important.

Concerning my experience with patients, the examples that I had with Mr. Adrian Marston and later on when I finished my residency during my period at the Mayo Clinic were steps that were especially important in the way I understood how critical it was to establish this special relationship with the patients.

It is no understatement to say that what I learnt with Professor Cardesa was crucial in my desire to follow academic surgery.

I remember that I used to meet with Professor Cardesa once every 2 weeks in his office. At that time, I admired him because he was able to write abstracts, to write the papers in English. So, I thought at that time I would like to be able to write in the future a paper in English, in good English, an abstract. And sometimes it was in the middle of the residency. Sometimes I had been on call during the whole night. I was tired. And then Professor Cardesa, the week before, he told me you should make this modification, these corrections, and you should work on it for the next meeting. And I was tired. I didn't work enough for the paper. And the day we had the meeting, he told me, 'Manuel, I think you haven't worked enough on the paper. So please work a little bit more and we will see each other next week'. So, these are the kind of things that will make you grow. Well, you know how important working hard is, being meticulous and the way that you learn and have a good mentor.

I also had other mentors during my careeer.

Yeah, that's right. Concerning my experience, I can tell you that even more than during my residency, our department became one of the most important departments in Spain. My father was able to recruit young surgeons when he arrived in Barcelona. Many of them then became professors. He provided another view about how to practice surgery in Spain, a more scientific, a more academic way.

I remember that one of my father's first books, because after finishing his residency in Santander in the north of Spain, he moved after his wedding to the United States for 1 year and visited Boston, the famous Lahey Clinic. He visited Philadelphia; they went to the Mayo Clinic, and that experience was very important. So, he was really affected by reading the book of [Francis] Moore, about the physiology of surgical stress. My father then wrote a book that became famous and was well received in Spain, on the fundamentals of surgery. At that time in the 70 s, discussing in Spain what we call the postoperative disease.

JM: Do you mean complications?

MP: The response to the operation was important because surgeons were more devoted to the practice, to the technique, and they didn't think about the pathophysiology and the surgical response and how to manage that.

JM: Are you talking about sort of the complications of surgery or more the long-term outcomes? Is it the long-term outcomes?

MP: What happens after the operation? No, {I am more] talking about wound healing, about renal failure, about nutrition, all these concepts that were not common, the things that affect surgery, but we don't think of them in the beginning when we're in the operating room. We don't think of those things, perhaps at the outset.

JM: I'd like to go back for a minute. You mentioned something about Mr. Marston in London, and you mentioned two words that come to mind. The first is the respect for the patient and the second is the idea of ritual. And I wonder if you could say a little bit more about those things, about respect and about ritual.

MP: The concept of ritual [involves] all the components I could dissect from the way he approached the patients. I remember those ward rounds, Mr. Marston surrounded by the house surgeons and the head nurse, etc. But how respectful they were when they approached the patient! And I remember talking to the patient, but first, [it was] 'Good morning, Mr. Taylor, etc'. The way they approached always, and how respectful they were when asking the patient, for me as a student, asking the patient whether they could start examining the abdomen or at that time, because it was vascular surgery, many patients with intermittent claudication, etc. And all these components that for me as a student made me think about how important the way is you approach the patient in the first encounter, but even later on during subsequent encounters.

JM: At what stage of your training was this? Was it when you were a student that you went to do this, or was this later?

MP: I was a student; it was at the end of my third and fourth years.

JM: What you saw there, how was it different from what you had seen before? Because it sounds like it made an impression on you.

MP: Yes, an impression, because I did not see the same in Barcelona. The way they approached the patients. I remember the University Hospital at that time, where patients were, it was a very old hospital, built in the beginning of the last century. Ramon y Cajal had been a professor in the School of Medicine. But at that time, there were very old wards, women, men, were separated. And I didn't have the same impression when we were making rounds on how our surgeons, seniors, mostly seniors, and even junior consultants, they approached the patients in the same way. Things have changed, but at that time, at least for me, I could see the differences.

JM: Would it be fair to say that this planted a seed that you might not otherwise have discovered on your own later on? Knowing who you are, but do you think this planted a seed that later grew when you returned to Spain?

MP: Yes, I could say that. And since then, well, I've tried to behave to see the patients in the same way I thought these patients were seen during my stay in London. But also, I think that after that, another fantastic experience was as a young consultant during my stay at the Mayo Clinic. At that time, that experience was fantastic. Because then for the first time, I saw that the patient was at the centre of the process. For me, it was fantastic. At that time, I was attached to the division of general thoracic surgery. And the way these patients were assessed [in a] multidisciplinary way by different specialists! I was not used to seeing that in Barcelona then. Things have changed. But at that time, patients were seen in Barcelona by an oncologist, then the surgeon, then the nutritionist, then etc. But at that time for me, I discovered that the practice of medicine could be done differently. And the patient was at the centre. And I still remember patients having the visit with the surgeon, the assessment before the operation, and just detecting something. And then the patient was seen immediately by the cardiologist or was seen by other specialists.

Since then, I think I've tried to manage in my area as a gastrointestinal surgeon with a special interest in esophagogastric surgery. I've tried to manage and to treat my patients in the same way. For instance, at present, I try to visit and to see patients jointly with the oncologist or jointly with other specialists. I still see that in our days, patients have scheduled visits 1 day with the oncologist, 1 day with the surgeon, 1 day with the nutritionist. And just in 1 week, they are seen three times. They must go to the hospital three times. I don't believe this is the way to manage and to treat our patients.

JM: So do you think that seeing the patient as a person or this respect that you talk about, which I know is very important to you and something that you talk about and you want to teach about, do you think this comes naturally to students or do you think it has to be somehow shown or brought out of them? What do you think about this? How do we encourage this in students?

MP: Well, I think that students can learn about how to approach and how to deal with the complex relationship with patients and other team members in a specific specialty. They can learn, but they should have innate skills in this area, but I think in my experience I see the importance of the role model. You can teach everything, you can show to our students well, you can explain how you should approach the patients, the importance of different components of what we call the 'bedside manner', but if you don't, if they do not see how you behave in front of a patient, how you behave when you are making rounds and how you try to explain for the patients facing a very complex problem, uncertainties, but at the same time provide confidence to the patient. All this, the importance of the language, all this can be taught by example and I know that because my students tell me, 'Dr. Pera, for the first time, I am very grateful for having the experience of being with you, seeing this patient because I have realised how complex it is to approach a patient that is coming to your office with concerns, with uncertainties', etc. So, I think that it's important to provide this concept during the undergraduate period, but the experience [of being] close to a mentor is fundamental.

JM: One of the things we talk a lot about in our meetings and that the meetings have addressed is the role of outside disciplines in trying to foster this kind of understanding of people. Now, from what you've described, it sounds like it really has to be demonstrated by a master surgeon, a faculty person who understands what an operation entails, someone who understands the patient and who has the respect and the attention of the students. It seems hard to believe that others can influence this and yet…what do you think about this? Where do people get the necessary sort of cultural formation to be able to appreciate these aspects of human character, of your patient's character, of yourself? I guess what I'm getting at is the relationship of the technical versus the humanistic aspects of our education. Does this question make sense?

MP: Yes, in my case, I've been fortunate because at home, my father has been what we could say was a humanistic surgeon. He′s a person that probably has a library with more than 3000 books and at home, we were surrounded by books. At home also, we have very interesting conversations with my brother Cristobal, who lives in the United States, an editor, and my father about literature and philosophy. Also, I think it's important to appreciate the importance of the language. It complements your practice. It's very important. I try even with my residents or my students, to translate to them the idea that they must enrich their inner part, their soul, with these other disciplines.

JM: Do you speak to your students specifically about these kinds of ideas? Or do you allow this to come out on its own? How do you do this? Do you talk to them directly? You're saying things about enriching the soul or enriching character.

MP: During the clerkship period there is always the opportunity to talk about it. Even when I give a lecture, I coordinated the subject, the Fundamentals of Surgery. There is always the opportunity to incorporate some of these aspects. When you are talking about the origin of surgery and you talk about mythology and you can explain about Chiron and the wounded centaur, and you talk about the concept of the wounded surgeon. There is always the opportunity. And, while visiting patients when you explain to your students how important it is when you are talking to a patient about a very complex problem, you have to use a very rich language. It's impossible to discuss this very complex problem with very simple language. So, you have to temper your language with these other disciplines, at least in my experience, and I try to translate this concept to our students, to make it easier.

JM: I wanted to get back to some of the memories that you had about your grandfather and your father, because you mentioned in particular the grandfather who would share the room with you. He would tell you stories. What were these stories like? What do you remember? What do you remember from the details of what he told you?

MP: He practiced in a small village. So, everyone knew him and the way how people were so grateful to his practice, how he treated them. So, mostly the idea he told me was how happy he felt by practicing in this way.

JM: Did you actually ever go to the operating theatre with him to see him work or go to the hospital to go on rounds with him? Or are these memories of what he told you and how you saw that people reacted to him?

MP: Well, the memories of my grandfather,... he retired when I was 7 years old. But concerning my experience with my father, sometimes he used to take me to the hospital. And that time there were nuns in the hospital. And he left me with the nuns. And they showed me those very old wards. And, well, it was an experience, but sometimes at home, together with my parents, they would talk about their experience in the United States. Just after my parents got married, they went to the United States by way of Gibraltar because of the political situation in Spain at that time, and my father continued his training in different institutions in the USA, in Boston, Philadelphia and Rochester. And so, for us, it was like a big adventure, certainly a big adventure.

JM: I'm curious, since we're trying to talk a little bit about some more details, if you remember, perhaps specific patients that stand out in your mind, specific experiences, either in the operating room or with people that you took care of. There are people who sort of you carry with you in memory or that you think of from time to time.

MP: For sure. Yes, I can tell you that in the hospital and in our department, I am known because I remember the names and last names of most of my patients even though I sometimes have problems remembering my own mobile telephone number.

And also, I remember the context and the experiences around the lives of many of my patients. And for me, this is important when I see my patients in follow up visits in the outpatient clinic. Many times, when you start your conversation with the patient by asking about the son who now has started studying engineering or talking about the mother who was a few months ago admitted to the hospital. So, talking about these other things, not only the main problem of the patient, but also those aspects that surround the life of the patient is important. I remember, well, stories of what happened with, or how difficult it was to...

I always say to my residents that, that when you are in charge, you have the responsibility with a specific patient, you have to work hard because sometimes you have a complex operation and it takes a long time to be close to the patients, to follow the patient during the whole postoperative course. You have to spend a lot of time and to be present, to be present with your patients. So, this is something that is important; it is important. And many times, patients and their relatives, when I see patients, even years after the operation, they remember how, you visited this patient on a Sunday morning or how you approached and saw your patients.

JM: Can you say something about the Gimbernat Surgical Society? Because I know this is a very important part of your work. And if you could say a little bit more about what it is, how it came to be…

MP: The Gimbernat Surgical Society, well, I didn't know what a Student Surgical Society was until probably 13 years ago when I visited my friend Derek Alderson, the former editor of the BJS, the British Journal of Society. At that time, he moved from Bristol to Birmingham to be full professor there. And then I had a young trainee that, as part of a grant, she could spend 3 months in the United Kingdom. So before sending this resident to Birmingham, I asked Derek, and he offered a position there. And then I visited Derek there.

One day he told me, 'Manuel, I have a meeting with students from the School of Medicine. If you want, you can join us'. And then I saw that they were talking about, organising a skills lab, lectures, surgical anatomy lectures, etc. Then he explained that those were members of the Birmingham Students Surgical Society. After that meeting, he allowed me to have a meeting with those students. And then I understood better and learned more about these surgical societies, the activities they organise. And so, I thought that was a very good opportunity to introduce for our students to promote interest among our students to the surgical speciality. So, when I returned to Barcelona, I talked to a small group of students, the fourth-year students. And then I asked them whether they would be interested in starting, organising, or founding a society, a Student Surgical Society. And then at that time we, we choose the name Gimbernat. We started as a small group 12 years ago and we have also included as a main goal to introduce our students to the humanistic part of medicine through conferences or lectures in medical humanities. I remember that for one of the first lectures, I asked a well-recognised philosopher from Catalonia, Rafael Argullol, to talk about 'The Wound as a Philosophical and Literary Metaphor'. And it was one of the first lectures. And since then, well, the society now has almost 100 members and they have a beautiful website in English and they have links with other surgical societies, mostly in the United Kingdom. In addition to all the lectures, etc., during the summertime and through my connections with good friends, professors of surgery in different prestigious institutions, since the beginning, I have sent more than 40 students to very prestigious surgical departments: Trinity College in Dublin, Imperial College, King's College in London, University of Edinburgh, Karolinska, etc. It's been a great success.

I can tell you that a few weeks ago, they organised the 'Scalpel Symposium'. Five years ago, we started organising this 2-day symposium, where we organised almost 15 skills labs, vascular surgery, urology, cardiac surgery, how to replace a heart valve, dermatology, etc., ophthalmology, and also conferences. And this year, 200 students attended the symposium, students from all around Spain, Europe, and even from Latin America. And it was a big success. And I can tell you what makes me even more happy about this experience: the members of the society, especially the members of the committee, it's amazing how professional they are in organising all the activities. They acquire the capacity of leadership, of ways to organise. It's amazing. And for instance, I sent an email to the members of the committee saying that I was very proud about what they have done. And a few days ago, I received an email after the Scalpel meeting saying, 'Thank you, Professor Pera, because you've been a fantastic mentor for us, and an example, and you have helped us a lot during all these years'.

So, for me, this is the most important, even though it is a lot of work for me because sending emails, trying to get those electives in other universities, but in the end, seeing these young students, how they progress through the years, and when they are finishing, they are more mature. So, it's been a great experience for me.

JM: It sounds also as though you have recreated something that you had described from your earlier medical school days of that special surgical programme that you had to take the examination for, that gave you an extra dimension of education and an early exposure to surgery based on the interests that perhaps your grandfather and your father had added to stimulate your own natural interest. You've recreated that in a way. But you also did something that I think is very unusual in bringing a philosopher in, and I'm just curious about this topic, the philosophy of the wound. Is that something that you suggested or that your colleague in philosophy suggested?

MP: No. This was a sentence that Rafael Argullol, included in a beautiful text he wrote for one of the most prestigious newspapers in Spain, El País, when he was asked to write a review about the book that my father had published a few months before.

JM: You mean like a book review? He was reviewing your father's book. -

MP: Yes, my father wrote a beautiful book, The Wounded Body, a philosophical dictionary of Surgery.

JM: That was the title of his book, The Wounded Body?

MP: The Wounded Body. Yes. He wrote a beautiful review, and in that he discussed the concept of the wound, and he also discussed the thinking that leads to surgery. He tried to relate surgery, the ways of surgery, the technique, the dissection, all the parts, the components that are within the surgery, how the thinking, when we are talking about the surgery, when we start thinking, the process of surgery. You have to dissect, you have to analyse, there is critical thinking, and in that text he also tried to discuss how the wound had been used. He used the concept of the surgical wound as a metaphor in philosophy, and also in literature. It was Rafael Argullol, but we also invited one of the most important philosophers in Spain, a good friend of my father, Emilio Lledó. He's now 96 years old, and he also spoke about 'A Philosophy of the Body'. No PowerPoint, no slides, it was pure conversation with our students, fantastic. The whole room was full of students, almost two hundred, and it was also a very good experience. So, I think this is another way to enrich the extra-curriculum, or as David Kopacz calls it, the counter-curriculum.

JM: Personally, I find the idea of having conversations and sessions on philosophy of the body and philosophy of the wound completely consistent with how I think about surgery. I'm not sure everybody does, some people may be a bit more concrete and do perfectly good work, but this aspect, this extra dimension, is very enriching, and such conversations might draw other people into the field that otherwise might not think about it.

MP: Yes.

JM: What do you think about the current world of surgical education compared to what you went through? I know that we're both a bit older, we probably went through very demanding residency programmes, training may have changed, and I wonder how you see the present world of surgical education. Do you think it's as good as it can be? You've already done a great deal with the Gimbernat Surgical Society, I just wonder what other things you think would be helpful, what would draw people in, intelligent people, people who are good with their hands, people who want to make a difference for the physical needs of others, what do you think about this?

MP: Well, I think now, at least in Spain, we are seeing a decline in the interest of our students in surgical specialties, at least some specialties, not, for instance, plastic surgery, maybe urology, well, this is a demanded specialty, but at least for specialties such as general and digestive surgery, the interest has declined. Our students, now see these specialties as being too demanding. You have to spend many hours, [accept] responsibility, you have to be on call, etc. Now I think that it's difficult to share what at least I see in our residents, in our young residents, how much they value the quality of life and the way they want to live and how much effort they have to put into their practice. And now we have a shorter time to train our residents because now they leave the day after they have been on call. Now it's becoming a little bit more difficult. It's very difficult to find now residents that are interested in pursuing an academic career. It's very difficult. Now they want things that can be achieved immediately or that will not take too much time; for us being involved in a project would take 2 years or 3 years. There's no interest in this kind of dedication.

JM: It seems that what you are describing are general social changes that might be specific not only to medicine, but more general, affecting all different professions and walks of life. But what will this do, you think, to the quality of surgical work, both the technical quality and the human quality of surgical work? How do you see the future?

MP: Well, I think concerning the training in surgical skills, I think now there is a lack of time. And also, we have to develop all the simulation systems and procedures in order to provide all the expertise and skills in the surgical techniques for the patient. And this kind of training has to be developed in our hospital. But at the same time, we have also to be better in teaching and training our residents in clinical judgment. I see that, at least in my residents, there is a need, because a clinical judgment is a combination [of skills]: you have to have knowledge, but in combination with experience, the way you have been taught. And it's a combination that gives you the skills to deal with both complex and less complex problems. But I see a lack of these skills. Now we expect that especially images, CT scans, all these different techniques will give us the diagnosis. And we have to improve in our residents how to deal with all the information in order to reach a better diagnosis and also to establish the best decision for our patients. Sometimes they are not able to synthesise the whole information in order to decide the best option for the patient. And sometimes it's not just to decide to operate, it's to decide not to operate on a patient.

JM: I would say based on what you've told me, it sounds like the key ingredients are a mixture of experience and mentorship so that you provide not only experience and responsibility for what they do but allow them to see good people do the work. And those good people themselves had to learn from other good people. So, there's a tradition of handing it down from one generation to the next. On the one hand, you reinvent it in every generation, but on the other hand, there has to be a sense of continuity. There's something continuous, longitudinal in the profession, in spite of the progress in technology, instruments, diagnostic skills and all the rest.

MP: Yes, for sure.

JM: We've been talking for a long time and I wonder if there is there anything else that you would like to add right now that's been stimulated by this conversation before we finish today?

MP: Well, you know, as a surgeon know this too, I always felt the responsibility. How much responsibility I have when treating a patient, because in surgery, you assume the whole responsibility for the patient. So, I don't know about other surgeons, but since the beginning, I have always kept in my mind the responsibility I have with a patient. Sometimes it's difficult to deal with that because sometimes, at least in my experience, sometimes if you are concerned about, well, a complication of how the patient is progressing during the postoperative course, your doubts or your concern, sometimes for me, it's difficult to forget all these feelings, even when you are at home, no? But at the same time, the great satisfaction you have when even after a complex procedure and your concern, your doubts, uncertainties, you see that the patient is progressing well. So it's a combination of concern, but at the same time, the great satisfaction you have when you see the patients at the end of the postoperative course, and you see the patient in the outpatient clinic after the operation. And so it's a mixture of feelings that maybe other surgeons, I don't know, the way they see this, well, they feel this, but in my case, sometimes I feel stressful about that, but at the same time, it's what makes me continue in my practice; seeing how the patients are so grateful when they see the results, the final outcome and how they have seen my dedication and presence and the way I've been close to them.

So, I don't know, but in my case, the way I always feel the responsibility with my patients, sometimes it's stressful, but at the end there is great satisfaction when you see that your patients are doing well. So, it's a mixture of feelings.

JM: Not everything that happens in surgery can be put into words. As you, I think, well know, given the chapter that you're contributing with Jonathan on The Word and The Hand. But we've covered a lot in language, and I think it's not always easy to do that. These kinds of conversations, I think, are very enlightening, very helpful. They're not over. I think we have to have more conversations about this, not just the two of us, but more people in surgery need to talk about these things because we spend so much time physically working and I think many things are generated in the mind, but often we don't have enough time to just share that among ourselves. So, thank you very much. We'll stop at this point. I think we've had a long morning for me, for you, but we'll continue. We're not done with everything.

MP: Okay, Jacek, it's been a great experience. Thank you so much. Yeah, it's really great.

JM: And you made it very easy for me, so I appreciate it.

Chapter 5
Caring for Others Through Relationships: Pedagogical Approaches Inspired by Narrative

Ana Filipa Cardoso

Telling stories, listening to them, being moved by them to act are recognized to be at the heart of many of our efforts to find, make, and honor meaning in our lives and the lives of others.

—Rita Charon

5.1 Caring for Others Through Relationships: Pedagogical Approaches Inspired by Narrative

Health is currently understood as a value that contributes to human development. It is highly sensitive to the social dimension. Person-centered care is the art of embracing the person as an equal partner in the design and co-production of care [1]. Therefore, a key component of health systems, and it is an indicator of quality of care by ensuring that people have access to care of the quality and appropriateness they need. It focuses on respecting and responding to a person's care needs, preferences, and values in all clinical decisions by delivering care through a range of activities and includes working with the person's beliefs and values; engagement; having a sympathetic presence; sharing decision-making; and providing holistic care [2].

Healthcare system agendas have firmly affirmed the need to focus on people's experiences. The call for person-centered care is not new, yet despite a high priority over many decades and numerous frontline interventions, a lack of person-centeredness care persists [1]. If on one hand, the focus is on respecting the uniqueness of the person, promoting autonomy, self-determination, equal participation in decision-making, and empowerment, on the other hand, there are some barriers to

A. F. Cardoso (✉)
Nursing School of Coimbra (ESEnfC), Coimbra, Portugal

The Health Sciences Research Unit: Nursing (UICISA: E), Coimbra, Portugal
e-mail: fcardoso@esenfc.pt

J. McFarland et al. (eds.), *Humanism in Surgery*, New Paradigms in Healthcare,
https://doi.org/10.1007/978-3-031-86018-8_5

person-centeredness care and communication that may distance professionals' practices from rituals of caring for the person and strips them of their dignity.

Both person and clinicians have repeatedly voiced a concern that healthcare systems do not sufficiently respect the individuality and human dignity of persons who seek their help [1]. Although the intertwined nature of the person and the body is well understood, in understanding a health problem, the clinician often ends up ignoring identity and personality. Ignoring the person in the person is a deeply worrying phenomenon [1].

For example, the study by Agledahl et al. [3], which aimed to study how doctors care for sick people, both medically and as human beings, found that even though doctors were concerned about the person's health, the focus on the clinical dimension often overlapped with existential elements. Doctors attended to people courteously, showing a polite and friendly attitude and emphasizing the relationship between them, but they actively shifted the focus from people's existential concerns to the medical facts and rarely addressed the personal aspects of the person's condition, treating them in a biomechanical way.

It is still necessary to help link the gap between the theoretical and philosophical perspective and the daily philosophy of care, where it is unequivocally emphasized that people have the freedom and power to be involved in the decision-making process so that their life projects can be realized. This reality can be transformed by a deep reflection on the healthcare education models that have been developed over the decades. At present, the deficit model dominates thinking in the health care system. In part, this is due to the prevalence of the biomedical model [4].

However, the biomedical model has become a reductionist approach in which persons are reduced to, and thought of, in terms of their body parts: "the diseased heart," "the malfunctioning lung," and "the pain in the stomach." The healthcare model need not be a deficit model. Clinicians can diagnose and treat problems and also have a strong perspective and practice whole-person care [4]. People's personhood does not need to be ignored, and their strengths should not go unnoticed.

Thus, the fact that the health system sees its responsibility only as re-situating and reforming the dysfunctional body represents the positivist understanding of the human being and the concept of health and, as we can see from the crisis, does not act well in re-situating nor can it understand human suffering and existential illness. Because when it is impossible to re-situate the deficient function, clinicians don't have much to do, and the person's existential suffering would remain neglected [5].

Perceiving health as relational means to set up connections among all stakeholders and recognize the impact of their interactions on each one of them. Re-thinking the meaning of care as healing integrates personhood into "patienthood" [6]. This philosophical perspective prompts us to consider the importance of recognizing people as distinct and exceptional beings who, when they fall ill, also undergo a range of transformations in their lives that extend beyond the physical symptoms of the illness itself. Illness disrupts most of the person's previous possibilities as if the person has been thrown out of everydayness [5]. Illness disrupts the idealized life, and people may live an unprecedented and unknown vulnerability as they must lead with the undesirable consequences, uncertainty, and dehumanization due to the illness or treatments.

It implies changes in self-perception, protection of self-identity, adaptation to the social world, redefinition of people's competencies as social actors, and demanding new ways of harmonizing with the environment and social dynamics. Illness is, in this sense, a biographical disruption [7] and it calls for a new awareness of oneself as a person, a new identity that integrates this new reality, the biographical work of the illness.

Illness experiences are not solely confined to the physical aspects of the body but are also influenced by the personal meaning it holds for each individual and the cultural and environmental factors surrounding them. It is essential to understand how the person experiences pain and illness [8]. Illness intensifies the routine drives to recognize the self. It is when one is ill that one must decide how valuable life is, which relationships are most meaningful, and what terrors or comforts the end of life holds. When people become sick or disabled, they question their existence in new ways [9].

When experiencing illness and vulnerabilities, Watson calls attention to the confirmation of the persons as a person. It's a way of proceeding in human relations that is based on both respect for the other person and an understanding of who they are and what they experience. It consists of recognizing the person as a human being, as a valid person who is given importance. This attitude manifests itself first and foremost through listening. Listening to a person and confirming their existence, showing them that they are important to us gives them back their power. One of the ways to do this is to consult them, to ask their opinion, but it is also to give them importance.

I would like to share a story. It's about an elderly man named Basílio who was in his mid-70 s. He must have faced many challenges throughout his life, but unfortunately, I don't remember much about his story. At the time, I was working as a young nurse and my focus was limited to the specific body part that needed to be fixed. I lacked the maturity to care for fragile human beings and understand the ethical responsibility that comes with caring for a vulnerable person in suffering. Perhaps I had read about it in books, but I had not yet fully embraced it.

> One day, while working in a surgery ward, I met Basilio who had been diagnosed by the medical team with ischemia in his lower limbs. However, I don't think that was the term he used to describe his condition. The healthcare team recommended amputation, but he refused and decided to go back home. Sadly, he returned a few days later, feeling hopeless and devastated, not because he had accepted his fate, but because he had no other choice. Eventually, his leg was amputated, and his journey towards recovery began.
>
> The day I approached him to suggest that he improve his body hygiene, he looked at me with indifference, which made me feel like my efforts were not appreciated. He only replied in short, one-word answers to some of the suggestions I was making. It seemed like all his anger was transferred to me. Despite this, I persisted, perhaps because I believed that improving his hygiene was important. However, I soon realized that I was wrong.
>
> As I reflect on the situation, I realize that I was wrong to assume that Mr. Basílio needed to comply with my wishes or the wishes of our team and institution. At the time, he was in a state of despair, and what he required was beyond the scope of what we could offer. What was the point of washing his body when it was broken and incomplete? Even though he did not express it in words, his silence and demeanor made it clear that he had difficulty looking at his leg. Instead of looking at it, he would turn his head and gaze at the cold, dark blue tiles

on the wall of my ward. To help him confront his fears and discomfort, I suggested that he touch his leg. However, he refused my suggestion.

I proposed that we could together and make this discovery of new limits of his body. And so, it was. I suggested that he put his hands on top of mine and top of the sheet. And that he would go as far as he dared. He accepted. But every time he got close to what was left of his leg, he avoided it. I used to stare at him from a distance, in the doorway of the room. And there he was, looking the other way and trying to reach the end of his leg! He managed to touch what was left of his leg 3 days later…

Now that I look back, I realize how far I didn't go. My priority was the need to respond to some kind of service standard, to day-to-day routines, and all these powers took precedence over my ability to interpret what wasn't being said, but which was evident in his blue eyes, which stared at the cold dark blue tiles every time he uncovered what was left of his leg. I realize that his long silences communicated much more than all the monosyllabic sentences he uttered to answer questions about futile things. Now I understand that Mr. Basilio was not that diagnosis! That the name of the treatment: amputation, gutted him as a human being!

That his identity vanished with the removal of that leg to an uncertain place! That the pompous name for his illness was something else: suffering! I realize now that I was unable to accept his vulnerability, his suffering. Perhaps because I had difficulty dealing with it! I can't remember many of the words I said to him, but I believe they amputated him even more. At that time, I couldn't understand what it really…meant to him… What it meant not to have a leg: the impossibility of leaving the house to do what connected him to life, visiting his wife's grave in the cemetery.

I still vividly recall Basílio, and I feel remorseful for not having been able to help him as he deserved. I should have asked questions such as: "How are you feeling?" "What concerns you the most?" "How are you dealing with the situation now?" "What does it mean for you to lose a part of you?" or "How can I help you?" to understand his struggles and help to support the suffering.

But I lacked the basis, and the necessary resources to assist the human suffering and to be able to support people and to help the person to create meaning. Today, as a more mature human being I still reflect on the story of this man. He taught me a vital lesson. I learned that the stories we witness and the narratives we allow someone to tell can teach us more about ourselves and others, and they can also help in the healing process. Now as a nurse and a nurse educator, I feel that I have an opportunity to make a difference in so many other Basilio's lives; by helping students to develop the self-knowledge and resources they need to assist the suffering of other human beings and their selves. Next, I will present some pedagogical approaches that I implemented inspired by Narrative Medicine in the training of nursing students, for more empathetic and humanizing care in a relationship-based healthcare perspective [6].

5.2 Narrative Medicine

When we get to know narrative medicine, a whole new world of perspectives opens. I came to know narrative medicine through the hands of the inspiring Dra. Susana Magalhães. I pay tribute and thank her for leading me through this inspiring world and that help me to gain a new vision on the humanization of care and pedagogy. I've been using her inspiring exercises in my classes ever since.

Rita Charon's book title "Honoring the Stories of Illness" shows us the way to rescue the person and nurture their humanity in rigid healthcare contexts. The competence to recognize, absorb, interpret, and be moved by the stories of illness, is at the heart of the medicine narrative [9]. It is an approach to relational ethics, that allows cooperative mutuality to flourish [10]. As it claims the relational, intersubjective dimension of clinical practice [11], narrative enables clinicians to rescue the thickness of healthcare anchored in three pillars, the three Rs of healthcare: Relationship, Recognition of one's own and of others' Vulnerability, Refection (or, we shall say, Responsibility, Respect, Reconciliation) [6].

This was a great challenge since the curricular unit in which these strategies are applied is the first year of the Nursing course and therefore, the students had no experience of clinical practice. They must imagine sick and vulnerable people and make them intrinsically want to care for others, to be attentive, to be empathetic and good listeners, to nurture relationships that care for people they don't know, who are strangers to them, who are from a distant and impossible time to imagine. I came across another challenge which was how to create meaning and how to get them to value things that are new to them, like touching, feeling, expressing emotions, and saying words that connect with other people.

Besides Rita Charon, I also come across Francisco Mora's reflections in his book "Neuroeducacion." He says, "You can only learn what you love." So, curiosity must come to the classroom, because curiosity ignites emotion. And with emotion, the windows of attention are opened. I've realized that it's important, more than just sharing knowledge about how clinicians can establish relationships with people, that each student may experience emotion, which allows them to have the curiosity to seek more knowledge about themselves and others.

As previously discussed, the clinician's education is still often guided by a disease-centered perspective. Sadly, health care professionals are not equipped to listen to such telling of the self with a diagnostic and interpretive ear, so too soon, the narrative is derailed by such questions as, "Is the pain sharp or dull?" or "How long did it last?" [9].

Caring is characterized by the attitude toward otherness. It is a result of reciprocity and a balanced relationship that is mutually beneficial and involves different roles, toward acknowledging each other's vulnerabilities. We are all vulnerable, and we all have relationships of dependence. Therefore, we must consider each other as complete individuals and protect every aspect of our uniqueness [12]. In caring, the relationship between the subject of care and the otherness being cared for is central. It's not about prioritizing the subject or the object of care, but rather about the connection between them as human beings [12].

Costanzo & Verghese [13] highlight in their paper "The Physical Examination as Ritual" the interesting concept of ritual. The ritual typically signifies a rite of passage, the crossing of a threshold, or a sacred event that is marked in contrast to events that are either quotidian or profane [13] in contrast to a routine that can be defined as a regular sequence of actions. The authors focus on the importance of rituals at the bedside (setting, appearance, tone of voice), suggesting that such words and rituals of the therapeutic act may change the chemistry and circuitry of a person's brain [13, 14].

Rita Charon draws attention to the fact that person-centered care and relationship-centered care require respectful authentic relationships with the person that come about through attentive and creative listening [9]. More genuine efforts to teach clinicians to listen to persons who need care include sophisticated training in self-awareness and mindfulness [9]. Clinicians can increase their awareness through a variety of approaches. Most involve reflection about past and present experiences, in solitude or with others, and often require time set aside from the usually hectic pace of training or work life [15].

In the caring process, self-awareness, introspection, and reflection should be a ritual. Self-awareness is a personal, professional, and conscientious attribute, the significance of self-awareness for nurses, self-aware nurses and its impact on personal care, behaviors, and actions signifying self-awareness, and what is needed to enhance self-awareness [16].

Self-awareness enables clinicians to recognize their emotions, temperaments, and potentials, ultimately assisting them in understanding the strengths and limitations of their persons and helping persons recognize their strengths [17]. Haley et al. [18] in a study developed with nurses, identified that greater self-awareness in nursing students resulted in increased empathy and improved person-centered care. And so, it is vital to encourage nurses to develop self-awareness as an essential competency [17, 18]. Improvement in active listening and self-awareness may lead to improvement in empathy, and, in turn, improvement in person-centered care [18].

5.3 Once Upon a Time

Considering the relevance of self-awareness skills development, the students are invited to practical classes, to develop a self-reflexive exercise. Because everyone has a story, in practical classes each student is invited to reveal themselves as a human being but also listen to the other colleagues. The personal narratives are shared in the classroom so that students can have a voice, feel heard, or feel acknowledged as a person and reflect on the way they feel doing it. They can reflect on their narrative, their journey, their singularities, and what makes them special. They do this from the prompt: "What makes me special and a unique human being?" Each student begins the exercise by saying: "Once upon a time…" remembering Dra. Teresa Temudo [19]. This exercise evokes interiority but also the possibility of getting to know the idiosyncrasies, what is common to each person, but also what makes them different from other colleagues. I remember one student saying, "It's the first time anyone has taken an interest in us as people, and that's great!" this exercise also appeals to the sense of empathy. Having the experience of feeling recognized as a person makes them aware of how important it also may be for the people you care for. To care for someone, one must understand and interpret how they tell their story.

The stories that people tell are expressions of their inner experiences, unique, intersubjective, and contextual and it depends on the meaning they attribute to their experiences, and not on the experiences themselves. Storytelling is a fundamental human need, just like eating, and it is what makes us human (Kearney & Ricoeur cit. by Casal, 2015). Narrating is a way that human beings must search for meaning in our existence and suffering. It is also an opportunity to communicate and understand someone else's suffering and find a story that gives it meaning [8].

The task of clinicians such as Billeri et al. [12] consists precisely of recovering the threads of the person's identity, helping him to express his history of illness, and his symbols, rewriting together a new healing story, or, where unfortunately this is not possible, to give back to the person an idea of his own coherent and unitary experience so that he can reach the end most consciously and serenely possible. It is rather an understanding of people as a total being, who needs to achieve their balance and health not only thanks to the use of specific biomedical therapy but also to the creation of a bond and positive communication with the caregiver [12] and this has an intrinsically therapeutic value.

Hermeneutic skills, such as attention, interpretation, representation, and imagination are essential to avoid what Fricker calls Epistemic Injustice (testimonial injustice and hermeneutic injustice) [20]. This process requires the professional to remain connected to the other person's story, enter their world imaginatively, interpret it from their perspective, share their understanding, and act together to alleviate their suffering.

5.4 Tell Me More About Yourself

The students are also invited to develop their skills of attentiveness, active listening, presence, and empathetic presence. They are invited to explore the narrative of another colleague. With this exercise, they experience some initial difficulties in exploring the story of a person they don't know, and in establishing bridges with them. A simple prompt such as "Tell me about yourself. How would you describe yourself?" or "This is the first time we've been together, what can you tell me about yourself as a person? What do you think we need to know to look after you?" can often be sufficient [21].

This exercise is inspired by the "Tell me more," an approach for person-centered interviewing developed by Platt et al. [21] This strategy was developed to assist clinicians in effectively communicating with the person. It is common for clinicians to find it difficult to choose the right words to make the most of each interaction. This tool is particularly useful in helping clinicians understand the persons, as well as to aid people in effectively managing their illnesses [21].

When treating an illness, it's important to consider the person's unique experience, including their values, desires, thoughts, feelings, and how they experience the illness. It is important to train physicians in in-person interviews with a refined vocabulary. No single phrase as "Tell me about yourself" works equally well for all clinicians and persons, and a skilled interviewer will adjust the language based on the individual and situation [21].

Nevertheless, Nakagawa et al. [22] add to this question other questions that allow exploring persons' values are: "Tell me more," "Why?" and "What else?" These three questions can be asked repeatedly or in combination to form a clear picture of a person's personality. This process also enables surrogates to contemplate the person as an individual, which allows them to provide more meaningful responses to specific opening questions [22].

To assess the person's experience of illness, the focus may also be on four dimensions—Feelings, Ideas, Function, and Expectations. The acronym FIFE can be a useful reminder [23]. Platt et al. [21] made it clear by developing core questions to help clinicians address who the person is, and the concerns, impact, feelings, ideas, and expectations the person has.

At first, it is relevant that clinicians know who this person is. Phrases like: "We should take a little time to get to know each other since we will be working together now. Let's start by asking you to tell me about yourself, and later I'll be glad to answer your questions about me" may be helpful [21].

Exploring concerns may be the first step: "What are you most concerned about?" "Do you have any specific fears or worries right now?" Exploring the person's feelings is important in assessing the emotional burden and psychological impact of the illness. How this person experiences this illness is another relevant issue. It can be addressed by questioning: "What has this illness been like for you? I can imagine that this illness has been disruptive of your life. Can you tell me about that?" [21].

Questioning the person's ideas about the illness is another relevant dimension. "Well, I may have some ideas, but I need to understand as well as I can what you think about what is wrong with you. Then we can discuss our ideas together" [21] and what are their main feelings about the Illness: "How does that make you feel? What's the feeling that goes with that? You know, the emotions?" [21].

The expectations that people have from the clinicians and the illness may be addressed with questions like: "What do you expect or hope I can do for you today?" "What are your expectations about what might happen with this illness?" [21, 23]. Explores the impact of the health condition on their daily life may be addressed with: "How has your illness affected you day to day?" or "How does this illness affect important people in your life?" [21]

At the end of the exercise, each student could present their colleague's narrative in their own words. With this exercise, each student becomes aware of the responsibility of being o interpreter of someone else's narrative. This implies the ability to interpret people's words and select the appropriate words to respect the shared reality. In this sense, one student referred to:

> This exercise made me reflect on the responsibility of selecting the right words to tell the Other's story.

5.5 My Story Through an Object

Students are also invited to tell their story through a special/symbolic object or artifact. The prompts usually used are: "Sometimes people have special objects or artifacts that are very special and talk more about the personal narrative. Tell me more about yourself by telling the story of this special object/artifact." Lots of beautiful stories emerged: The heart tattoo of a student that represents the love of all women in the family, namely her grandmother who was a mother to her or the student who left an African country in search of education against his mother's will, who keeps the photograph she gave him thinking she would never see him again. Through the stories of their colleagues, students could be touched by other stories, discover emotions, mirror suffering, and gain awareness about who they are as listeners. With this reflectional exercise, they discover a common ground: vulnerability.

In addition, with this exercise we can reflect that when caring, we move through a forest of symbols and may reflect on the importance of taking care of the person's symbols, such as the rosary, pictures, and draws that often are kept on the bedside table and can be the only connection to their memories, to their loved ones, to their hope or life and raise awareness of rituals of presence in person territory. It brings deeper reflection on the importance of developing non-verbal communication skills, such as competence when approaching people's territory and personal space when in the hospital or other institutions.

The literature emphasizes that actions such as removing people's belongings, or artifacts of one's identity imposing hospital clothing, or imposing restricted monitoring of actions normally taking place with some degree of privacy, including eating, and using the bathroom; imposing difficulties to rituals associated with values and beliefs; generally requiring people to lie in bed may annul the uniqueness of the person and its dignity. This is one of the aspects that must be considered to minimize the sense of aggression, since that evidence shows the attitudes of the staff, such as touching the person's possessions without permission and exposing the person, causing discomfort, and violating the person's privacy. People who were lonelier and had more privacy at home perceived a greater invasion of their territorial space by the nursing professionals [24].

These behaviors reduce the uniqueness of the person. With a certain degree of similarity, Goffman's perspective of healthcare institutions as total institutions. They are characterized by the bureaucratic control of the basic human needs of a group of individuals. The totalizing practices provided are those in which, through mortification of self, a person within an institution exercises little control, and is essential to serve the needs of the institution [25]. Mortification of self happens when individuals lose their roles, identities, and autonomy they have on the "outside." The degree of autonomy given to individuals also determines the degree of mortification [25].

5.6 I Am a Person, Not a Number

When caring for someone we should recognize them as human beings [26]. Clinicians need to respect a person's individuality in the care context by addressing them by their names and not by their problems. When clinicians focus on the problems of their persons, they tend to frame their behavior negatively [4]. When the process of diagnosing is generalized to the person, it becomes problematic. This means that the person is reduced to their symptoms as if the symptoms can exist separately from the person. Instead, the person should be viewed as a person who is experiencing an illness or symptom [4]. To put it simply, referring to a person as a mere number, such as "Bed 41," or by their condition, such as "That one's the hypertensive," or even worse, referring to their body parts, like "The prostate of bed number six," shows a deeply concerning perspective of viewing people as objects that exist solely to serve the institution, rather than as individuals with inherent dignity and value [4].

Travelbee [27] also considers that people are unique irreplaceable individuals: "a one-time being in this world, like yet unlike any person who ever lived or ever will live" and argues that "patient" is a stereotype and category. In this sense, the term "patient" should be abolished. There are no "patients." There are only individual human beings in need of care, services, and assistance of other human beings. This claims the need to identify permanence and confirmation [27]. The students are also invited to call people by their names or acknowledge their individuality by addressing people by their professional titles. It can help to restore a sense of dignity and importance, thereby making them feel valued and respected [28]. One effective way to show respect for others is by calling them by their preferred name. The "#CallMe or The Call Me Because Names Matter" campaign strives to encourage the use of person' preferred names in healthcare settings. This practice helps to create cultural awareness and demonstrate respect toward the persons. Using people's preferred terms of address in healthcare can offer them dignity, kindness, and respect. It is also essential to seek the opinion of others and acknowledge their value, which can often be overlooked in the face of illness and the hospital environment [29].

Students are invited to use person-first language or person-centered language because it may help distinguish an individual from their diagnosis or impairments. Using destigmatizing language is also a relevant recommendation in the NICE guidelines [30]. When communicating with others, it is crucial to show respect and empathy toward them. Using person-centered language is an effective way to display sensitivity and good manners, and it can also help to avoid labeling people. According to the NICE guidelines, it is recommended that we should prioritize the person over their clinical conditions. It is important to describe what a person has, rather than what they are [30].

Another important ritual is sharing their names with the persons. Evidence shows that commonly healthcare professionals tend to forget to introduce themselves, which can negatively impact the person-provider relationship. Dra. Kate Granger shared a true story of her journey as a person with terminal cancer, where she observed that many staff members did not introduce themselves before delivering care. As a result, she started a campaign to encourage and remind healthcare staff about the importance of introductions in healthcare. The "#hellomynameis" campaign [31] was initiated to establish a human connection between a vulnerable individual who is suffering and someone who wishes to offer help. The primary focus of this campaign is to foster therapeutic relationships and build trust in challenging situations. I challenge all to remember those words of Dra. Kate Granger.

5.7 Assessing People Suffering

Costanzo and Verghese [13] propose that the primary ritual professionals must automate is the process of attuning to the person's suffering [13]. Assessing a person's suffering should be viewed as an essential part of providing care and personal writings by sick people and healthcare professionals can contribute to this.

Inspired by Charon's perspective, autobiographical writings, or videos of people's narratives ("human library") of person, health professionals' reflective writing, and students' writing in Parallel Charts are shared with the students to promote the development of interpretative skills. Also, stories such as Maria's letter to her son Martin, who she had to say goodbye to when he was 6 months old...The story of Rui who was admitted by Covid to an intensive care unit... or the story of Alexandra, Rui's wife who tells the part of Rui's story that he doesn't remember, and the loss of their son while he was hospitalized. By analyzing and looking carefully into these stories students may have a deeper look into the illness and suffering narratives of people. This exercise has a deep impact on students. It helps them to anticipate experiences with people and establish bridges with reality unknown. In their reflections, they say:

> It made me realize that everyone feels things differently, but that we all feel something. These stories bring reality to us it was the first time I heard the 'voice' of the people we care about! says Adriana, a first year nursing student.

The CARE approach is an interesting resource for person-centered communication and a very useful resource to automate is the process. It involves listening attentively and adopting a holistic approach to gain a comprehensive understanding of the person's situation, perspective, and emotions, including the meanings they attach to them. Clinicians can achieve this by actively listening, showing a genuine interest in the person as a whole person, and fully comprehending their concerns. In the process of assessing, clinicians need to ascertain what aspects of the person's life are important to them and what values they hold dear. It is also essential to understand how the person makes sense of the situation they are facing [32].

Another person-centered interviewing strategy is BATHE. It can be viewed as an informal screening test for emotional problems. "B" stands for background: the question "What is going on in your life?" will elicit the context of the person's visit. Alternative opening questions can take the form of "Tell me what's been happening since I saw you last." It is useful to connect with persons in this personal way at each visit. "A" stands for affect. "How do you feel about that?" or "How does that make you feel?" allows the person to report the current feeling state [33]. "T" stands for trouble. "What about the situation troubles you the most?" helps both the clinicians and the person focus on the subjective meaning of the situation. "H" stands for handling. "How are you handling that?" assesses functioning. "E" stands for empathy. A response such as "That must be very difficult for you" legitimizes the person's reaction [33]. These strategies are also used in role-play scenarios, where students are asked to assume the role of the ill person and the professional role.

5.8 Healing by Presence

A meaningful way of offering support is by being genuinely present. Presence can be a valuable resource to alleviate people's suffering. Presence is a reciprocal and healing relationship between the healthcare provider and the person receiving care. It is not a solitary experience, but rather a connection achieved through a compassionate exchange of the human experience [34]. Presence is a purposeful practice of awareness, focus, and attention with the intent to understand and connect with the person [35]. Everyday practice or ritual supporting these strategies could support physician self-care as well as physician-person connection [35]. Presence does not necessarily require more time, but a complete focus on the person's needs without interruption to allow for the sharing of the human experience [34] The study by Zulman et al. [36] identified evidence-based practices that foster this time-honored ritual between physicians and persons to create connection, particularly in the first moments of a clinical encounter.

This practice comprises two components that comprise physical and psychological preparation for a clinical encounter: [1] personalized preparation for the person and [2] taking a moment to pause and focus [36]. The recommended clinician practices to foster connection with the person are organized by: Preparing with intention, Listening intently and completely, Agreeing on What Matters Most, Connecting with the person's story, and Exploring emotional cues. Some examples are the Warm-up act, Hand on the doorknob, or reflection about bias [36].

5.9 Being in Other's Hands

Dr. Susana Magalhães introduced me "Hands" by Moya Canon. I have used this and other poems to reflect on human vulnerability using metaphors to reflect on the mystery of being dependent on the hands of others who care for us. Students are invited to do close reading and reflexive writing and share stories of vulnerability after reading the poems starting with the prompt: "The hands that hold me that day…." This is a powerful exercise that also helps students make the connection between caring and being cared for and the power of the human touch. This is also a strategy that calls for self-knowledge and introspection. In one of these exercises, Inês, a four-year student, shared a story about one of the most important moments in her academic path, which made her rethink her future career. She wrote:

> The day I first saw a person I cared for leave, in a room with three beds and no privacy, I tried to hold her hand, not realizing that I, Inês, a nursing student, for the 1st time at the hospital, also needed to be held in mine. After all, nursing is about being. And I had to be. And on that day, when I almost gave up, not because of the contact with death, but because of the conditions in which it was happening, I was embraced and comforted by the person who most needed a lap that day: the mother of the girl who had just passed away. It was at that moment that I realized that I don't have to annul myself as a person to be a good professional.

5.10 Personal Narrative Writing

It is also relevant that students have opportunities to develop themselves as persons and share their own vulnerabilities and suffering when caring for someone. Many clinicians and educators have been attracted to narrative writing as a road toward empathy and reflection in clinical work. Nursing students keep reflective journals as they proceed through clinical training [9]. During the internship students are invited to write about the person's life and also to do a reflective writing is called: "I need to talk about…."

The students are invited to describe an experience of care that has been memorable for them and reflect on the emotions and feelings that they lived during that moment. After thinking about that relevant moment, they are invited to write about: "what was most challenging," "how I felt about this experience," and "what I discovered about myself in this experience." A fourth year student described her experience with this reflection exercise, emphasizing its positive results:

> (…) because when we think about and express such strong clinical experiences, we realize things that until then we did not know about ourselves, such as vulnerabilities or strengths" or "(…) just the fact that we have someone who understands 'our inner world' tell us that they understand us and that what we feel is all normal, makes this last phase of ours more fluid and full of richness, due to this sharing and mutual help.

5.11 Our Bodies, Our Selves

Our Bodies, Our Selves is the title of one of the chapters of Rita Charon's book [9]. The care provided by nurses often involves caring for people's bodies. However, sometimes we assist dehumanizing practices when the person is objectified. Illness causes two stories of the self to be told at the same time, one told by the "person" of the self, and one told by the body of the self. How the body communicates its story is very mysterious. Although the body is material, its communications are always representations, mediated by sensations and the meanings attributed to them [9].

Sometimes it's as if the body speaks a foreign language, depending on other bilinguals to translate, interpret or, in some way, make transparent what it wants to say [9]. The self depends on the body for its presence and its location. Without the body, the self cannot enter relations with others. Without the body, the self is an abstraction [9]. Rita Charon says that accepting the power and privilege of touching another's body, interfering with it, hurting it, or perhaps healing it incurs in health care professionals' profound duties to acknowledge the inviolability of the person's body as a locus of the person's self. While doctors and nurses might breach the body's unity, we do our best to maintain the "wholeness" of the person. The body is the proxy for the self, and demeaning or disrespecting the person's body demeans and disrespects the person's self [9].

The body is the story of the person. The telling need not even be in words. These Rita Charon reflections inspired me to develop another exercise. At first, students are invited, in pairs, to explore the body of another colleague (less intimate areas of the body, such as arms, legs or back with the due consent). They also explore the narrative "written" in the body of the colleague, by scars, tattoos, etc. This exercise helps to promote awareness to ask questions about meanings.

In my experience as a supervisor, I found that many students still found it very difficult to touch other people or use less humanizing forms of touch, such as clamped hands or claws. The care we provide as nurses also involves touch, often in situations that make people even more vulnerable, such as bathing. In this sense, students are also challenged to create rituals of respectful touch.

Once I asked the students: "does anyone ever try to understand what people may feel when they are bath by a stranger." They said, "I have never thought about that, but it must be very violent." In this sense, students are also invited to "bathe" their classmate's body (less intimate areas of the body, such as arms, legs or back with the due consent). In pairs, and seated front to front, the one's who are bathing can train safe, respectful touching rituals that promote the dignity of the other. Those being bathed keep their eyes closed. Both have experienced the discomfort of being touched or cared for by others, or touch; reflect on being ashamed, feel safe in the hands of a colleague, or put themselves in a place they had never even imagined.

Students are also encouraged to abandon forms of "imperfect care," of heavy, clenched, clawed, or pincer hands, to make them soft and safe, and to create rituals of touch that promote the dignity of the person by having the teacher and their colleague's feedback. In the end, they reflect on their feelings and emotions of touching and being touched by someone they don't know so well and prepare themselves for using the touch as a powerful communication resource. This exercise helps the students to reflect on the intention of touch as a communication strategy: "What do you intend to communicate to the other when you touch someone?"

5.12 Feeling Vulnerable

Students are invited to create rituals of trust. This exercise also allows each student to feel vulnerable at the hands of others. Students (if they are comfortable with the request) put on a blindfold, other students act as their careers and help them carry out simple activities, such as sitting in a chair or going for a walk. With eyes closed, like vulnerable people in care, they experience the need to be cared for by another college. Their stories usually reveal emptiness, powerlessness, discomfort, and despair. At this point, without the blindfolded student realizing, I invite the student carer to "abandon" the person they are caring for. Ana, a first year student, wrote a very deep reflection about this:

> Being abandoned by my caregiver I felt even more disoriented and lost than I was initially being guided. When I realized I was abandoned I started to go into despair, because I don't like being alone. Not all people are the same, but I think that nurses must keep in mind that they are afraid of being alone, even more so in a place unknown to them. Once again, I mention that for me it was a very distressing experience, because despite knowing the space I didn't know where I was and didn't know what to do to find the safe harbor. (This experience lasted 2 minutes) I believe that other people may feel this way, being left in the hallway, waiting for us to gather materials at the time of a procedure.

5.13 Empathetic Words

Empathy is a pivotal issue in the path toward the humanization of care and is one of the cornerstones of narrative medicine. Yet, in the social context we are today, rather than empathy we are most often forced to speak about the lack of empathy [37]. Person-centered communication requires empathetic approaches. Empathy is a complex, multi-dimensional concept and involves an ability to; (a) understand the person's situation, perspective, and feelings (and their attached meanings); (b) communicate that understanding and check its accuracy; and (c) act on that understanding with the person in a helpful (therapeutic) way [38]. Empathy can be shown in various ways, both verbal and non-verbal.

The students are also invited to have a more focused perspective on how they gaze, touch, and/or use gestures. Empathy don't require more time. For instance, sitting next to the person can increase the perception of person-centeredness. The literature reveals that simply sitting instead of standing at a person's bedside can have a significant impact on person satisfaction, person compliance, and provider-person rapport, all of which are known factors in decreased litigation, decreased lengths of stay, decreased costs, and improved clinical outcomes [39].

To develop a sense of presence, and by the principles of listening intently and completely (Sitting down with the person) and connecting with the person's story [36], the students develop exercises that allow them to train more effective forms of non-verbal communication. I would like to highlight one exercise, which I have entitled: "I have time for you." The student starting from the trigger phrase: "Now that I have time for you, tell me something about yourself that we don't already know." This exercise is often implemented in clinical settings to reduce the person's burden of loneliness and to increase knowledge about the person.

It aims to increase the feeling that the clinician is available to listen and put into practice some person-centered communication strategies such as NURSE [40]. NURSE strategy is a very powerful and useful tool for understanding the person's perspectives and views of his or her illness. The person's perspective includes feelings, ideas, concerns, impact, and expectations as described above. NURSE comprises: Naming: "It seems like you are feeling…," "I wonder if you are feeling…" (…), Understanding: "I can understand how that might upset you," "I can't imagine what that would feel like!," "This has been a hard time for you." (…) Respecting: "It must be a lot of stress to deal with…," and "I respect your courage to keep a positive attitude despite your difficulties" (…), Supporting: "Please let me know if there is anything I can do to help," "I will be with you in this difficult time" (…) and Exploring: "Tell me more about what you were feeling when you were sick." "How are you coping with this?" (…) [40]

Narrative medicine can inspire us in so many ways to promote humanizing care. It is in our hands to be a part of a shift from a disease focus to relationship-based healthcare that implies recognition that a person is a unique human being who has the right to be treated with respect and dignity. Narrative rescues the humanity in all of us, so, as clinicians, we should all be narrative interpreters.

Acknowledgments I would like to express my deepest gratitude to:

Jonathan McFarland (Associate Professor, Faculty of Medicine, Autonomous University of Madrid, Madrid, Spain; Sechenov University, Moscow,)

Susana Magalhães (Unit for Responsible Conduct in Research, Institute for Research and Innovation in Health, University of Porto, Porto, Portugal).

References

1. Berntsen GR, Yaron S, Chetty M, Canfield C, Ako-Egbe L, Phan P, et al. Person-centered care (PCC): the people's perspective. Int J Qual Heal Care [Internet]. 2021;33(Suppl 2):ii23–6. Available from: https://academic.oup.com/intqhc/article/33/Supplement_2/ii23/6445897
2. Mccormack B, Borg M, Cardiff S, Dewing J, Jacobs G, Janes N, et al. Person-centredness—the 'state' of the art. Int Pract Dev J. 2015;5(Suppl 1):1–15.
3. Agledahl KM, Gulbrandsen P, Førde R, Wifstad Å. Courteous but not curious: how doctors' politeness masks their existential neglect. A qualitative study of video-recorded patient consultations. J Med Ethics. 2011;37(11):650–4.
4. Gottlieb LN. Strengths-based nursing care health and healing for person and family. Springer; 2013.
5. McFarland J. Health humanities for quality of care in Times of COVID -19 [Internet]. In: Marini MG, McFarland J, editors. Health humanities for quality of care in times of COVID -19. Cham: Springer; 2022. (New Paradigms in Healthcare). Available from: https://link.springer.com/10.1007/978-3-030-93359-3.
6. Magalhães S. Looking behind the veil: why narrative medicine matters in times of uncertainties. In: Health humanities for quality of care in times of COVID -19. Springer; 2022.

7. Bury M. Illness narratives: fact or fiction? Sociol Heal Illness. 2001;23(3):263–85.
8. Frank AW. Just listening: narrative and deep illness. Fam Syst Health. 1998;16(3):197–212. https://doi.org/10.1037/h0089849.
9. Charon R. Narrative medicine: honoring the stories of illness. Ann Intern Med. 2007;146. 152 p
10. Barbosa A. Ser pessoa, Vulnerabilidade e sofrimento. In: Manual de Cuidados Paliativos. Lisboa: Faculdade de Medicina de Lisboa; 2015. p. 978.
11. Casal T. Narrativa e Medicina: A perpectiva da primeira pessoa no encontro clínico. In: Narrativa e Bioética. Lisboa: Faculdade de Medicina de Lisboa; 2015.
12. Billeri I, Dadà S, Giunta F. Chapter 7: The medical doing on the person. In: Pingitore A, Iacono AM, editors. The patient as a person [internet]. Cham: Springer; 2023. (New Paradigms in Healthcare). Available from: https://link.springer.com/10.1007/978-3-031-23852-9.
13. Costanzo C, Verghese A. The physical examination as ritual: social sciences and embodiment in the context of the physical examination. Med Clin North Am [Internet]. 2018;102(3):425–31. https://doi.org/10.1016/j.mcna.2017.12.004.
14. Verghese A, Brady E, Kapur CC, Horwitz RI. The bedside evaluation: ritual and reason. Ann Intern Med. 2011;155(8):550–3.
15. Novack DH, Suchman AL, Clark W, Epstein RM, Najberg E, Kaplan C. Calibrating the physician: personal awareness and effective patient care. JAMA. 1997;278(6):502–9.
16. Younas A, Rasheed SP, Sundus A, Inayat S. Nurses' perspectives of self-awareness in nursing practice: a descriptive qualitative study. Nurs Health Sci. 2020;22(2):398–405.
17. Eckroth-Bucher M. Self-awareness: a review and analysis of a basic nursing concept. Adv Nurs Sci. 2010;33(4):297–309.
18. Haley B, Heo S, Wright P, Barone C, Rao Rettiganti M, Anders M. Relationships among active listening, self-awareness, empathy, and patient-centered care in associate and baccalaureate degree nursing students. NursingPlus Open [Internet]. 2017;3(November 2016):11–6. https://doi.org/10.1016/j.npls.2017.05.001.
19. Temudo T. Era uma vez um menino. Visão [Internet]; 2019. Available from: https://visao.pt/opiniao/2019-08-12-era-uma-vez-um-menino/
20. Fricker M. Epistemic injustice: power and the ethics of knowing. Oxford University Press; 2007.
21. Platt FW, Gaspar DL, Coulehan JL, Fox L, Adler AJ, Weston WW, et al. "Tell me about yourself": the patient-centered interview. Ann Intern Med [Internet]. 2001;134:1079–85. Available from: patient-centred interview
22. Nakagawa S, Callahan ME, Berlin A. Patient values: three important questions—tell me more? Why? What else? BMJ Support Palliat Care. 2023;13(3):363–4.
23. Ambuel B. Fast facts and concepts #17—Patient-centred interviewing. 2015.
24. Marin CR, Gasparino RC, Puggina AC. The perception of territory and personal space invasion among hospitalized patients. PLoS One. 2018;13(6):1–9.
25. Jenkins D, Burton C, Holmes D. Hospitals as total institutions. Nurs Philos. 2022;23(2):1–6.
26. Entwistle VA. Treating patients as persons: a capabilities approach to support delivery of person-centered care. Am J Bioeth. 2013;13(8):29–39.
27. Travelbee J. Interpersonal aspects of nursing [Internet]. 2nd ed. Philadelphia: F. A. Davis Company; 1971. Available from: https://nursology.net/nurse-theories/interpersonal-aspects-of-nursing/
28. Salazar H, Duarte J. A comunicação em cuidados paliativos: uma estretégia fundamental. In: Lidel—Edições Técnicas L, editor. Intervenção psicologica em cuidados paliativos. Lisboa: Pactor; 2017.
29. #CallMe in a nutshell [Internet]. Available from: https://callmebecausenamesmatter.org/
30. NICE National Institute for Health and Care. Talking about people [Internet]. Available from: https://www.nice.org.uk/
31. The #hellomynameis Campaign [Internet]. Available from: https://www.hellomynameis.org.uk/key-values/
32. Bonner P, Devince A, Herman-Smith P, McCardie S, Cotton P, McNeney F, et al. The CARE approach. A learning tool for healthcare professionals.

33. Stuart MR, Lieberman J. The fifteen minute hour. Efficient and effective patient-centered consultation. CRC Press; 2019.
34. Hessel JA. Presence in nursing practice. Holist Nurs Pract. 2009;54702:276–81.
35. Brown-Johnson C, Schwartz R, Maitra A, Haverfield MC, Tierney A, Shaw JG, et al. What is clinician presence? A qualitative interview study comparing physician and non-physician insights about practices of human connection. BMJ Open. 2019;9(11):1–8.
36. Zulman DM, Haverfield MC, Shaw JG, Brown-Johnson CG, Schwartz R, Tierney AA, et al. Practices to Foster physician presence and connection with patients in the clinical encounter. JAMA—J Am Med Assoc. 2020;323(1):70–81.
37. Marini MG. Narrative medicine. Springer; 2016.
38. Mercer SW, Reynolds WJ. Empathy and quality of care. Br J Gen Pract. 2002;52(Suppl):9–12.
39. Swayden KJ, Anderson KK, Connelly LM, Moran JS, McMahon JK, Arnold PM. Effect of sitting vs. standing on perception of provider time at bedside: a pilot study. Patient Educ Couns [Internet]. 2012;86(2):166–71. https://doi.org/10.1016/j.pec.2011.05.024.
40. Fortin AH, Dwamena FC, Frankel RM, Smith RC. Smith's patient centered interviewing: an evidence-based method. McGraw Hill; 2018.

Chapter 6
Conversation with Surgeon 3—William Reiner

Jacek Mostwin

Interview Dr. William Reiner March 7, 2024 by Zoom at his home in San Diego, CA.

Abbreviations that follow:

JM: Jacek Mostwin
WR: William Reiner

JM: I'm going to record this because we'll need a transcript later, just to let you know. So, I hope that's all right with you, otherwise I'd be scribbling furiously. Where are you now? You are somewhere in California, right?

WR: Yeah, I'm in San Diego County, North County. It's called, the town is called Escondido. So, it's in a little valley surrounded by hills. We're actually on one of the hills, so it's straight up or straight down, depending on which way you want to go.

JM: And have you been relatively free of all these horrible weather situations that we've been exposed to, that you've been exposed to? It's mostly hit north.

WR: I mean, we've gotten more rain than usual, but Los Angeles and Orange Counties, but especially LA County and north of there have gotten hit the hardest. We really haven't had that kind of rain. We're a little south and actually east. I mean, we're farther, we're so far east that the storms tend to curve around and then go north and miss us.

JM: Well, here we are aging in place. Definitely aging. The only thing we have left to add is our memories. So, in all fairness, I should tell you how this all came about. I got involved in this group called the Doctor as a Humanist, which is sort of a, I don't know, sort of a loose affiliation of people with similar interests, mostly physicians, some not. I somehow got roped into one meeting and

J. Mostwin (✉)
Department of Urology, Johns Hopkins Medical Institutions, Baltimore, MD, USA

J. McFarland et al. (eds.), *Humanism in Surgery*, New Paradigms in Healthcare,
https://doi.org/10.1007/978-3-031-86018-8_6

then I got roped into sort of a strategic position. And they were going to put on a conference about a year ago on humanities in surgery. But, you know, there's kind of a push, particularly from the people on the humanities side to get funding because medical humanities gets more funding than straight humanities. But this is how it was with ethics: a gold mine for the philosophers. So, what I suggested was that we change the title of the conference to Humanism in Surgery, because my approach is not that we need to add more to the curriculum and have people, you know, becoming poets, although that would be fine, but rather to look at the real humanism that already exists in surgery and bring it more to light, let it shine a little bit.

WR: Right.

JM: So, that conference took place, and it led to the idea of having a book. And initially I was just asked, would you like to contribute a chapter to this? And could you also find some other people who could contribute chapters to this? And I suggested to the other editors, that you might have a physician join you as co-editors of this book. Oh, that's a great idea they said. So, next thing you know, I'm one of the co-editors. Then I suggested it might be a good idea if we had some interviews with real live surgeons who have done striking or unusual things that reveal this theme of the human side of surgery.

WR: Right.

JM: Oh yeah, they said, that's a great idea. So here we are. You were right at the top of my list because of your very unusual professional course in life: starting in urology and moving to psychiatry, but still focused on urological patients. And that's a very unusual thing that you've done. And I also recognize that today it's an extremely delicate, and I would say, contentious topic. We don't have to get into all of that. We'll see how the conversation goes, but really, I'm more interested in how it all came about for you and how you made that move. We've talked about it so many times, but perhaps we could just start from the beginning. Your father was a physician. Is that right?

WR: Yeah, my father and his identical twin brother were both surgeons.

JM: Oh, you have an identical twin brother.

WR: No, not me. He did. He did. Oh, they were both surgeons.

JM: I see. Right. Well, can you go back a little bit and talk about some of those earlier days and, you know, how things got started for you and how the medical seed got planted?

WR: Well, yeah, I was actually in humanities and didn't have any intention of going...well, I did have an intention of going into medicine because of the expectations of the family, but that vanished in college, and I went into the humanities. And when I got out of college during the 1969 recession, no one was hiring. I didn't know what I wanted to do. I did not want to get a PhD in humanities. That part I had learned. And ultimately, I decided to go ahead and try myself at medicine. So, I applied and was admitted. And that's, that's really how it started. It was a bit accidental, partly to do with the times.

JM: When you say you majored in the humanities what particular humanities were you interested in at that time?

WR: Well, I was actually a history major with an emphasis in Russian history and a sub- emphasis on India and Indian history,

JM: Is that American Indian or subcontinental India?

WR: Subcontinental Indian. I had a phenomenal Russian history professor who really got me interested and that's how I started. But when I finished, it was not something I wanted to continue. I saw what he did in terms of his own research and his own publishing. That path really didn't interest me. I was really more interested in dealing more directly with people and interacting with people, something that I could carry out where I would be interacting. And that's really how I got into the medical field. So, I kind of came about [it] outside of the family expectations and then back into it on my own.

JM: When you were growing up, did you have much contact with your father's work or your uncle's work?

WR: Oh, my father was not my uncle at all. My father and my uncle became estranged, interestingly. My father was a distant father. He spent most of his time away, most of his time working. So, we really didn't see much of him. I didn't have much exposure, [just] a little bit of exposure in high school and a little bit of exposure in college, but not, not very much. I had enough exposure that I actually was interested in his field of orthopedics. I saw what he could accomplish in before-and-after situations and how he could improve the lives of people, especially the elderly people with joint replacements and the like. That did spark an interest in me and that interest continued.

JM: So, at some point you had to do the necessary sciences to get in. Did you complete that as an undergraduate or did you have to do what we call a post-baccalaureate program after graduation?

WR: Well, I was actually in the inaugural class of UC San Diego, University of California, San Diego, and the inaugural school there, the first college was Revelle College, which was science and engineering. So, I didn't have a lot of choice; besides, it was required. So, I completed everything in college required as a minor, biochemistry was my minor, biology we called it there.

JM: Before we leave your college days, when you think of like-minded people, colleagues, friends or people that you associated with, were they more in the sciences or more in the humanities or a mixture?

WR: The majority of the students there were interested in the sciences and engineering. I was focused on my final year especially on the humanities, simply by the requirement of my major field of study. So ultimately, it was a mixture.

JM: And then when you got to medical school, there was no more Russian history. What was your medical school experience like?

WR: Well, it had its ups and downs, and I wasn't sure what I wanted to do. I began with an interest in internal medicine until I had my first rotation and decided that was not going to interest me, that it was going to be too, too, how do I put this tactfully, boring for me. But I had a mentor in the surgical field, an older fellow who had gone to medical school and then he was drafted and spent 4 years in the military and then came out to do his residency. [He was an] older fellow from my standpoint at the time, probably in his mid-thirties, but at any rate, he mentored me and and got my interest going in surgery. And then I became interested in urology because the urologist there did the kidney transplants. And I really wanted to be a transplant surgeon when I finished my medical school and thought that's what I was going to do.

JM: Had you been involved in any of the kind of research that some of our more ambitious medical students today will pursue?

WR: [It was] simply because I was interested. I got involved in nephrological research at Cedars-Sinai and spent 3 months there. Mostly what we actually were doing was artificially obstructing one side and then measuring the excretion patterns in the obstructed side versus the unobstructed side.

JM: Were these animal experiments that you were doing?

WR: These were all animal experiments.

JM: Do you recall what animals they were?

WR: They were dogs. They were not a certain breed. They were mostly mongrel dogs.

JM: I used to be very sympathetic to lab animals until I got bitten by dogs and then I changed my mind. How did you feel about, how did you feel about those, those dogs that you had to take care of? If you can use that term.

WR: I had mixed feelings about them. They were actually nice dogs, by and large. I was overexposed to animals in my youthful days. I grew up on a farm. We had, well, my mother was, how does one put it, my mother was obsessed with horses and earlier with dogs. So, we had dogs and horses and cattle and... you name it, we had it. And they were always unusual animals. Most people might have chickens on a farm, but we had fighting cocks and hens, which were nasty birds. So, I had mixed feelings about animals going into medical school and mixed feelings about dealing with dogs in the laboratory as well.

JM: Most of my work was with Guinea pigs and then with real pigs. Guinea pigs are much cleaner, of course, and easier to hold in your hand. But when the time came, I was ready to let that go and concentrate on people. So, in medical school, you got interested in urology and you got interested in nephrology. And so, when the time came, how did you make your choices? Did you go right from medical school into your residency?

WR: Yes, I did. I got interested in pediatrics as well. So, I really was interested in pediatric urology with the idea of doing transplant surgery and pediatric urology. That was sort of a mixed bag. That wasn't going to work, but I didn't realize that at the time. We had to do 2 years of general surgery prior to our urology residency, as you recall, in those days. And my experience in the transplant team was just a lot of heartache and not quite the joys and successes that I had hoped for. So, I got discouraged about that, but still interested in the pediatric aspect. I was still interested in urology. So, the pediatric urology was a bit of a focus, even in my first 2 years, although I didn't have the chance to have much exposure to it at all. And of course, pediatric urology wasn't really much of a field in those days. Really, it was after that that it developed.

JM: When I came there [Johns Hopkins], you had been there for a few years. I came from Michigan where I'd done my general surgery. Did you do general surgery at Hopkins, or did you do it elsewhere and then came to the program?

WR: I did my general surgery at UCLA and UC Irvine, and then went to the program. Right.

JM: And [Patrick] Walsh had been at UCLA, so he already knew the system you were coming from.

WR: Yes, correct. Right.

JM: So, once you got to Baltimore, we were both residents in the same program together. You were a few years ahead of me. Thank God I had the good fortune of working with you. Otherwise, I don't know what I would have done. So, I'm still very grateful for that and remember many fine moments.

WR: That goes both ways, by the way. You haven't even described this in this interview, but we had some wonderful moments.

JM: And it kind of worked out the way you had expected in terms of going on into pediatric urology.

WR: Yeah, what happened was I was set up to do a pediatric urology fellowship in England. Bob Jeffs helped set that up for me. And then I got married and then, inadvertently, my wife got pregnant. And the team at England, when they found out I was married, they said, "Oh dear, that will be difficult. It's doable, so you can still come." But when they found out my wife was pregnant, they said, "No, that's not possible. There's no way you can handle a wife and a child in the living quarters here. It won't work." So, I had to scratch that idea and decided just at that point to go into practice. And I went to an area where there were no pediatric urologists between San Francisco and Los Angeles. So, I got a huge amount of exposure to pediatric urology in my years of practice there.

JM: And of course, you had had more exposure to pediatric urology being with Bob Jeffs at Hopkins than you might have in another residency somewhere else. So, you were sort of automatically the local expert when you got there. How did it progress then, your practice? Was it really a large pediatric practice in addition to whatever else you did?

WR: Yes. My interest in major birth defects was piqued by Bob Jeffs, certainly bladder exstrophy being the key one for him, but other birth anomalies as well, including the intersex population. So, when I went into practice, I started drawing patients who were 20 years old, 10 years old, 5 years old, and then new, young patients. So, I saw new ones and all the other people's older patients who may or may not have been doing well.

JM: By this you mean patients who may have undergone reconstructive surgery or intersex surgery earlier in life and now needed care.

WR: Correct. Or they didn't undergo it, but wanted to undergo it, something along those lines. Yeah, I saw a number of adults actually who had pediatric problems that had never been diagnosed or corrected. So those I was able to correct and those were very gratifying cases. But I ended up with about 40% of my surgical practice being pediatric urology. I would have preferred to have a higher percentage, but the demands were such that I had to do adults as well. I don't mean the financial demands. I mean the demands of the region. We were short of urologists. So, I kind of didn't have a choice in that regard.

JM: Were you in a urological group practice at the time or were you working solo?

WR: No, I was solo until the last 2 years when I joined a large multi-specialty group in order to have a partner, because, in fact, that's really what I was looking for. And they had a urologist. So we worked together. And then at that point, that's when I made the decision to change careers.

JM: From my perspective, one of the potential advantages of the way you worked is that you were able to see, as we used to say, children of all ages, without restriction. The arbitrary line that's drawn between children age 18 or 21, at which point they transition from pediatrics to adults is, I think, a big problem still today, and it's a topic of great discussion in urology and probably other specialties as well: how to deal with children who grow up once they've undergone all these big procedures or these initial problems. They don't stop living and they're still living with these problems.

WT: That's right. That's right. And I did, of course, continue to see them because I saw everybody. And I watched these children and listened to these children. And, well, they weren't all children at that point. Some of them were adolescents, some of them were young adults. They would come to me with questions and developmental issues, developmental problems, and they wanted to know what to do about them. And so did their mothers. The mothers, well, I should say, their parents, but let's be honest, it was mostly mothers, the questions they asked, I couldn't answer. I thought, well, you know, those are great questions. I don't know the answer. I didn't learn any of that in my training. And I went to the books, to the journals, and I really couldn't find much in terms of those questions and those issues and research. And that began to really pique my interest. I mean, why hadn't people done research? And there was a lot of work that had been done in child development, but it was all in general child development, not in children with major medical or surgical anomalies. There was a little bit of work done up at Seattle in craniofacial anomalies, more than in most places in most areas. But craniofacial anomalies, although there are some similarities to major neurological anomalies, there also are some huge differences.

JM: Well, the craniofacial is right there. You can see it. Other things are concealed by clothing, but only in part. Sooner or later, those things do come out. And perhaps as a result, they're intimate in a different kind of way.

WR: Well, one of the interesting points is that the children grow up just about at any age. If you could get them to talk about it, you realize that they think everybody knows they have, let's say, bladder exstrophy. [They'd say] "Everyone knows that I have bladder exstrophy." And I'd try to point out to them, you know, I'd say, just stand up and turn around and tell me what you think I'm looking at. And they would say, well, you're looking at somebody with bladder exstrophy and blah, blah, blah, blah. And I'd say, I'm looking at a boy who's four feet two and weighs 80 pounds and has dark brown hair and is wearing a shirt and a pair of shorts and socks that don't match. And other than that, I don't see anything, which they didn't really follow.

JM: Can you recall some of the questions that these families would have for you? You mentioned questions in general terms. Can you describe one or two that stick out in your mind?

WR: The biggest questions from the mothers were, how are these children going to function sexually and how are they going to deal with relationships? The mothers focused on the social issues and very human issues. The fathers were interested in those issues but tended to go to work and let the mothers deal with the problems that were going on. The children, as they got older, asked more questions in terms of their identity, of who and what they were. And those were very tough questions because again, I would have a solid notion of who or what a given child was. And the child didn't necessarily have that notion at all.

The most startling case to me was a 14-year-old girl who came to me and said, I'm not a girl, I'm a boy. And this was a child with an intersex condition, not a transgendered child in the current sense, by any means. And this child didn't say, I want to be a boy. This child said, I am a boy. In fact, the child had quit school. And the child quit school because they put the child in girl's physical education and girl's chorus. I thought it sounded wonderful myself, but that was a personal issue. And this child quit school because of that. And that was probably the most momentous aspect of my desire to change careers when I saw this child and dealt with this child over the next 5 years and realized what he was going through and what he had to go through because he was having negative responses from everybody, including his parents about this. They already had two boys. They didn't want another boy. They wanted a girl. Well, he wasn't a girl and didn't see him.

JM: Is this a boy who had undergone a gender reconstruction in infancy or early childhood because of disconnection between genotype and phenotype?

WR: This was a child who was born in a foreign country and wasn't examined and wasn't looked at until they came to the U.S. and someone, somehow had managed to avoid looking at their genitalia. I don't know that this child had ever had his genitalia looked at.

JM: I see. Before we get into the question or the theme of your professional transformation to which you've been giving hints as to how it came about, let me ask: for most of these children, were the questions somehow related to genital identification or was it a broader or a deeper psychological identification?

WR: That's an excellent question. And it's very difficult to dissect the two from each other because the genital identification and the sense of identity played such a key role together. It only was when I began to realize...they had both a genital identification issue and they had an identity issue. And we can talk about gender identity, but it's more than gender identity. It's full- blown identity. It's who and what am I? And this child came out and told me...this was a very quiet child, but boy, very, very firm in his statements.

JM: Can you remember the exact words that this child used in presenting this question to you? What was the way in which it was framed? Can you recall?

WR: Well, this wasn't a child that presented with questions. This child presented with an answer. This child came and said: this is who I am and I'm not going to school because they're looking at me as a girl and they're going to make me do girl things and I'm not a girl, so I'm not going to do them. So, I'm not going to go to school. So, when I finished my evaluation and the workup, I said to this child, okay, I mean, you've got an intersex condition. I didn't say it in those terms, but I said, you have an intersex condition that in fact, you could have been raised male. Turned out later that most of these children do see themselves as male, no matter how they're raised. And I said, what's going to happen to you? Because he agreed if he was changed to male, he'd go back to school. And I said, okay, we can convert you to male socially, we can get your parents to agree, which was difficult, but they ultimately did. And we can surgically reconstruct to a limited point. And I said, but what's going to happen when you go back to school, and the other children talk to you about that? What are you going to say to them?

He said, well, I'm not going to say anything. And I said, well, what if they ask you, we thought you were a girl, why aren't you a girl? And he looked at me very quietly, clenched his fist and said, "I'll beat the shit out of them". And I said, okay, that's pretty much establishing the identity here.

So ultimately this child went back to school as a boy and ultimately fell in love with a girl. And the last I saw of them; they had lived together for 2 years independently. He was a very independent child.

JM: So many people who would consider themselves surgical specialists or people whom the world would consider as surgical specialists when confronted with situations like that might say, you need to see a psychiatrist or that's outside of my specialty, but you didn't do that. And even at that time, even though perhaps you had not consciously decided to move into psychiatry, you were already interacting with this patient at a different level than just the technical surgical level.

WR: That's right. I hadn't thought about psychiatry at all at this point. It was only in the next, well, probably a good 3 or 4 years after this child, before it really started to hit me that that's what I was really interested in doing. Yeah. This listening to the children, and when I say listening to them, you can ask questions of children, but you don't know what the answers mean. Especially adults...[they] tend to ask yes, or no questions of children and they get yes or no answers, but you don't know what it means. Children have a tendency to answer the way they think you want them to, or the way they think mom and dad want them to, and they'll look for clues and cues from their parents. I learned long ago that if you just pull a child in front of their parents, so their chair is in front, that they don't tend to look for the cues and clues the way they do otherwise. At any rate, what I would do is comment to the children, sometimes make observations that often were completely wrong, totally off base. Actually, those sometimes were the most useful because if you make a comment that are off base, the child almost always responds that you're wrong in some fairly firm way. If the child's having a tantrum and they finish their tantrum, you can say, "Well, gee, you seem like you're really, really mad." If they're not mad, if it's something else that's going on, they can blur it out, "I'm not mad." "Oh, you've learned something." This is information. These are data that are coming in, but you have to listen to the child, not to correct them or contradict them. That's what I seem to have a natural ability to do. I learned that when you listen to children and adolescents and young adults, for that matter, young adults are much easier, but when you listen to children and adolescents, then they begin to spontaneously provide data, if you will, if you want to sound more clinical. They provide information that can be very useful to understanding who this young person really is. They're not adults, and they don't think like adults, but they are people, and they can communicate. The advantage of spontaneous communication from them is that they're not very likely to create, to confabulate, if you will, to create stories that may not be real, but that they want people to hear. I'm not saying it doesn't happen. I'm just saying it's less likely. When they're spontaneous, it's less likely.

JM: When these experiences began for you, were you looking either for other resources or other people who might've had similar interests, other information, something that would boost your knowledge or give you support or allow you to speak about what it was that you were finding?

WR: Well, that's what I went to the literature for, and I went to the literature over and over again. In those days, we didn't have computers. We had the Index Medicus, which was a bit daunting, but I would go through it, and I finally decided that I must be just terrible at coming up with indexed keywords because I could never really find very much on these kinds of children until I finally realized there probably wasn't very much on these kinds of children, these kinds of developmental issues. I'd ask other people in the field. I'd go to the meetings and see the people that did the pediatric surgery and the pediatric urology and ask them for help and for questions and for suggestions, but they didn't have a lot of suggestions for me. I think partly, especially with the older crew, they weren't as.... the older generation, and I am an older generation now, so I feel like I can say this,...they weren't as open to just listening to children and paying attention. They were more attuned to the parents, and there's nothing wrong with being attuned to the parents, but it's not enough.

JM: You say that it takes time to listen to children or listen. You've mentioned that several times. Was that time built into your work, or did you somehow just pull it from your work? Shall we say, steal it from your work so that you would have the time? On a practical level, just how much time are we talking about in terms of these conversations with children?

WR: Yes, that was a very difficult problem because I was very short of time. Since the area I was in was very understaffed, the demands on my time were high. They were all legitimate demands, and the adults as well as the children all needed help. They all had questions and problems. I pulled the time from my time. Unfortunately, of course, that meant I was pulling it out of my family's time because I would end up working until 7.30 and 8 o'clock at night. Then I'd rush home quickly to see the kids before they went to bed and try to do something for my wife because she was being beaten to death by two young children, two very active young children. Then I would go back to the hospital and make rounds. It was very trying. It was very difficult, but I really felt the need to take that time with the parents, the mothers, and the children to listen to them and learn from them because I had learned a great deal from them.

JM: You encountered surgeons in the past who spent time the way you're talking about spending time with patients?

WR: Well, Bob Jeffs certainly did. He would spend a great deal of time with patients and a great deal of time with parents. I think Bob listened to the children. He didn't spend as much time as I did, but I don't know that he had...he had the demands on his time as well, probably more demands. I learned from him in that regard, although I would have to say that it was natural. I spent time with counseling kids when I was in college. I was a mixed-up college kid, but nevertheless, I counseled younger kids. I worked with a Boy Scout troop in the slums of South Philly for my first year in college when I was back east. I was in Philadelphia for my first year. I learned from all of those experiences. I learned from my own younger cousins who all needed counseling as well. I didn't know how to counsel them, but I listened to them. So, I had experience doing it. I mean, Bob Jeffs was a big stimulus towards that.

JM: There is this quality in the good physicians who take care of children, this ability to see the person in the child in a way that I think others, even parents sometimes, but certainly many adult physicians and ordinary adults, seem to forget: children are human beings and have a world all of their own and are worthy of respect and attention, just as adults are.

WR: That's right. I think that the pediatric urologists of the last generation and this generation are really very unique in the surgical world in dealing with children. They're very attuned to the child as well as being very attuned to the mothers, much more so than I think the people that dealt with the surgical aspects of pediatrics in the more distant past. I think that they learned from people like Bob Jeffs, and I think they've paid great attention to the changes that have occurred in the research and in the literature, that's come out over the last 25 or 30 years about the developmental issues that their young patients go through. They're very interested in that. It's quite remarkable, but it's also, it's very pleasing to me to see how the pediatric urologists, and it's not just in the US, I've gone to other countries and watched the pediatric urologists there and they seem to be the same. They seem to be very keyed into, very tuned into their kids and to their patients.

JM: Now, at the time when we were at Hopkins and still in our training program, John Money, a name familiar to the world, had generated a theory about gender identification. When you were seeing these children, both whether they had or had not had operations, if it was a genital reconstruction, it would be one thing, if it was exstrophy, it was another.

WR: I'm not sure that John would have been dealing with that, but he had created a certain sort of expectation and a sort of paradigm that existed at that time.

JM: And you were seeing these children and trying to make your decisions and recommendations against the background of this accepted paradigm directing how children should be treated.

WR: Right. It's about 3 years before I saw this one young patient that I mentioned, who told me that she wasn't a girl, she was a boy. I had a Hispanic family, Mexican family farm workers, who spoke no English. So, I had a translator, which is always difficult, but they had a little boy, a little baby, that was their seventh child. And he was born with a micropenis. And the training, of course, that I had was to convert these children to female, to castrate them and raise them as female. So, I carefully went over this, and my interpreter was excellent, a very bright, capable woman. My interpreter was lovely in how she related to me, but at the end, the father basically told me, he said to her that this guy's an idiot, I'm not going to do anything he says. And they walked off and she said to me, what's going to happen? And I said, well, this kid's going to be a disaster for them. Well, 3 years later, I had the next big experience, which was the boy that changed from what the world expected of him and became a boy. And then I began to watch the other kids and deal with them. And I realized in looking back that these Mexican farm worker parents who were uneducated, although they hadn't been to school, were not dumb people. They were bright. They had six other kids as examples. And they said, what do you mean? I mean, this kid may be born with a micropenis, but he's a he. So, I began to question that paradigm and began to say, how can we be so rigid in making this decision when again, we haven't really listened to the children. We don't know what happens to those children when they grow up, which is interesting because, of course, in Money's PhD dissertation, he looked at, I think it was about 273 or so cases of adults with various intersex conditions. And to oversimplify his summary, his findings, they actually did okay. And basically, none of them had undergone surgery. So, I began to question, although I didn't know that at the time, but I began to question this paradigm because I just found it too rigid. I found myself too rigid. And I began to question my own thinking processes. I said, I must be thinking this through wrong. If this 14-year-old kid can come in and tell me that I'm wrong and prove to me that I'm wrong, then I'm not looking at these questions in the right way, I'm going to have to reassess. So, this is why I say that listening to the children had profound effects on my ultimate career and my career choices.

JM: So how did it come about then? Because we're getting close to the point where you walk through one door. You didn't really leave behind the country of surgery because you really can't leave it behind. You can leave the OR, but the world of surgery that you knew and the experience that you had, you carry with you. So, at this point, how did it come about that you decided to make this transition?

WR: Yeah, that's a complex personal story that I don't want to get too much involved in, but I will say.

JM: Anything you want can be off the record. So, it's not a problem because you'll have a chance to review everything.

WR: What happened was that my father died in the midst of a series of difficult problems. All the urologists in the area where I was had either died or had liver transplants or retired. I suddenly found myself massively overworked. And at the same time, my father died and I just sort of threw up my hands and said, "This isn't going to work. I don't want to do it anymore." But I do want to do something that doesn't distance me from the surgical world, because I had a rich involvement in the surgical world. And I had looked into, I had thought of the ideas of child development fairly extensively. I hadn't investigated it. I didn't really have the time, but I had thought about the ideas. And it was about that time after my father died that I ultimately said, I'm going to go back to retrain. I want to carry on my work, but not in the OR. I want to carry on my work in an outside laboratory, not on an inside laboratory, so to speak. And also, I wanted to be able to provide the mothers and the children with a clinical education, with the clinical background that I needed to have to be able to answer those kinds of questions that they presented to me, these developmental questions.

JM: Some people might've gone to the laboratory to study the genetics of these conditions, but you chose to go back to deal with people face-to-face.

WR: I learned in my college days at UC San Diego that although the laboratory is fascinating in its results, I'm not a laboratory man. I don't have the obsessiveness that you really have to have in a laboratory. I don't have that kind of obsessive quality to carry out good laboratory research.

JM: And yet you had the discipline to listen to those children, go home, and then go back to the hospital and stay up late and work extra hours compared to others. So perhaps it's a different form of that kind of intensity. But tell me now, when you went back to, because you went back to Hopkins, was it the only place you wanted to go or had you explored others? And then what was that like, those encounters with the psychiatrists when you first knocked on their door, said, "Here I am, I'm Dr. Reiner. I've spent X number of years doing children's urology and I want to be one of your residents." How did that come across?

WR: Well, most of them seemed to look at me like, "You must be crazy," to be honest with you.

JM: Coming from a psychiatrist, that's a dangerous opinion.

WR: Exactly, precisely. But actually, they were all very interested. I looked into six different programs from the West Coast to the East Coast, but I really always wanted to go back to Hopkins because I knew Hopkins, number one and number two, I knew the kind of expertise that you find there. Not that you don't find it elsewhere, but I didn't know how to find it elsewhere. I didn't have enough sophistication. And then I interviewed at Hopkins with Paul McHugh and Philip Slavney, those were the main interviewers I had. Well, I had others, but those were really the main ones. I realized that these people were bright, educated, well-read, and they had a real idea of how to educate people in a very complex field that was changing. It was just at the beginning of real change, very much the way urology was when you and I started off with Pat Walsh. It was at the beginnings of great change. And I watched that great change and participated in it as you did with Pat Walsh. And then afterwards, well, the same thing was beginning to happen in psychiatry. Most of the programs I went to, the people, the chiefs of the department, the chairman would say something like, "Well, we have an eclectic education here." And I thought, "Well, I don't know. What does eclectic mean?" I mean, it sounds to me like that means you don't know exactly what the field is. Well, that wasn't my experience at Hopkins. And Paul McHugh used to get a great deal of criticism because people saw him as very biologically oriented and very rigid. But in fact, they really misunderstood Paul. Paul was very oriented towards the aspects of education that allowed his residents to be able to adapt to the changes that he knew were occurring and were going to occur over the next 10–20 years, very much the way Pat Walsh did with us in urology. We were prepared for those changes as they occurred through our education. And Paul McHugh was the same. Well, he's retired now, but he prepared his residents for that very kind of change in a very exciting way, a very exciting man.

JM: Can you recall any of the conversations that you might've had with Paul or Phil when you came back for that interview? The people who would be reading a transcript from this conversation may or may not know who Paul McHugh or who Phil Slavney are. Of course, these are legendary names, and they're very interesting people, very intelligent people. So, I'm just trying to picture what this conversation might've been like.

WR: Well, very different with Paul and Philip. Their approaches were very different in talking to me. But Paul was extremely interested in my background, extremely interested in my training and my experience in urology. And when I discussed with him the very kinds of things we're discussing, I mean, he really, he sort of brightened, he sort of lit up in a way to use the vernacular. And he explored some of those ideas with me. And then he discussed his approach to education, which was, in a sense, it sounded like he was presenting a paradigm of his own and actually told me to read his book, his book, his and Phil Slavney's book on the four principles of psychiatry, the four perspectives of psychiatry. And I thought, well, this is a cookie cutter kind of an approach, but he was so bright and so... he was a fascinating man. And I thought, you know, this guy's got his rigidities, but then I've got my rigidities. I don't mind a few rigidities. I mean, that's not the point. Well, then I read his book, and I thought, whoa, this is not a cookie cutter approach. This is a broad-based approach to prepare residents to move on to excellence as the field changes. And that was really that.

JM: It had not occurred to me until just this moment when you were speaking about how Paul lit up about this, but later he became a serious investigator into the psychological outcomes of gender transformation surgery. And I just wonder how much of that might've been triggered by his early experiences with you and your interests.

WR: I don't know if anybody talks about that. I didn't realize it at the time, but I think it was. And as I got into my studies and then we actually presented a grand round, and he wanted child psychiatry to present. And I was called on because I was the junior member of the faculty. So, you know, I had to present, and I presented one of the cases where a child had been born with normal testes and was a normal male but had basically an absence of the penis or near absence of the penis and was castrated and raised female and converted at the age of five. This was the old Money paradigm.

JM: John Money?

WR: That's correct. Yeah. This is a child from another state, not from, not from Maryland and our teams there had not been involved with this child before I saw him. And so, I presented this case, and Paul interviewed the parents, and it was a fascinating interview. The parents were fascinating.

JM: The interview took place there at the presentation?

WR: Yes, in Hurd Hall, and yes, Paul said afterwards, it was the best, the best grand rounds he had ever conducted. He was quite ecstatic about, about the results. And then he followed me, I think more closely at that point in my research.

JM: So, you came with the intention, I think, of specifically taking care of these patients and learning more about them and providing more clinical care for them. Would that be a fair statement?

WR: Absolutely. My intention was to take care of pediatric urological patients in child psychiatry.

JM: So, it was not only your own education, if you will, but you actually were carrying these patients, their memories and future patients like them into this field. This was more than just, shall we say, your interest in that you were already carrying a whole family of patients, if you will, of memories and experiences into this field. And when you first started doing this, because you stayed on faculty there for a while after you finished your pediatric fellowship...I mean, we're going over 4–5 years of very serious work. How old were you at the time, if I may ask?

W$R: Oh, my goodness. I must've been 48 when I started on the faculty.

JM: So that's quite unusual. I mean, people do go into psychiatry after some experiences in life, but still, this must've been very demanding on you to be in this position at this time.

WR: Well, it was demanding. Yeah, of course it was. But on the other hand, it was exciting to me. It was, it was challenging. It was fun, but fun in an exciting way because I was really excited for the, for the families, for the kids. And the fact that I was, I was building up a practice because I think I had something to offer. And what did I have to offer? Well, I had the experience or the experiences of all of the patients whom I had seen before a given patient and family came in. And that was the kind of offering that I think that they were really hungry for.

JM: So, you had the kind of authority that a surgeon who understands the condition would have because you had, quite literally, gone beyond the surface. You had done the reconstructions, you'd seen the complications, you knew what people go through. No one has to explain this to you. And when you see these patients, they know that about you. And probably just in the first few words of conversation, they know this about you.

WR: Oh, they figured it out. The children themselves would figure it out very rapidly. And it was amazing how it altered the relationship. They, they would open up from the very first meeting in ways that kids don't generally open up like that. I mean, kids will open up to me in my first meeting with them, but not, not opening up, you know, with, with intimate details, they'll open up, but it's superficial. You have to get to know a child before they open up and you can get into any of the intimate aspects of what's really going on in their head, in their brain, really. But these kids would open up from the beginning.

JM: So, Paul was a supporter right from the start for you?

WR: Oh yes, yes. Paul and...

JM: At some point, you probably were presenting materials from your research about these children. You were presenting this material at conferences or meetings. Am I correct about that?

WR: That's correct.

JM: And what kind of reception did you receive?

WR: Well, the first the first report that I gave was at a NIH, really an NICHD meeting, co-sponsored by the NICHD and the University of Pennsylvania CHOP, Children's Hospital of Philadelphia, their pediatric urology group. It was in Dallas. I was one of, oh, I think probably a dozen speakers. I presented my initial data, which I hadn't published yet, but it was, gosh, I think 10 or 12 patients. Well, I presented children who who were genetic males but raised female because of some major anomaly with the genitalia. And the pediatric urologists were stunned. And yet they were fascinated. I mean, to the point that one very well-known pediatric urologist got up to the microphone and said, well, if I've been doing this all wrong all these years, what have I done to these children? And I said, no, no, no, you haven't been doing anything wrong. You've been doing what you were taught to do, and you've been doing it well. If indeed, I said, my research carries through and it looks like it will, I said, you just need to go to these people and say, look, I've been helping you all this time. I'm going to continue to help you in any way that I possibly can. They were very open to that approach. I really thought I was going to get thrown off the stage, to be honest with you.

JM: This is very interesting because when people present controversial or challenging opinions, you can expect to get a broadside in return, but it sounds like instead what happened here, you had an open conversation, a truly educational and formative experience.

WR: Oh, it was, well, again, to use the vernacular, it was mind boggling. I was so surprised. I really thought I was going to have, I thought some people would listen and be interested. I think that the CHOP people who had already had a preview of my data were actually very interested, but I thought they would be unusual, but they weren't. It turns out that the audience was very, very interested. I mean, there were, don't misunderstand, there were negatives. There were people who challenged what I said. I said, well, I don't have answers. All I can do is present the data and then it's up to us to follow through with the data and continue to do the research and draw inferences from the data.

JM: And did you have other experiences where you presented your findings? You could say as a summary thesis that the surgical transformation of phenotypic abnormalities that are incongruent with the genotype doesn't really address the deeper psychological issues that may be related to genetic imprinting in utero, that we need to examine this a little further. If you presented this material to other audiences, were you met with similar sympathy or did you get different responses?

WR: Well, how do I put this tactfully? I didn't receive from the other pediatric subspecialties; I didn't receive the openness. There was interest and there were people who were open to what I was saying, but I did not have the openness that the pediatric urologist showed. And by the way, it wasn't just at the US because I also presented at the European Society for Pediatric Urology 3 years later and had a similar response there. But it was clear to me that the pediatric urologists were much more open to what the effects were on the children and on the parents and on the growth and development of the family than, well, I don't mean to say the other fields weren't, but the other fields were more rigid about the teaching. Now they've changed, I think. Certainly, pediatric endocrinology has changed, but it took more time.

JM: But I'm thinking now of speaking outside of our own immediate specialty to people who may be a bit resistant to the fact that you're coming from urology, psychiatry, and not from their tribe, if you will. What about the general psychiatric community, particularly the pediatric psychiatric community? Did you have a chance to present or share your information with them? And what sort of responses did you get?

WR: Yes, I presented symposia at three of the meetings of child psychiatry. I didn't present at any of the adult groups, but I did in the child group. And there was interest, but I was surprised at how small the interest was because I had speakers from diverse areas speak, including people in child psychiatry, as part of the symposium and there were 80 or 90 people at the meeting. I thought it would draw far more, but it didn't. I never was able to generate the interest in the urological fields within child psychiatry that I thought that I needed to generate.

JM: Well, not many people had the kind of experience that you did. I mean, perhaps there might've been others in orthopedics, there might've been others in neurosurgery, but urology is unique in what it deals with. So perhaps your situation was very unusual for most people in the field.

WR: Yeah. It is. Urology is a very unique field. And yeah, the subject matter that the patients come in with, if you will, is intimate and private and enshrouded with guilt and shame sometimes.

JM: And surgical all at once.

WR: And surgical all at once.

JM: That makes it a very unusual and unique kind of situation. Now you've stepped away from clinical work for some time, haven't you?

WR: Yes, I have.

JM: And how many years do you think you spent in clinical surgery and then in clinical psychiatry related to your earlier work? What percentage of your time had been devoted to each area; would you say? How much of your time did you spend in the early days in urology? And then later on, starting from the time when you made the change, how many years would you say?

WR: Well, my total experience in urology, counting surgical training was 18 years. And then I started in my psychiatry training in '92, so I retired in 2016. So, what does that come to? That's 24.

JM: So a little bit more, almost 50/50. It's almost an evenly split career. And by the time you stepped away, I think that... I wasn't sure whether I should bring up the current gender issues, because they're different than the sorts of matters you dealt with, but have you felt in any way inclined to participate in the ongoing conversations? They do seem somewhat political. I just wonder if you have any thoughts about them, or we could keep it totally off the script if you wish.

WR: It's a risk of the area that I've been involved in. It's become incredibly politicized, and when it becomes political, then it becomes non-clinical. And I'm interested in the clinical. I'm interested in child development. I'm not interested in politicizing these things. I'm not interested in pushing children one way or the other. I want the children to be able to develop in their own way and to tell us who and what they are. Now, for some children, that's going to be very, very difficult, but for the majority, I think for a large percentage of children, if you leave them alone, so to speak, and give them an adequate, safe environment, they'll be able to tell you who and what they are, and ultimately be able to communicate what they need.

JM: When you started doing the kind of work that you ended up doing in psychiatry, you were probably one of a very small group of people, if not the only one who was really doing this. Today, do you think it's similar, or do you feel now that there's a broader interest? You mentioned that in the profession and pediatric urology in general, there's much more sensitivity to children's lives. Do you feel that this is fairly represented in some of the difficult politicized situations that we're facing?

WR: I think the field of endocrinology, urology and pediatrics have gotten overwhelmed with the politicization and don't know what to do with it. I think that the pediatric urologists are very open to having social workers, psychologists, psychiatrists working with them. They would encourage it, along with endocrinologists as well. That, I think, is beneficial overall, but what do we do with the politicization? How do we handle it? I don't have an answer for that.

JM: That goes back to your own original experience, which was that, as a surgeon, you could easily have brought in all those experts who may or may not have been able to help your patients the way you did, but you chose to pursue this on your own. It takes us back to the meaning of the word clinical, because when the average person hears the word clinical, they think of people in white coats who are distant and objective and are observing in laboratories and things like that. I believe that when you say clinical, you're saying something different. You're saying being at the bedside, being face-to-face with people.

WR: That's right. That's exactly what I mean. In terms of the white coat, just to give you an example, I never wore a white coat once I left my residency, because I found it a turnoff, even to some degree a turnoff for adults, but certainly a turnoff for children and for the mothers, I think. I did have the experience, though, once of spending 45 min explaining a very complex birth anomaly that a little infant had that needed to be repaired. Really, it was a ureterocele, but it was a complex ureterocele. After I finished the training, it was very early in my practice, I said to the mother, "Now, you must have questions. Please feel free." I had drawn pictures and written notes. She said, "I only have one question." I said, "Okay, sure. What's that?" She said, "Are you old enough to be operating on my baby?" I looked at her eyes. I said, "That's a hard question."

JM: If the world could only see how many things we have to do alone with our patients in the operating room and all the rest. There's a pressure to build medical teams, if you will, which is very fine. Of course, one needs the support of many others. If I think back, and I'm sure if you think back, on the many hours you spent face-to-face solo with people, listening to them, operating on them, I think this is something that's very difficult to share with the rest of the world. It's a very personal experience. I know it has been for you. It's been for me. I think when you scratch the surface and you talk to people who have done this kind of work, you realize just how deeply personal it is.

WR: Yes. That's, I think, why surgeons, why I think all physicians, but surgeons in particular, take malpractice suits so personally because each of us as a surgeon invests far more than just time in our patients. We have an emotional investment. Of course, they have an emotional investment. When they are upset with something in some way and they sue, it's very harsh, being pierced with a very sharp and harsh arrow. Yes. Many of us, unfortunately, know that feeling, but somehow, we just keep going. That's right. You have to. One lawyer said to me, "Well, getting sued is the price of doing business." I thought, "Well, but I don't really do business. That's not what I'm doing."

JM: We're not only getting to the end of the natural flow of this conversation but getting to the end of something else as well. When you look back at it all, when you sit back, you don't have to go to work in the same way now, you don't have to deal with highway driving to make it to the operating room at six in the morning, et cetera, what kinds of things come back to? What do you remember that comes back with either fondness, or with relief that you don't have to deal with it anymore?

WR: Well, the six o'clock part, I definitely have gratitude for not dealing with that anymore because I'm not a morning person. That was hard, starting with college. Well, no, starting in high school. Everything started at the very latest at eight in the morning, usually earlier. That I don't mind being done with. In terms of things that are memorable, my memorable moments are all dealing with patients. They all have to do with individual patients who struck me in some way or touched me in some way that I found either deeply moving or that I learned profound things from them. There's probably a handful that I could come up with in a few minutes, but a much larger number if I spend some time. I can't talk about my patients even in the abstract because they all have such rare conditions. They'll figure out that it was them. Even if it's not that particular patient I'm talking about, they'll think I'm talking about them. I don't do that because I feel that their privacy is very precious. I would never invade their privacy. That's where the memorable times in my career all come down to patient interactions. For the most part, adolescent patients. I really learned a great deal from adolescent patients, just remarkable aspects of human development. We talk about child development, but it's really human development we're talking about.

JM: You think it's possible for people in surgery? I still consider you a person who was very deeply involved in surgery. Even when you were in psychiatry, you never really hung up your gloves, shall we say. Do you think it's possible for people in surgery to really share the depth of what they go through with the rest of the world or with others in any way? Or do you just go home and then get up the next day and go back to work?

WR: In casual conversation, in the cocktail kinds of conversations, people will sometimes ask questions that really do involve the personal aspects that surgeons go through, the incredibly emotional aspects. I'll try to give them some feeling for what that really is and what it means to a surgeon. It's very difficult to convey in a short time, especially in a more public way.

I think that the closest I've ever seen it being depicted was in the TV show M*A*S*H, that displayed the emotional aspects and the difficulties that surgeons have and the trauma that they go through in dealing with the trauma that they went through. That probably did it much better than I could ever do.

JM: M*A*S*H was written by, I think, originally as a short novel by an American surgeon serving in Korea, Richard Hooker. He wrote from the perspective of the radio operator. If I understand correctly, if Wikipedia is correct, he sold the rights to the book for the TV series for just a few hundred dollars and never got another penny out of it. I think he was very bitter about it afterwards. Then of course, a movie adaptation was made as well. The series was a fortune maker for these people, and he never got anything out of it.

WR: I found that the TV series was much more powerful than the movie. The movie was misogynistic and pretty harsh, but the TV series really got to what the surgeons and nurses deal with and what they go through. Of course, they were dealing with terrible traumas, but surgeons and nurses deal with terrible traumas as well as minor traumas and moderate traumas.

JM: We've known each other for many, many years. Many of the things that you've talked about, I've heard before, but you've presented it in such a clear way. I think that when the transcript comes out, people who read this will be able to see who you were, who you are, the kind of work that you did. It's not just about you, it's about the work that you did, how valuable and unique that was, what that says about people in surgery, what they're capable of, when they really, as you say, listen to those patients, when they look and see carefully just what they've been exposed to. Without that, you cannot understand. You can't understand what it's like unless you've been through it yourself.

WR: I think that's absolutely right. It's a little bit like a man trying to understand pregnancy and childbirth. We can have women explain it to the nth degree, but we're not really going to be able to feel it because we can't go through it.

JM: We're coming to the end of our recorded session. Is there anything else that you wish you had said or would like to be sure gets down in print? Once we review the transcript later on, you can always add or amend whatever you want.

WR: The one thing I didn't mention that I didn't think of at the time, but at the end of my surgical career, and this was partly what was happening to me at the end that helped to push me out of surgery and into psychiatry, people would ask me, "How do you operate on people?" I'd say, "Well, you don't really operate on people. The person you see in the pre-anesthesia room, or you see them in your office, of course, but when you get in there, you put drapes on and you're operating on a small square or rectangle that's going to be whatever organ you're going to operate on." But at the end of, and I sort of believed that, I think, during my career, but at the very end, I began to see the people I was operating on as people, and it actually made it much more difficult. It almost made me, what's the word I want? I almost became phobic about surgery at the end because I was seeing the infant I was operating on or the little kid or the young woman or whatever.

JM: I've heard doctors who become parents, surgeons who become parents, look at children differently after their own children are born.

WR: Oh, yes. Oh, yeah.... Well, no...I mean, just having my children born during my residency, I, well, my first one was born during my residency. I mean, the first thing I did was a urological exam. I counted fingers, toes, and genitalia, and then I looked to see if he was breathing.

JM: Well, it's good you did that. Not everybody would do that. And maybe, say you had some patients where somebody didn't do that, or they did and they didn't know what they were looking at... another problem.

WR: Actually, a lot of patients [were] that way. That was unfortunate.

JM: Our era of medicine is changing and becoming different. And when you and I are patients or may already be patients, we look around to see if when someone listens to our chest, they will first ask us to take our shirt off. I don't know how many experiences you've had with people listening to your chest and heart through clothing. And I remember what a forbidden thing that was when I was a student.

WR: Oh, yes. No, no one has asked me to remove any clothing except for the dermatologist.

JM: Well, I'm going to stop the recording in a minute. But I can say is that it's absolutely wonderful to see you.

WR: Oh, it's great to see you. It's been so long. And I'm glad I did this.

JM: At least we had the Zoom and not a phone call because at least we can see each other face to face. It's been an absolutely fabulous opportunity to hear your story in a formal kind of way, but at the same time, just to reconnect and revisit it.

WR: Well, you know, your questions, your questions are probing and important. I mean, you really asked the key questions, I think. So, this is great. This was wonderful, wonderful.

JM: You'll get you'll get a recording, a transcript and a recording so you can have it as well. You know, I started out to be a psychiatrist when I first went to medical school.

WR: I didn't know that. Oh, yeah. That was my original interest. I thought I could never make it with those other guys who were studying comparative anatomy in college, I couldn't take that. I had to go to the philosophy classes. I couldn't take those guys. But somehow it all worked out.

WR: Well, I'm going to the philosophy classes now.

JM: Which ones, if I may ask?

WR: Well, I've joined the OSHA group. You know, there are lifelong learning groups that are attached to major universities. And we can actually go to all kinds of courses at UCSD. I do it through UCSD. It's really nice. But they also have speakers that come from the university and other places also.

JM: Any particular kind of philosophical courses you're taking?

WR: Well, recently I've been listening in and going to the astrophysics or whatever they call them now. What are the astronomers today aren't called astronomers anymore. They're astrophysicists. So I recently read the book and then heard the lecture by Brian Keating, you know, who's looking for the for the microwave coming from the few seconds right after the Big Bang. If, as he says, if there was a Big Bang or if there was only one Big Bang. The Big Bang. You know, you can have a really interesting conversation about this.

JM: We can talk about all the unusual things I heard that link philosophy and science. There was a presentation by Luc Montagnier, Nobel laureate for his HIV discoveries. It was at the Shrine at Lourdes, and it was 2012. We were having a symposium on what does it mean to be healed today. Montagnier spoke about the memory of water. Now regarding these ideas, he's a sort of a maverick scientist, one of a small group of people who have done intense dilutions of substances, including nucleic acids and water. And if you dilute it down to the point where no other assay can identify it, MRIs that were done before will be identical to MRIs that are done after the dilutions, suggesting that the water itself retains a memory of what was dissolved in it. Put two and two together with, the frozen ice tails of comets and I don't have to say any more. It's linked to what's called the panspermia hypothesis, like some big fish in the universe just released all these eggs and seeds and some landed here on Earth.

WR: One landed in my backyard. There it goes. Well, there's Stuart, Stuart Kauffman and his organic molecules studies... a theory, you know, where everything is built into the organicity and it's going to occur because it's going to occur. I mean, it's mechanistic, but also, it's very philosophical in many ways. So, there's some fascinating work going on.

JM: Just before we finish, I'm going to I'm going to remind you of something I didn't really want to be on the record, but when you were chief resident....

WR: I do remember!

JM: I remember so distinctly: it was it was actually on one of the CMSC (Children's Medical and Surgical Center) wards where we were making rounds. I'll never forget that moment. It was great. We got to get together face to face again. It's been so long.

WR: It's been so long. I really miss you. And it's wonderful to see you.

JM: Oh, it's wonderful to see you. I'll make the effort to come there for no other reason than just to see you. Any chance you could be coming out here?

WR: There's always a chance that I'll make it to Baltimore. I've got so many connections. But if you want to go to San Diego while it's snowing in Baltimore or while it's storming in Baltimore, that's always a good thing. Right.

JM: Well, is it still raining in San Diego?

WR: The mudslides are over now. Oh, the sun's not shining, but it'll be out within a couple of hours. We haven't had any mudslides. Those are all up in L.A. They've really gotten hammered.

JM: I'm going to turn off the recordings and say say goodbye for the time being. Jen sends her love. She's she's downstairs working on her stuff. We were sort of late getting started, so she had to go down to join a webinar. But she said, send Bill my love. I think of you so often and we speak about you a lot.

WR: You know, you're oh, I speak about you, too, and your and your kids. Well, I really only know one kid. I really only know one of your kids. Oh, well, that's a good reason.

JM: Maybe we should all come out there. I've got a bit of travel fever myself and I would love to come out and just spend a couple of days doing nothing except hanging out with you.

WR: Well, that'd be great. It'd be fantastic. All right.

JM: Be well, stay well. And thank you so much for this. I think a lot of people will get an inspiration and hope from the things that you've said. And when you see it in writing, I think you'll agree you really said quite a lot.

WR: Oh, thank you. I appreciate it. And I appreciate the opportunity as well.

Chapter 7
Art as Medicine

Ana Zão

7.1 Art and the Person-Centered Approach

Art can be defined as the expression or application of the human creative skill and imagination, to produce works that may be appreciated primarily for their beauty or emotional power [1]. It is the ability to express the emotions, and it includes a variety of languages such as literature, visual or fine arts (painting, sculpture, drawing, …), and performing arts (theater, cinema, dancing, music, …) [1].

The definition of art remains controversial throughout the centuries. Even more challenging and personal is the interpretation of art itself, for the meaning and emotions brought by art are influenced by the individual's circumstances, past experiences, and personal, environmental, and contextual factors. The individual experience of art reinforces the much-needed individualized and person-centered approach when addressing health problems using art as medicine, as it will be explored below.

Evidence on how art promotes health, and well-being has grown in the last decades [2–4].

The person-centered care is in line with the current statements of the World Health Organization (WHO), which define Health as a "state of complete physical, mental and social well-being, and not merely the absence of disease or infirmity" [5,

A. Zão (✉)
International Center of Arts Medicine, Porto, Portugal

Physical and Rehabilitation Medicine Department and Chronic Pain Unit, Centro Hospitalar Universitário Santo António, Porto, Portugal

School of Medicine and Biomedical Sciences (ICBAS), University of Porto, Porto, Portugal

RISE Health, Porto, Portugal

Instituto CUF Porto, Porto, Portugal

European Commission—Expert Group Culture and Health, Porto, Portugal

J. McFarland et al. (eds.), *Humanism in Surgery*, New Paradigms in Healthcare,
https://doi.org/10.1007/978-3-031-86018-8_7

6]. As also stated by the WHO, well-being encompasses quality of life and the ability of people and societies to contribute to the world with a sense of meaning and purpose [5–7]. The focus on well-being and in an equitable accessibility to culture-based initiatives and dissemination of art-based interventions supports the overall thriving and sustainability.

7.2 Art as Medicine: Art Prescription, from Health Promotion to Prevention and Treatment

Art promotes a stimulating and enriched environment with a healing power.

The benefits of arts for health are well-recognized, whether for prevention and promotion of health and well-being, or in the management and treatment of several diseases (with a comprehensive spectrum of action from neurological and mental health problems to chronic disabling pain and developmental disorders, for example). Evidence is also increasingly robust on the benefits of using the arts, particularly music, preoperatively, intraoperatively, and postoperatively.

7.2.1 Music as Medicine

Music is one of the richest cognitive, sensorimotor, and emotional experiences of the human being, which involves hearing, seeing, moving, coordinating, remembering, and feeling different musical elements [3].

The connection between medicine and music is already ancestral (they even shared the same God in Ancient Greek—Apollo) [8]. In fact, music has been used for therapeutic purposes for several centuries, but initially its use was empirical. With the advent of functional imaging and other recent technologies, it has been possible to better understand and prove its effectiveness [2].

7.2.1.1 Music Neurophysiology

Music is a complex temporally structured sound language that stimulates and integrates neural networks in a very specific and unique way (including sensory-motor and language processing, cognitive, memory, and emotional components), allowing access to functions not accessible by non-musical stimuli [2, 3, 9]. Listening or playing patient's preferred music is even more powerful, for it seems to grant easier access to these brain functions [2].

Thus, music can elicit deep cognitive, emotional and sensorimotor responses because it stimulates different brain regions such as the auditory cortex (responsible for perceiving the basic acoustic features of music such as the frequency, duration and loudness), medial orbitofrontal cortex, midbrain, amygdala, nucleus accumbens, cingulate cortex and other limbic and paralimbic areas (experiencing pleasure, motivation to listen to or to engage in any musical activity, sense of reward and music-evoked emotions), inferior and medial prefrontal cortex, premotor cortex, anterior and posterior parts of the superior temporal gyrus and inferior parietal lobe (important for the perception of higher order musical features such as harmonies, intervals, rhythms, chords, ...), dorsolateral prefrontal cortex, cingulate cortex and inferior parietal areas (engagement of the attention and working memory system for continually keeping track of the music), hippocampus, medial temporal and parietal areas (involved in episodic memory, for hearing music that is familiar to the patient from past experience), lingual gyrus on occipital lobe (for music reading and dance expression, for example), cerebellum, basal ganglia and motor and somatosensory cortices (responsible for perceiving the rhythm of music, moving to the beat, tapping in synchrony with an external pacemaker, such as a metronome, coordinating or producing music) [2–4, 9–12].

As stated by Altenmüller et al., the multimodal effects of music, including the music's ability to tap into the emotion and reward system in the brain, support the therapeutic use of music by enhancing the rehabilitation process and restoring neurological dysfunctions and impairments of acquired or congenital brain disorders [3].

The neuronal circuits activated through music and the competencies acquired when performing music-based interventions can be transferred to non-musical functions when the stimulus of music is not present [2, 3, 11, 13].

Music-based interventions, even music listening, activate a wide-spread network of brain regions on both hemispheres (connected by corpus callosum), related to sensorimotor functions, attention, semantic processing, memory, creativity, and emotional processing [3, 14].

Several studies have shown how musical training shapes the brain and stimulates structural and functional changes, such as the enlargement of primary motor cortex and corpus callosum [12, 14], thus encouraging some authors to also describe the musician's brain as a model of neuroplasticity [14].

Recent studies using functional imaging have demonstrated that listening to one's favorite music may effectively increase pain thresholds and might strongly affect pain perception, possibly by enhancing descending pain inhibition and reducing the activity in ascending pain pathways, and through modulation of pain-related responses in the anterior cingulate cortex, respectively [15].

Therapeutic instrumental musical performance and other music-based interventions where the patient has an active role performing musical therapeutic activities or exercises have also proven to have a significant neuromodulator effect, as facilitator of sensorimotor, emotional, and proprioceptive integration, promoting the recovery of multiple domains, leading to neuroplasticity [2, 3, 12, 13].

Music training and the participation in music-based activities, also have positive effects on social bonding and interpersonal relationships, as have been shown by studies on Dance for Parkinson Disease [16–18].

Understanding the potentialities of music as medicine involves not only knowledge on the neurophysiological phenomena of music, but also on musical identity and musical perception. Musical perception, the ability to perceive and identify sound waves as part of a musical language, can be influenced by several factors such as biology, culture, contexts, education, state, traits, competences, and previous musical experiences. The specificities of the different musical elements (timbre, tonality, melody, harmony, rhythm, dynamics…) and the individuality of each person, will contribute to the attribution of meaning to this sound language and will promote the blossoming of a wealth of emotions, making the perception of music a unique experience.

7.2.1.2 Music Therapy and Music Medicine

Some controversy still exists concerning the term music medicine and the distinction between music medicine and music therapy.

Music therapy is defined by the American Music Therapy Association, as the clinical and evidence-based use of music interventions to accomplish individualized goals within a therapeutic relationship by a credentialed professional who has completed an approved music therapy program [19, 20].

Although some authors advocate that music medicine refers strictly to listening to pre-recorded music for health-promoting goals or the use of music by medical doctors that have not acquired certification as music therapists[19, 21], I consider this a narrow view of the term Music Medicine that is based on the assumption that doctors cannot have training in music therapy, which may even lead to some bias in the interpretation of results from comparative research studies.

As a medical doctor and a musician, with training in music therapy, conceptually I would propose a broader view of the Music Medicine term as a medical field (more than a specific intervention), comprising all music-based interventions (structured and non-structured) to promote health, prevent, treat or manage health problems, connecting Medicine/Health and Music.

Thus, it includes:

- Structured music-based interventions ((both music therapy and structured music-based interventions imply a therapeutic relationship and the music therapist/health professional should have knowledge and training on applying music-based intervention):
  - Music therapy: music-based interventions to accomplish individualized goals within a therapeutic relationship by a credentialed professional who has completed a music therapy program. These interventions may be performed as isolated interventions—unimodal intervention (i.e., the patient does not engage in any other therapeutic modalities integrated into the same therapeutic medical plan, for example, physical, occupational, or speech therapy), through music therapy sessions, where the patient is evaluated by a music therapist who is responsible for the hole treatment plan regarding music ther-

apy (both prescription and application). When music therapists are integrated in Healthcare Institutions (for example, a Physical Rehabilitation Medicine Department or a Chronic Pain Medicine Unit), those interventions may be included in a broader therapeutic plan within a multiprofessional and multidisciplinary team. In this case, it may be considered a music-based structured intervention (as described below).
  - Structured music-based interventions integrated in a multimodal medical plan: structured music-based interventions prescribed and applied by a health professional with training in music therapy, integrated in a holistic and multimodal medical therapeutic plan, typically coordinated by a medical doctor with robust knowledge and experience on music-based interventions. For example, the integration of music-based interventions in a rehabilitation program comprising other modalities on physiotherapy, occupation therapy, speech therapy, exercise, orthosis or pharmacological prescription), coordinated by a Physical and Rehabilitation Medicine specialist with expertise in music-based interventions.
  - Music Prescription: refers to the prescription of specific types of music or structured listening experiences by a health professional to achieve therapeutic outcomes, or for prevention or health promotion. As with other forms of cultural prescription, it typically involves the intervention of cultural mediators.

- Music participation or engagement: other music-based interventions that applied or developed on a healthcare context, within the Community or other settings, which are not structured for a specific therapeutic purpose, or not prescribed or applied by a music therapist or a healthcare professional with robust knowledge on music-based interventions. Typically, they involve active participation in musical activities (for example: playing a musical instrument, singing, dancing, …) or receptive music engagement (for example, listening to music, attending concerts, …) and are primarily focused on Health Promotion and Prevention, though they may also have a therapeutic effect.

Therefore, Music Medicine may focus on health and well-being promotion, prevention (from primary to quaternary prevention), or treatment and management of health problems (Fig. 7.1).

When prescribing a music-based intervention, two important aspects should be considered: the musical identity of the person and the specific aims of the intervention. Regarding the aims of the intervention, it should be discussed with the person, and their specific needs and expectations should be considered when defining the treatment plan.

Several modalities have been proposed as effective music-based therapies.

Music listening, a perceptive modality, has been one of the most known and implemented interventions [2, 4, 17, 22]. It seems to facilitate the recovery of cognitive and neurobehavioral functions (attention, memory, learning ability, executive functions, mood) in several clinical conditions, such as stroke [18, 23–25], disorders of consciousness/traumatic brain injuries [26, 27], and Dementia [28].

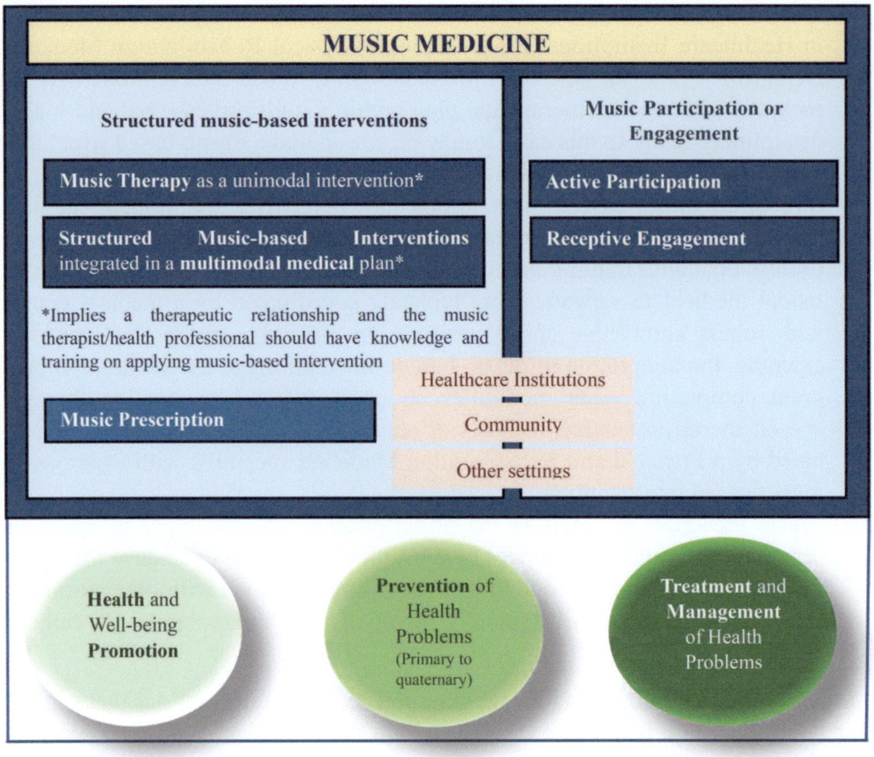

Fig. 7.1 Conceptualization of music medicine field

Regarding pain management, music-based interventions have demonstrated interesting results, compared to conventional treatments alone, including for the improvement of pain and associated disability, mental health and well-being, physiological parameters (regulating vital signs and increasing dopaminergic activity), and sleep quality, increasing patient motivation, social engagement, social support and therapeutic alliance, as well as contributing to a significant reduction in analgesic consumption [29–31]. Studies have shown superior results when using the most significant music for the patient [15, 29].

However, several other structured music-based therapeutic interventions have been proposed and proven to be effective [4, 16–18, 28]. Music therapy can improve motor control, speech, language, and memory in stroke and Parkinson's disease patients [4, 16–18]; it can trigger memories and improve mood and socialization in Dementia patients [28], and it can also reduce pain, anxiety, depression, and quality of life in cancer patients [31, 32].

These modalities should be integrated into a rehabilitation program and seem to have additional clinical benefits in several domains (when compared to the standard treatment), such as clinical and functional outcomes, health-related quality of life, and well-being [4, 17, 18, 28].

Rhythmic auditory stimulation is one of the most commonly used interventions [33]. It consists of a rhythmic synchronization of the movement taking advantage of the physiological effects of auditory rhythm on the motor system to improve the control of movement in rehabilitation and it may be used in different contexts, for example, to potentiate the gait training in stroke patients, Parkinson, or for patients with lower limb chronic pain and kinesiophobia [33]. This modality is usually integrated into a broader rehabilitation program or other multimodal plans and seems to have additional clinical benefits (when compared to standard treatments) to improve mobility, sensorimotor coordination, gait pattern (speed, cadence, step length, stability, symmetry, velocity,), proprioception, balance, mood, and fatigue. It also positively influences the quality of life and interpersonal relationships (particularly when performed as a group activity, also promoting social bonding and emotional well-being) [2, 33–36].

In Dance, the individual has the opportunity to express themselves through body motion/movement, as response to a music stimulus. Dancing also seems to facilitate bonding, produce positive emotions, and improve coordination, cardiopulmonary function, and endurance [2, 17, 37].

Another example is the Therapeutic Instrumental Music Performance (TIMP) [33]. The use of TIMP is based on the assumption that the music performance and training require multimodal processing, involving the integration and cooperation of visual, motor, auditory, affective, and cognitive systems. This intervention stimulates functional movement patterns and has been most commonly applied for neurological rehabilitation and chronic pain management, with significant improvements in pain, mobility, strength, fatigue, dexterity, coordination, neuromotor control, balance, gait pattern, functionality, quality of life, emotional status, self-esteem and the sense of well-being, enhancing the patient's reintegration into their different contexts [33, 38, 39]. Several instruments may be selected in a therapeutically meaningful way (being the most common the piano or other keyboards, guitar, and percussion) [33, 39]. Sometimes, the barrier to the implementation of TIMP is the limited access to these instruments, whether in health institutions, in the patient's home, or in institutions in the community. In this case, it may be pertinent to create collaboration protocols with academic or professional artistic institutions (eventually also the involvement of their professionals for developing some music-based interventions in the community), as is already practiced in some countries as local or regional initiatives.

Several singing-based therapies have also proven to be beneficial, such as the therapeutic singing (with an adding value in interpersonal relationship and mental health when performed in group-group singing), melodic intonation therapy (for patients with motor aphasia), musical speech stimulation (for dysarthria) and other singing interventions which not only positively impact speech or language disorders but also improve pulmonary function and capacity (for example after cardiothoracic surgeries) and swallow [17, 33]. The performance of wind instruments also seems to improve these outcomes [33].

Peripartum singing (including singing for the infant) has been used to promote well-being and improve mood during pregnancy, as well as for the prevention of postpartum depression and to strengthen the bonding between mother and infant [2, 40–42]. Music therapy also seems beneficial in reducing postpartum anxiety and pain levels [40].

During childhood, music-based interventions also improve the development of behavioral, cognitive, emotional, physical, and social domains, as well as executive functions, memory, language processing, and communication, promoting mental health across the lifespan [2, 43–45]. In pediatric health care, the highest quality of evidence for the positive effects of music therapy refers to autism spectrum disorder and neonatal care [43, 45]. However, music-based interventions also have been explored in other pediatric contexts and their efficacy has been proved (epilepsy, children with different disabilities or under neurological rehabilitation, pain, anxiety, and stress in medical procedures, pediatric oncology, or palliative care) [2, 45].

Studies focused on mental health also have shown a statistically significant reduction in depression levels, as well as improvement on participants confidence, self-esteem, or motivation after listening to music (CD recording or live music), singing, playing, or improvising with instruments [46]. And the improvements were even more significant among elderly participants [45].

7.2.1.3 Music as Medicine in Surgery

Evidence is increasingly robust on the benefits of using the arts, particularly music, in surgery settings in pre-, intra-, and postoperative contexts.

Several systematic reviews and meta-analyses have demonstrated the statistically significant effects of music interventions in patients undergoing surgery in decreasing emotional distress, pain, anesthetic use, opioid, and non-opioid intake, as well as improving vital signs, behavioral cognitive disorders, fatigue, mobility, strength, coordination, dexterity, balance, walking endurance, gait pattern, and quality of life, enhancing the patient's reintegration into their different contexts after surgery [2, 47, 48]. The improvement in patient satisfaction, well-being, and self-esteem is also reported [47]. Some authors also have shown significantly greater benefits when the music is chosen by the patient or when the patient's preferences are taken into account [49–52].

Regarding neurosurgeries on musicians, for tumor resection or surgical treatment for epilepsies involving eloquent areas, an intraoperative musical performance (played by the patient) is an important intervention which allows a more accurate monitoring of complex function, rather than the simple finger exercises and movements [53].

Music also has proven to be beneficial for patients undergoing minimally invasive procedures, such as listening to music during ultrasound-guided injections or other pain medicine procedures, during urological procedures, biopsies, cardiac procedures, endoscopies, cystoscopies, hemodialysis, and local anesthetic procedures [2, 48, 54]. It appears to reduce pain, anxiety, procedural satisfaction, and the patient willingness to repeat the procedure [55, 56].

7.2.2 Other Art-Based Therapies

Art, whether music or other forms of art, is a vehicle to communicate, reconstruct, and heal pain and emotions triggered by the disease. The arts empower patients and stimulate creative expression, resilience, and body and mind flexibility.

Studies have demonstrated the benefits of several art-based therapies in the management of different health problems, from oncology to pain disorders, improving pain, anxiety, depression, hope, and quality of life [57–60].

Literature, an art which puts in words what we feel, our frustrations, and our emotions, and helps us organize our thoughts, also capacitates medical doctors, improving their methods of inquiry and thought, and the power to invigorate the spirit [59]. The creative writing has been explored as a vehicle for coping, healing, processing emotions, and understanding the patient's own feelings, emotions, pain, disease, and disability [58]. Poetry intervention has also been explored in hospitalized pediatric patients with promising results, reducing fear, sadness, anger, worry, and fatigue [60]. Our poets also portray in words their feelings, their pain, and their difficulty in dealing with and being understood in the suffering and restlessness that the disease causes them.

Guided museum visits may explore the clinician capacity to look at the patient beyond the most obvious signs, to improve the details of their descriptions in clinical reports, to think creatively, to solve problems, to communicate and appreciate other perspectives [59, 61], because the viewing and appreciation of art works, such as painting, activates not only systems involved in the visual representation and recognition of objects, but also brain areas related to the emotions and cognition [59, 61].

Drawing is also an interesting tool for studying, as illustrated by the anatomy books and, for example, by the DRAWinU Project (Drawing Across University Borders), where drawings of medical students, teachers, and doctors were exposed in a museum. As a Professor of Anatomy, I have experienced the usefulness of drawing to teach and to learn anatomy and other disciplines. The capacity to translate learning into drawings implies a deep knowledge of the underlying anatomical concepts, including the three-dimensionality of the human body, movement, and functionality. As a medical doctor, I also take advantage of drawing, during my consultations, as a useful tool to promote health literacy and educate patients about health, illness, and treatments (it can be therapeutic and facilitate doctor-patient communication).

7.2.3 Culture Prescription in an "Artificial Intelligence World"

Art is a cultural expression and a tool for social transformation and evolution. Through culture, art finds its meaning and purpose, allowing us to develop our inner resources so that our emotions, imagination, and intellect may support and enrich each other. Our positive feelings give us strength to develop our rationality and hope for the future to sustain us in adversities [62].

New technologies have allowed the expansion of ways of applying art-based interventions and the diversification of music-based stimuli. It has also been fundamental in facilitating access to the arts, namely through online resources (guided visits to museums through videoconference), attending concerts virtually, online music therapy sessions, the use of digital tools and mobile phone applications (such as a metronome, a digital piano keyboard, or percussion instruments).

However, special attention must be paid to this technological evolution and exponential development of artificial intelligence, so that their added value is filtered without allowing them to completely subdue emotional intelligence, the importance of contact, physical presence, and relationships, whose healing effect is not negligible. Cultural and social prescription and a more humanistic medicine are increasingly needed to balance the (also needed) progress of technologies and to not let the art of caring fall.

7.3 Art and Medical Training

Physicians may also benefit from music listening to or practicing music or other art [63]. In the particular surgical context, listening to music seems to have a calming and relaxing effect, decreasing the anxiety and stress levels, and enhancing the accuracy and the speed of the surgical task performance [63]. Nonetheless, noise (not music) in the operating room can have distressing effects on surgeons, jeopardizing the patient's safety [64]. Other studies reinforce that listening to preferred music in the operating room may have a positive effect on trainees' microsurgical performance [65]. The preferred music significantly improved speed, knot quality, and performance [66].

Furthermore, the practice of a musical instrument by physicians seems to improve skills such as manual dexterity, neuromotor coordination, and the ability to concentrate, which are essential for surgical practice [66].

However, the benefits of Arts in Medical Education go beyond the acquisition of motor skills. The arts foster communication and relational skills stimulate empathy, facilitate understanding of the patient in their individuality, and help to regulate emotions (with a significant impact on the doctor's mental health) [59]. The arts and humanities also enrich the lives of healthcare professionals and contribute to a more critical thinking.

The promotion of Education on arts and humanities in Medical Pre and Postgraduate training is essential to capacitate medical doctors for the holistic and person-centered approach previously underlined. The introduction of Courses on art in Biomedical Faculties is already a reality, such as, for example, the Course on "Medicine, Music and Mind" (lead by me) included in the master's in medicine at School of Medicine and Biomedical Sciences—University of Porto (ICBAS) and the Course on "Cultural Prescription" of the University of Porto. But more courses on these topics, as well as on, social prescription and narrative medicine should be implemented for medical doctors, other healthcare professionals and cultural mediators to create synergies between culture and health [59]. More certified courses on music therapy and art therapy are also needed, to ensure more health professionals are qualified to develop and implement art-based therapies.

7.4 Medicine—The Art of Caring for Others

Being a doctor is also a form of art: the art of caring for others and showing genuine concern and compassion. Art fosters creativity and enhances our ability, as doctors, to listen, understand, communicate, and express, promoting a rich and healthy doctor-patient relationship and a person-centered care. In the art of Medicine, a deep knowledge of diseases and their associated structural changes is not enough; it is necessary to understand the patient, to know their contexts and circumstances. The art of medical practice also encompasses the clinician's behavior and communication with the patient and family [59]. In fact, the interaction of all members of the multidisciplinary team (not only clinicians, but also nurses, therapists, and other healthcare professionals) may promote or limit the healing process [59].

So, in an era of artificial intelligence explosion (with all its undoubted benefits), emotional intelligence and empathy will continue to be powerful weapons in the art of caring and managing human life and society.

Recalling the motto of the ICBAS, inspired by Abel Salazar, "A doctor who only knows Medicine, doesn't even know Medicine," it is important to highlight that art can also be a source of physician enrichment and a vehicle of communication, helping him to understand the patient in his individuality and in a holistic way. Likewise, Sir William Osler's inspirational phrase ("Listen to your patient; he is telling you the diagnosis"), draws our attention to the importance of a comprehensive "looking" (and "listening"), focusing not only on the disease and its sequelae or deficits, but on the individual "as a whole" (with their contexts, personal and environmental factors) to better recognize the impact of these health/illness states on their ability to carry out the most diverse activities that are significant to them and on their ability to participate in their different contexts (personal, family, professional, vocational, ….) [67]. The same medical doctor described the practice of medicine as an art based on science and reinforced the importance of the person-centered approach. Goldman and Dennis also described that the art of caring and comfort, guided by millennia of common sense as well as a more recent systematic approach to medical ethics, remains the cornerstone of medicine and emphasizes that without these humanistic qualities, the application of "modern science of medicine is suboptimal, useless, and even detrimental" [68].

The art fosters the patient to achieve the best outcome, increases patient's motivation and engagement on its treatment process, and stimulates a proactive behavior, autonomy, dignity, and education for a healthier lifestyle.

From another point of view, doctors also have an important role in understanding art, valuing its importance and potential in the healthcare, as well as promoting the health of the artist, so they can develop their art with the minimum limitations and explore their maximum artistic potential.

7.5 Conclusion

Music listening, artistic performance, and other artistic interventions are powerful tools (both for patients and for doctors) to engage multisensory and motor networks, induce changes within these networks, tap into emotions and reward system, and foster links between distant, but functionally related, brain regions. The neuromodulator effect of the arts, as facilitators of sensorimotor, emotional, and proprioceptive integration, promotes the recovery of multiple domains with long lasting effects and leads to neuroplasticity.

Art-based therapies are valuable tools for promoting health, and preventing or treating diseases, and can be applied in different settings (healthcare institutions, community, …), from pregnancy to old age.

To explore the full potential of art in healthcare, a specialized academic and clinical training is essential, as is a careful selection and application of the therapeutic intervention to fit the main therapeutic aims defined by the multidisciplinary team (where the patient plays an essential role).

Culture and Art promote healthier behaviors, emotional intelligence, and the ability to communicate, face challenges, and think critically, enabling people to reach their full potential. Art-based interventions will positively impact not only the patient or the healthy individual but also health and culture professionals, caregivers, and the community, leading to a happier and more productive, empathetic and united society, fighting social isolation, with an expected positive economic impact.

Consequently, it is important to promote more education and training on culture/art for health; to develop, implement and disseminate new and improved art-based initiatives for clinical practice and community interventions (creating cross-sectorial collaborations between Health, Cultural Institutions, and the Community); to develop multicenter and multinational research studies for monitoring not only the efficacy but also the cost-effectiveness of these different art-based interventions, to produce guidelines and to show to policy makers its added value in order to increase their support, creating synergies between culture and health sectors and humanizing the healthcare.

References

1. Oxford English Dictionary. Available from: https://www.oed.com/search/dictionary/?scope=Entries&q=art. Accessed Mar 2024.
2. Zaatar M, Alhakim K, Enayeh M, Tamer R. The transformative power of music: insights into neuroplasticity, health, and disease. Brain Behav Immun Health. 2023;35:100716.
3. Altenmüller E, Schlaug G. Apollo's gift: new aspects of neurologic music therapy. Prog Brain Res. 2015;217:237–52.
4. Altenmüller E, Schlaug G. Neurologic music therapy: the beneficial effects of music making on neurorehabilitation. Acoust Sci Tech. 2013;34(1):5–12.
5. Callahan D. The WHO definition of 'health'. Stud Hastings Cent. 1973;1(3):77–88.
6. Nobile M. The WHO definition of health: a critical reading. Med Law. 2014;3(2):33–40.
7. Schramme T. Health as complete well-being: the WHO definition and beyond. Public Health Ethics. 2023;16(3):210–8.
8. Cartwright M. World history encyclopedia. Available from: https://www.worldhistory.org/apollo/. Accessed Mar 2024.
9. Särkämö T, Tervaniemi M, Huotilainen M. Music perception and cognition: development, neural basis, and rehabilitative use of music. Wiley Interdiscip Rev Cogn Sci. 2013;4(4):441–51.
10. Salimpoor VN, Benovoy M, Larcher K, Dagher A, Zatorre RJ. Anatomically distinct dopamine release during anticipation and experience of peak emotion to music. Nat Neurosci. 2011;14:257–62.
11. Warren J. How does the brain process music? Clin Med (Lond). 2008;8(1):32–6.
12. Olszewska AM, Gaca M, Herman AM, Jednoróg K, Marchewka A. How musical training shapes the adult brain: predispositions and neuroplasticity. Front Neurosci. 2021;15:630829.
13. Chen WG, Iversen JR, Kao MH, Loui P, Patel AD, Zatorre RJ, et al. Music and brain circuitry: strategies for strengthening evidence-based research for music-based interventions. J Neurosci. 2022;42(45):8498–507.
14. Münte TF, Altenmüller E, Jäncke L. The musician's brain as a model of neuroplasticity. Nat Rev Neurosci. 2002;3(6):473–8.
15. Antioch I, Furuta T, Uchikawa R, Okumura M, Otogoto J, Kondo E, et al. Favorite music mediates pain-related responses in the anterior cingulate cortex and skin pain thresholds. J Pain Res. 2020;13:2729–37.
16. Machado Sotomayor MJ, Arufe-Giráldez V, Ruíz-Rico G, Navarro-Patón R. Music therapy and Parkinson's disease: a systematic review from 2015–2020. Int J Environ Res Public Health. 2021;18(21):11618.
17. Barnish MS, Barran SM. A systematic review of active group-based dance, singing, music therapy and theatrical interventions for quality of life, functional communication, speech, motor function and cognitive status in people with Parkinson's disease. BMC Neurol. 2020;20(1):371.
18. Zhou Z, Zhou R, Wei W, Luan R, Li K. Effects of music-based movement therapy on motor function, balance, gait, mental health, and quality of life for patients with Parkinson's disease: a systematic review and meta-analysis. Clin Rehabil. 2021;35(7):937–51.
19. Association AMT. AMTA official definition of music therapy 2024. Available from: https://www.musictherapy.org/about/musictherapy/. Accessed Mar 2024.
20. Bruscia KE. Defining music therapy. 2nd ed. Gilsum: Barcelona Publishers; 1998.
21. Gold C. All those things with music. Nord J Music Ther. 2009;18:1–2.
22. Baylan S, Swann-Price R, Peryer G, Quinn T. The effects of music listening interventions on cognition and mood post-stroke: a systematic review. Expert Rev Neurother. 2016;16(11):1241–9.
23. Tsai PL, Chen MC, Huang YT, Lin KC, Chen KL, Hsu YW. Listening to classical music ameliorates unilateral neglect after stroke. Am J Occup Ther. 2013;67(3):328–35.
24. Long J, Zhang Y, Liu X, Gao Q, Pan M. Music-based interventions for unilateral spatial neglect: a systematic review. Neuropsychol Rehabil. 2023;33(9):1462–87.

25. Särkämö T, Tervaniemi M, Laitinen S, Forsblom A, Soinila S, Mikkonen M, et al. Music listening enhances cognitive recovery and mood after middle cerebral artery stroke. Brain. 2008;131:866–76.
26. Kotchoubey B, Pavlov YG, Kleber B. Music in research and rehabilitation of disorders of consciousness: psychological and neurophysiological foundations. Front Psychol. 2015;6:1763.
27. Grimm T, Kreutz G. Music interventions in disorders of consciousness (DOC)—a systematic review. Brain Inj. 2018;32(6):704–14.
28. Gassner L, Geretsegger M, Mayer-Ferbas J. Effectiveness of music therapy for autism spectrum disorder, dementia, depression, insomnia and schizophrenia: update of systematic reviews. Eur J Pub Health. 2022;32(1):27–34.
29. Leis JA, Morrison CI. An integrative review of arts-based strategies for addressing pain and substance use disorder during the opioid crisis. Health Promot Pract. 2021;22(Suppl 1):44S–52S.
30. Garza-Villarreal EA, Pando V, Vuust P, Parsons C. Music-induced analgesia in chronic pain conditions: a systematic review and meta-analysis. Pain Physician. 2017;20(7):597–610.
31. da Silva-Santa IN, Schveitzer MC, Dos Santos MLBM, Ghelman R, Filho VO. Music interventions in pediatric oncology: systematic review and meta-analysis. Complement Ther Med. 2021;59:102725.
32. Li Y, Xing X, Shi X, Yan P, Chen Y, Li M, et al. The effectiveness of music therapy for patients with cancer: a systematic review and meta-analysis. J Adv Nurs. 2020;76(5):1111–23.
33. Thaut MH, Hoemberg V. Handbook of neurologic music therapy. Oxford University Press; 2014.
34. Tarr B, Launay J, Dunbar RIM. Music and social bonding: "self-other" merging and neurohormonal mechanisms. Front Psychol. 2014;5:1096.
35. Scataglini S, Van Dyck Z, Declercq V, Van Cleemput G, Struyf N, Truijen S. Effect of music based therapy rhythmic auditory stimulation (RAS) using wearable device in rehabilitation of neurological patients: a systematic review. Sensors (Basel). 2023;23(13):5933.
36. Ye X, Li L, He R, Jia Y, Poon W. Rhythmic auditory stimulation promotes gait recovery in Parkinson's patients: a systematic review and meta-analysis. Front Neurol. 2022;13:940419.
37. Carapellotti AM, Stevenson R, Doumas M. The efficacy of dance for improving motor impairments, non-motor symptoms, and quality of life in Parkinson's disease: a systematic review and meta-analysis. PLoS One. 2020;15(8):e0236820.
38. Yang S, Suh JH, Kwon S, Chang MC. The effect of neurologic music therapy in patients with cerebral palsy: a systematic narrative review. Front Neurol. 2022;13:852277.
39. Schneider S, Schönle PW, Altenmüller E, Münte TF. Using musical instruments to improve motor skill recovery following a stroke. J Neurol. 2007;254(10):1339–46.
40. Hakimi S, Hajizadeh K, Hasanzade R, Ranjbar M. A systematic review and meta-analysis of the effects of music therapy on postpartum anxiety and pain levels. J Caring Sci. 2021;10(4):230–7.
41. Wulff V, Hepp P, Wolf OT, Balan P, Hagenbeck C, Fehm T, et al. The effects of a music and singing intervention during pregnancy on maternal wellbeing and mother-infant bonding: a randomised, controlled study. Arch Gynecol Obstet. 2021;303(1):69–83.
42. García Gonzalez J, Ventura Miranda MI, Requena Mullor M, Parron Carreno T, Alarcon, Rodriguez R. Effects of prenatal music stimulation on state/trait anxiety in full-term pregnancy and its influence on childbirth: a randomized controlled trial. J Matern Fetal Neonatal Med. 2018;31(8):1058–65.
43. Swaminathan SSE. Musical ability, music training, and language ability in childhood. J Exp Psychol Learn Mem Cognit. 2020;46(12):2340–8.
44. Sharda M, Tuerk C, Chowdhury R, Jamey K, Foster N, Custo-Blanch M, et al. Music improves social communication and auditory–motor connectivity in children with autism. Transl Psychiatry. 2018;8(1):1–13.
45. Stegemann T, Geretsegger M, Phan Quoc E, Riedl H, Smetana M. Music therapy and other music-based interventions in pediatric health care: an overview. Medicines (Basel). 2019;6:25.

46. Leubner D, Hinterberger T. Reviewing the effectiveness of music interventions in treating depression. Front Psychol. 2017;8:1109.
47. Hole J, Hirsch M, Ball E, Meads C. Music as an aid for postoperative recovery in adults: a systematic review and meta-analysis. Lancet. 2015;386(10004):1659–71.
48. Yaluri N, Modi S, Kokkola T. Simvastatin induces insulin resistance in L6 skeletal muscle myotubes by suppressing insulin signaling, GLUT4 expression and GSK-3beta phosphorylation. Biochem Biophys Res Commun. 2016;480(2):194–200.
49. Kwong KC, Kang CX, Kaliaperumal C. The benefits of perioperative music interventions for patients undergoing neurosurgery: a mixed-methods systematic review. Br J Neurosurg. 2022;36(4):472–82.
50. Lin CL, Hwang SL, Jiang P, Hsiung NH. Effect of music therapy on pain after orthopedic surgery-a systematic review and meta-analysis. Pain Pract. 2020;20(4):422–36.
51. Chandrababu R, Ramesh J, Sanatombi E, Nayak BS, George A. Effectiveness of music on anxiety and pain among cardiac surgery patients: a quantitative systematic review and meta-analysis of randomized controlled trials. Int J Nurs Pract. 2021;27(4):e12928.
52. Patiyal N, Kalyani V, Mishra R, Kataria N, Sharma S, Parashar A, et al. Effect of music therapy on pain, anxiety, and use of opioids among patients underwent orthopedic surgery: a systematic review and meta-analysis. Cureus. 2021;13(9):e18377.
53. Scerrati A, Labanti S, Lofrese G, Mongardi L, Cavallo MA, Ricciardi L, et al. Artists playing music while undergoing brain surgery: a look into the scientific evidence and the social media perspective. Clin Neurol Neurosurg. 2020;196:105911.
54. Song M, Li N, Zhang X, Shang Y, Yan L, Chu J, et al. Music for reducing the anxiety and pain of patients undergoing a biopsy: a meta-analysis. J Adv Nurs. 2018;74(5):1016–29.
55. Wang MC, Zhang LY, Zhang YL, Zhang YW, Xu XD, Zhang YC. Effect of music in endoscopy procedures: systematic review and meta-analysis of randomized controlled trials. Pain Med. 2014;15(10):1786–94.
56. Agius M. Anxiolytic effects of intraoperative music therapy in adults undergoing local Anaesthetic interventions. Psychiatr Danub. 2021;33(Suppl 11):100–15.
57. Puetz TW, Morley CA, Herring MP. Effects of creative arts therapies on psychological symptoms and quality of life in patients with cancer. JAMA Intern Med. 2013;173(11):960–9.
58. Cronin M, Hubbard V, Cronin TA Jr, Frost P. Combatting professional burnout through creative writing. Clin Dermatol. 2020;38(5):512–5.
59. Dobkin PL. Art of medicine, art as medicine, and art for medical education. Can Med Educ J. 2020;11(6):e172–e5.
60. Delamerced A, Panicker C, Monteiro K, Chung EY. Effects of a poetry intervention on emotional wellbeing in hospitalized pediatric patients. Hosp Pediatr. 2021;11(3):263–9.
61. Vartanian O, Skov M. Neural correlates of viewing paintings: evidence from a quantitative meta-analysis of functional magnetic resonance imaging data. Brain Cogn. 2014;87:52–6.
62. Bettelheim B. The uses of enchantment: the meaning and importance of fairy tales. 1st ed. New York: Knopf: distributed by Random House; 1976.
63. El Boghdady M, Ewalds-Kvist BM. The influence of music on the surgical task performance: a systematic review. Int J Surg. 2020;73:101–12.
64. Fu VX, Oomens P, Merkus N, Jeekel J. The perception and attitude toward noise and music in the operating room: a systematic review. J Surg Res. 2021;263:193–206.
65. Shakir A, Chattopadhyay A, Paek LS, McGoldrick RB, Chetta MD, Hui K, et al. The effects of music on microsurgical technique and performance: a motion analysis study. Ann Plast Surg. 2017;78(5 Suppl 4):S243–S7.
66. Lies SR, Zhang AY. Prospective randomized study of the effect of music on the efficiency of surgical closures. Aesthet Surg. 2015;35(7):858–63.
67. World Health Organization. Towards a common language for functioning, disability and health. ICF [Internet]. 2002; Accessed Mar 2024
68. Panda S. Medicine: science or art? Mens Sana Monogr. 2006;4(1):127–38.

Chapter 8
Conversation with Surgeon 4—Christopher Wolfgang

Jacek Mostwin

Interview March 4th, 2024, with Dr. Christopher Wolfgang at his offices at the NYU Grossman School of Medicine, 550 1st Street NY, NY.

Abbreviations that follow:

JM: Jacek Mostwin
CW: Christopher Wolfgang

JM: It's so nice to see you again, Chris. I'd like to speak with you now a bit about who you are, where you came from, how you got into surgery, what you remember, your educational practice, guidelines and principles and things. Let's follow the conversation where it leads us. You started by saying that you grew up on a farm.

CW: I did. Yeah. So, yeah, for me, I had the best childhood in the world and I never really left the farm. I just found something else, but my heart is still on the farm. And I think that a lot of who I am now just goes back to my childhood. I had wonderful parents. My mom was, is the daughter, one of two from my grandfather on my mom's side, Conrads. And he was a physician. And my grandmother had also grown up on a farm. So we came from a very agricultural area. My grandfather was self-made and got into medical school on his own. He was the first in his family to graduate from college. Second, I guess you should know that his older brother also went to medical school. On my father's side, we had been farmers for years.

Growing up on the farm as kid is a great thing. I had the opportunity to spend a lot of time with my father and my mother. They were strict Pennsylvania Germans, but a very loving family. And I think that some of the things that it instilled in me was, number one, there was no entitlement whatsoever. You can do what you want or be what you want, but nobody is going to hand you any-

J. Mostwin (✉)
Department of Urology, Johns Hopkins Medical Institutions, Baltimore, MD, USA

J. McFarland et al. (eds.), *Humanism in Surgery*, New Paradigms in Healthcare,
https://doi.org/10.1007/978-3-031-86018-8_8

thing. You have to do it on your own. And then I think the second thing that was instilled into me was that it's a privilege to work and to do something that you're passionate about. So, whatever it is, just be passionate about it. And again, you know, work to your level of your ability. And so, I wasn't necessarily pushed in to agriculture and to farming, but those things were instilled in me in terms of work ethic. And then the other thing probably was cultural, our Pennsylvania German background. We were not very religious, but religion was a big part of our growing up. And it was basically "do unto others as you would want them to do unto you." We had a community in which we looked out for each other. If somebody was in need, we would help them. And so, I would observe my family being like that. And although I was not initially interested in medicine, those were the core values, I think, that were instilled in us as kids and that still provide my moral compass for what I'm doing.

JM: So, it was Pennsylvania?

CW: It was in Pennsylvania.

JM: Which part of Pennsylvania was it?

CW: I'm from a small town called Higgins, Pennsylvania. The town itself has maybe about 200 people in it. It's part of a larger region that is very Pennsylvania German. It's an isolated area. Many of the families in that region go back to the 1700s. My ancestors settled in that valley around 1760. They came to the United States in 1738 through Philadelphia, initially settling right outside of Philadelphia. The original farm is still there. It's now covered with highways. At some point between the 1740s and 1760s, they moved out to this area, which was a very isolated Pennsylvania German town. Interestingly, the son of the first generation, that would have been Michael Wolfgang, is buried in the graveyard of the church that my family still goes to, the Lutheran Church. For nine generations, we haven't really moved very far, and we were settled in that valley. That is my hometown where I grew up and that I consider that home. My father died young, he was 50, but my mom kept running the farm, taking care of it and overseeing it. And that's still, when the family gets together, we get together at the farm.

JM: When you were growing up, did you have much contact with farm animals or was it an agricultural farm?

CW: Early on, we had cattle, but later on we went to a grain farm where we grew, typically, corn: not the corn that you eat, but the dent field corn that goes into animal feed, soybeans, wheat, hay, and those types of things. And so, my father started with about 56 acres and built up a sizable farm. And we lived through that as kids and just sort of integrated into the farm and we spent time working.

JM: It's interesting that you had earlier mentioned that your daughter has chosen to be a veterinarian, an animal surgeon.

CW: Yeah. It's interesting because she's very, very bright. Getting into veterinary school is more difficult than medical school. And I'm very close with my daughter, but I'm not going to get any "father of the year" awards because she was growing up when I was a resident, and we ended up being very close. I think she became interested in the science and knew that she could do it. And I don't know if it was a conscious decision, but I think she saw the lifestyle of a surgeon and a surgical resident and she very much wanted to have kids and cared about family and decided to take a different path. I'm very proud of her. She's been very successful.

JM: At what point did medicine come into your life? How were you exposed to it? When did the idea that you might do this come around?

CW: So, I was very close to all of my grandparents, but particularly close to my grandfather on my mom's side, Joe Conrad.

JM: He was a physician?

CW: He was a physician. And that whole generation was great. He was born around 1918. When he was born, he didn't speak English. He only spoke German. That's how isolated the valley was. And the typical mode of transportation was horse and buggy. By the time he was an adult, they had somebody on the moon. So, it was an amazing generation. He and all of his siblings, including his wife and her siblings on my other side, fought in World War II. And that was that generation.

I was very close to him. He was a wonderful person, almost like another father to me, and very involved. Thankfully, he lived close by. And he had an immense work ethic. And his enjoyment was spending time outside, gardening, working on the farm and doing things. And I got to spend a lot of time with him. And I also got to see another aspect of him as a physician. He would take me as a young kid out to the hospital. After World War II, he specialized in radiology. I would go to work with him. And one of the things that was very meaningful to me was that when he would get on the elevator, everybody knew him. Everybody would tell me, "Your grandfather saved my life. Your grandfather delivered my baby." This is when he was in general practice. "Your grandfather helped me out." Just to see the number of people that he had helped. And then, even when I was young, he would sit with me reading the films.

He would explain things to me. And the surgeons would come down and visit him. He would spend time going over the films. He would connect me up and have me go to the operating room. And I think I was 12 years old when I watched my first operation, the resection of a large leiomyoma. I remember it like it was yesterday. And I was super impressed by that. At the time, I still hadn't decided on medicine. But I remember watching this operation. And the surgeon's name was Calussi. I still remember it very well.

His friend was a pathologist by the name of Russo. And he connected me up. I spent time in the pathology lab just watching all the pathology things. And I never at that time had decided I was going into medicine. But all of those things stuck with me. And the respect that he commanded! And the number of people that he had helped! It just was very inspirational to me.

I was the first one in the Wolfgang lineage to graduate from college. My father went to a trade school. He farmed. My parents were very interested in me going on to college. I loved farming. When I started in college, I went to Penn State, which was an agriculture school. That was the place to go. In the first year, I wasn't a serious student. I remember coming home and I had a GPA of 1.86, and my mom, my dad and my grandfather, were helping pay for school. My dad sat me down and said, you know, you're either going to come back and work on the farm or you're going to buckle down in school and start to focus on something. And it wasn't a conscious decision. I very much loved the sciences. I loved physics. I loved biology. And you know, without a lot of thought, I just focused on that. I started doing well, but I'd never given any thought to: what am I going to do? I even liked the agronomy classes that I had taken. And then just over time, I think it was not that my grandfather pushed me, but just the influence of my grandfather. Well, what am I going to do? And I decided that I would like to be a physician.

JM: Did he actually ask you about that or was it just his presence?

CW: It was just his presence. It was there to kind of nudge you along. It was just his presence. Like I said, I had the best childhood in the world. I was given a lot of support by my mom, my dad, my grandparents, but never was forced to do anything. They just wanted me to find my way and they gave me support no matter what I did. And so, it just sort of migrated toward that. Even when I came to that realization, I had 100% support from my father and my mom. Of course, my grandfather was very excited about it. And the other thing along with the sciences, as I studied the science, I also became interested in research. I may sound like it was a little diffuse, but I didn't want to only be a physician. I wanted to be able to do impactful research that actually made a difference in medicine. So, even before I went to medical school, I knew I wanted to do research and I then went into a combined MD-PhD program. My grandfather pushed a little bit, but I was very happy to go to Temple Med School, which is where he graduated. And one of my proudest moments and his was that (he was the first one to be able to do this) there was a tradition, if your parents had graduated from Temple Medical School, they could hand you your diploma. And I asked if my grandfather could hand me my diploma. And it was, like I said, one of my proudest moments. I still had tears in my eyes, and I think he had in his eyes when he walked on the stage and handed me that diploma.

JM: He was sort of your first teacher, your first mentor.

CW: Yeah, really. And he continued to be my mentor all along. I mean, whenever school would get difficult, you know, not that my mom and dad didn't care, but they really hadn't lived it. You know, my grandfather has an amazing story. As I told you, he was born around the turn of the century. And his mom died young. His father was not the most involved, and so all of his siblings took care of each other, and they helped themselves. And this is, it's just a great American success story. And I don't think it could be done today just because the opportunities are not there. But my grandfather and his brother, Chester, decided that they were going to go to medical school. And they worked as brush cutters and coal miners when they were young. This is when they were in their teens and early twenties. And they decided that first Chester was going to get into medical school. And then my grandfather was going to keep working. And then when Chester became a physician, he was going to help my grandfather. And that's exactly what happened. But the whole family was successful. Their sister was a nurse, and they helped her get into nursing school. And they all served in the military during World War II as either physicians or nurses. My grandfather was in the Pacific Theater as a physician.

JM: So that must have been quite something. They were German nationals fighting for the United States Army. I've read stories of Japanese nationals, one of whom wrote a very interesting book about his experiences with the surviving children of Nagasaki. He had grown up in the U.S. and was serving as a physician with the U.S. Army at the same time that his parents were interned in California camps that were created during World War II for Japanese Americans.

CW: It's interesting because the area was so isolated. All of my grandparents, when they were born spoke German in the household. And I remember my grandmother making fun of my grandfather when he was in primary school: he had to learn English and he couldn't pronounce milk "this is a mil-ik" and similar funny stories. But although they had that German heritage, I think that they had been in the United States for over 200 years as a family. They saw themselves as American. And the interesting thing, and I think it's a bit of a sad thing, is that when they came back from World War II, they said, that's it: we're not teaching the next generation German because they were a bit ashamed of that and very proud to be American and have fought, you know, in the war against Germany. And so, my parents' generation was not taught German. So, in a single generation the German language died out in our valley. When I was a kid, the newspaper called the Valley Citizen, had portions of the newspaper written in German. And now that no longer exists that's how quickly it sort of died out. So, I don't think there was any moral dilemma in their decisions. They saw themselves as Americans, but you know, still had that strong German ethnic background.

JM: So, one thing that comes out right away in our conversation is your link to multiple generations, your depth of connection to these people and the of pride and love that you have for them. When you mentioned your grandfather the physician who handed you the diploma, you said that he was a wonderful person. And the first thing you talked about had nothing to do with medicine. And then the second part included the conversations in the elevators and the viewing room. It's as though there were two dimensions that weren't really separable. The way you describe it, it sounds like one person, although we might separate the different aspects of it.

CW: That's an interesting way of thinking about it. To me, he was my grandfather and, you know, first and foremost, he was somebody I loved and respected, just like my grandfather on the other side had just as much influence on me and maybe gave me a hand because he taught me woodworking. And as I got a little bit older and then started going with my grandfather, I just saw this whole other dimension of him. He was just a good person in general. And it wasn't like he was Joe Conrad, the physician, he was Joe Conrad, the human. And it was just amazing to me to see this is my grandfather that all of these people depend on, he's helped so many people, an aspect that he never really spoke of when he was home. With us, he was just "pap."

JM: Did you carry his image with you then as you continued in your studies...? carriage return.

CW: One hundred percent.

JM: I see.

CW: In fact, in my office and in my house and pretty soon here as I hang my pictures, I have actually and literally carried his image with me. And I have two pictures of my grandfather when he was a physician, standing at the x-ray board and giving a lecture to a bunch of people.

And then, just him, sitting there: these are the old days where he sat in his office with his pipe and read films. And you know, when I, you know how it is in medicine, you get tired, you're wondering why are you doing this? And you know, you wish you had somebody, then I just look at those, that picture and I think of him and think about, you know, I'm here because of what he and what my whole family did for me. And it's inspiring and I think how lucky I am compared to what he went through.

JM: Once in medical school, you described a lot of interests: sciences, physics, wanting to do research and make a difference. And then you find yourself going in the surgical direction. So, tell me how that came to be.

CW: That was another thing. It was just sort of, I followed what I loved. I mean, I do and still very much love the sciences, and I still am very active in the lab and have a group. And to me it is, I think that there's all different personalities and there's sort of people who like doing a lot of different things and doing them well, but maybe not to the highest level. For me, and it's just a matter of personality, I want to pick one or two things that I really want to dive deeply into. And, as you know, my interest is in pancreatic cancer and pancreatic tumors. I specialize in that as a clinician and strive to be at the top of my field in the clinical management of those patients and then the technical aspects of being a surgeon. But just as important to me is that I want to be able to help the field in general. And so, I can take care of individual patients and that is very rewarding and very meaningful and it's an important aspect of what I do. But I can actually extend my impact on patients by trying to do things that will help everybody with these conditions, with pancreas cancer. Being someone who is involved in the clinical care of these patients, I know better than anyone who might be a scientist what are the exact problems that we face. What are the problems that we have to solve?

Pancreatic cancer, right now, if you have localized disease and you undergo an operation even in its earliest stages, 80% of patients will still get a recurrence. Why is that? The research then involves solving that very specific problem because if we solve that problem, the survival can go from 20% in 5 years all the way up to potentially even 100% if we solve this.

I just love studying. I was never one to look forward to getting out of school: "can't wait till school's over." Actually, when I was in college, I realized how great it was. When I was in medical school, I loved it and never wanted to lose that lifelong feeling. So, I do a lot of reading. I will read articles and just focus very much on the scientific aspects of what I do. It's very rewarding for me to still be able to do that now in an unstructured way and delve into the science of why these problems happen. But there's an outcome for "why it happens" because if we change it or we solve the problem, it'll actually impact the care of patients. And so being an academic clinician and specifically an academic surgeon, I think it's the best job in the world.

JM: You have picked, by any criteria, one of the hardest areas of surgery in which to work. The pancreas lives in a deep, deep cavity. Are these still open operations? Are you using the robot as much?

CW: Yeah. So, it's migrated to now where we do a lot of these robotically, but the impact of the robot or doing things minimally invasive is not as big as it is in other fields because it's still a big operation, whether we do it robotically or openly.

JM: But you have a lot of open experience from before the robot came around.

CW: Oh, absolutely.

JM: So, you're doing many of these operations which are very hard operations, by any criteria. I think you were at Hopkins for many years when it was an epicenter for this kind of surgery. So, you really, as you say, went deep. At what point did you start migrating in this direction? This is really complicated work. What drew you to this really difficult kind of work?

CW: Well, several things. My interest in the science, as my dad always says, "If you're going to try to solve a problem, pick a tough one to solve." So, this was a tough one to solve—and one that's going to make a difference, right? So many people do not survive the disease. If you make a difference, the impact will be huge. And so that was one of the reasons. The other area of surgery that I was sort of interested in was cardiac. And I know that the two are different, but there's a lot of things in the science of cardiac surgery: transplantation and artificial hearts, both of those things. But I tended just, again, because of my academic interest to be more interested in cancer biology. And so that's why I chose that. When it came to what field in cancer biology, I like working with my hands. Maybe this came from my other grandfather. I still do this. I enjoy woodworking very much. I like, you know, some people, I think that your hands are a manifestation of what goes on inside your mind (gesturing with his hands as he speaks).

JM: Just the way you are showing it now (referring to gesture).

CW: Yeah. And, you know, I like it. To me working with my hands is very satisfying because within a very short period of time, I can take a situation and if done right, make it better. And you see that within a single day. But there's just something natural about me working with my hands. I can give you some examples. One of my therapeutic activities, or one of my meditations, is when I do woodworking. My grandfather taught me woodworking. He was the fifth generation of woodworkers, and I still have some tools that date back to the mid 1800s. [He taught me] to be able to assemble a box with no nails, to do hand cut dovetails and those types of things. And there's just something about the focus and the precision in being able to do that that actually applies to surgery. Obviously, the stakes are higher. But my wife will probably not agree with this, but there's—I always joke around like I'll do the dishes, because I'm sitting there working with my hands. Or I'll do the woodworking because it's one of those opportunities where I can work with my hands, but the stakes are not high. It's very much my meditation. So, the nice thing about surgery is that I think it's, you know, one of my comfort zones. And so, to be able to have a job where it takes, where you leverage one of your strengths and are able to do something that is impactful…

JM: You refer to your comfort zones. When you say that, I naturally think of the operating room. Is that what you're thinking of?

CW: Yeah, absolutely. I love interacting with patients. I love all aspects of it. But if I—it's almost—I don't know how to describe it. It's almost like the fish in the water phenomenon. You know, some of the bigger operations that I do now involve a lot of vascular work and there's always a lot of planning to these cases and a lot of potential downsides. There's a high risk if things don't go well. And there's this little bit of tension. It's a good kind of tension. But then, you know, you get into the operating room and you put your gown on, the lights come on, you make the incision, and it just—there's this feeling of serenity, not being cavalier about it, but there's this feeling of like, "Okay, this I can do. This is, you know, my strength and this is what I can focus on." And to be able to have a job like that where you actually can—it's an outlet where you can leverage your strength and it's to the benefit of somebody. So, I say academics—for me, it's the best job in the world. I love the time I spend in the operating room. It's rewarding to be able to take care of patients and do something that is helpful for them.

Then there's the science aspect of it, you know, to bring all of those things together, I can honestly say I have the best job in the world.

JM: Did surgery come naturally to you when you started out?

CW: It always felt comfortable. But I always feel like—I think I'm a better surgeon now than I was 3 weeks ago. And so, am I where I want to be? I don't know if I will ever be, and I will always try to be better. But it always felt like it was, you know, the right thing. Right?…that I could do it. That would be another thing—well, I'd love to be an NFL football player. I played football in high school, right? And I'd love to be a running back. That would be great. But, you know, I could lift weights every day. I could run every day. I could, you know, study football tape. I could do everything. I'm never going to be an NFL football player. It's just not going to happen for me. Psychiatry was one of those things that there was some sort of innate interest or whatever. And I felt that if I focused on that, I could excel at it. And so, in that regard, it just felt right. Internal medicine—I loved internal medicine. I was one of those for whom every rotation was what I wanted to do. Even psychiatry. I loved psychiatry. But when I looked at what are my strengths and what are my weaknesses, you know, I—I think that for me surgery was the right thing.

JM: So, it's so interesting to hear you talk about all these specialties that you could have done, including psychiatry. I actually started out wanting to be a psychiatrist before I moved towards surgery.

CW: It was one of the most fascinating rotations I had ever done.

JM: Tell me something about your early experiences with surgery, your first operations, the patients that you took care of, that you were involved with. What sort of memories do you have of those times and experiences?

CW: First of all, going back to the older way of training, you know, you would actually spend a lot of your time not in the operating room until you were a third or fourth [year resident]. And actually, I don't think that was a bad thing. And I still enjoyed surgery very much. My goal was not to just be a technician. And so I actually enjoyed very much what I would call becoming a warrior: these patients would roll out of the operating room with a big heart operation or liver transplant or even a smaller operation and to be the captain of that ship and say, "I'm going to, you know, understand every detail about managing and being able to take care of these patients." So, my first memory of surgery was not being a surgeon, but it was becoming a warrior, that [sense of] "not on my watch" and nobody will be able to take care of these patients better than me if I learn and I strive. And so, in the beginning, it was just being able to take care of patients. And although I think I'm a very social person, being able to interact in a different way, being able to interact with patients, sit by somebody's bedside when they're not doing well, or sit by somebody's bedside when, you know, they've now just had a tumor removed or had a new liver transplant and have a new lease on life. It's a whole different type of interaction. And I think that you learn by being involved in that, but then also watching your mentors and people that you want to emulate how you interact. And so, my first memories of surgery were not the actual operations itself. You know, my first operations that I remember were doing inguinal hernias and stuff under supervision and just my hand shaking and thinking, "I'm never going to be able to do this. And I can't even do a hernia and they're doing these amazing operations. Will it ever happen?" But then understanding those weaknesses and going back and practicing and practicing and practicing. And again, I just, like, it seems like it's everything was rewarding, but that part was just to watch yourself grow and go from, you know, not being able to, you know, tie a suture without getting it tangled around your fingers to not even having to think about it, just through practice. And, you know, again, it gets back to nobody's going to hand you anything. You have to be able to do it on your own and being able to say, "Hey, I did this," through practice and hard work.

JM: It sounds like you learned a lot of this on your own and from your experience.

CW: I think we learn like any surgeon learns. If you pick a field that you think, you know, resonates with you, you don't have to be coddled. You're just given [the opportunity]. I'll be honest, I don't say I really did it on my own. I did it by being, you know, given the opportunities and having mentors who wanted me to do well, but they still can't do it for you. But actually, you know, endeavoring to excel at something and, you know, be given the support and the opportunity to do it.

JM: You mentioned watching your mentors. You already talked a lot about your grandfather. Are there people in particular, either during medical school, while you were a student or during your residency or both that stand out in your memory?

CW: Absolutely, the list could go on and on, but my grandfather was one. And I would even say my mom and dad were professional mentors too, because they would, you know, help me make decisions about what is going to make me happy in life. So, I think that they were important mentors. But with specific regard to surgery, when I first started one of the exciting things that I did was the trauma surgery service. And Bob Cooney, who's now the chair at Syracuse, was one of those mentors who had a way of being difficult, but also, you knew he cared and wanted you to do better. So, he wasn't going to coddle you, but though he didn't give you enough rope to hang yourself, he had really high expectations.

JM: How did you know he cared?

CW: Because no matter what, having high expectations was never a personal attack. At every step along the way, I think he recognized this was difficult, but then, he wasn't going to do it for you; he would continue to push and be there and pick you up when you fell down. And every once in a while, you needed to hear, "you can do it." And he would say that just enough: "you can do it." But then he gave me opportunities in the operating room. And I still remember when I had worked with him for a long time as an intern, and I operated with him a lot. And in the beginning, you're sort of just following what he tells you to do. And I remember the day we were doing a bariatric procedure, a gastric bypass. And he was demonstrating to me that "I think I can trust you." He wanted me to bring the Roux limb [tubular segment of intestine] up on this real heavy patient. And I brought the Roux limb up and I handed it to him. And we then sewed it [to the stomach]. And he looks at it, and after sewing the whole anastomosis, I had the Roux limb twisted. So, the first thing it showed me was a message, right? This is surgery. He gave me enough rope to hang myself. The patient suffered no harm. We took the limb down. I suffered the harm and then redid it. It was just as good as the first time. It was the perfect reminder that soon, somebody's not going to be looking over your shoulder. You're ultimately responsible. So, you better make sure that this was right. But the other thing is he, you know, did a little bit of ...whatever. And then he stood right there with me, and we did the case. And afterwards, it was no different than before. It wasn't like he lost any respect or hope for me. But I think it was a lesson, and I knew that perhaps he'd been there himself one time. And you know that lesson was something that I still think about it. Any small thing that you do is a double check, triple check. And the fact that he would have given me, you know, the opportunity to get it right, but I failed in that, was a message to me about how critical everything is that we do. He was one mentor, and he still is my mentor to this day. When we meet at the College of Surgeons, we go out for dinner. I will text him from time to time, you know, regarding leadership matters, ask him about his opinion. That list goes on and on. Robert Cilley was a pediatric surgeon. Unfortunately, he passed of pancreas cancer, but this was recent, not something that influenced me at the time. But he was somebody that I always wanted to emulate and still try and still don't know if I have met that metric. He was an amazing human being, somebody who really led from the front. Pediatric surgery was an extremely busy rotation, every other night call.

JM: Which location was this?

CW: This was at Hershey Med Center. And it was every other night call, a busy service. It was great to be on that service, but you know, when you were on call at night, it was busy. And then the next day, when you were post call, you would be rounding at nine, 10 o'clock at night. Now, you could complain about that as a resident. I mean, we loved it, but you couldn't [complain] because Robert Cilley was there too. This guy was there and maybe he didn't stay that one night, but he was there till 10 o'clock at night rounding. And one of the things that, you know, one of the mantras they always tell us is always do the right thing. And you know, it's an easy mantra to have, but sometimes it's hard to actually live it. And then you say, do people really do that? And it never happened, without fail. We were busy in the operating room. There was all of this chaos and we were taking care of all of these patients. And then we would do evening rounds and they would start at nine o'clock. And then we would go down and we'd round on the ward patients. Those were under our service. They were pretty much tucked away. Then we would go to the MICU [Medical Intensive Care Unit] and I pretty much guarantee we'd walk into the MICU at nine-thirty, ten o'clock at night. They would need what we called an L-Cath, they would need a a central line. They would need something. And he must've been tired: there's this whole other level of tiredness. You know, it's easy being a resident when you're ultimately not responsible, but he's the one responsible. We'd walk in and, and the, the MICU attending would come up: "we need a catheter on this patient." Right. And I knew the answer. He would just look at me and I'd run down to the operating room, grab his headlight, his loupes, the Jakes and the jewelers (small, delicate surgical instruments used in fine work), because I knew the answer was never going to be no, no matter what. And the other thing, there was a morning, it was a Saturday morning and there was a major, major snowstorm. And I was the chief on the service this time, not the intern. And Dr. Cilley was on for the service and he was rounding as the attending. And I knew it didn't matter if there was an earthquake or a fire or whatever, he was going to be there on time. And I had to be there on time. I remember I took my pickup truck and launched it into a snow drift and I couldn't get in there. I ended up taking off my clogs, putting on boots and walking to work and rounding on the patients. And sure enough, at six A.M. Dr. Cilley shows up. We were probably the only two in the hospital, but his dedication to patients and always doing the right thing has always stuck with me. No matter how tired, no matter how difficult, no matter how much you don't want to do it, if a patient needs it, that's the most important thing you have to do at the time.

JM: Is there any other of memory that you have of his interaction with patients that you witnessed or heard about that sticks in your mind?

CW: He just, he generally cared. He generally cared about about people. And he didn't do it because, oh, this is what I need to do. He did it because here's a mom with a, you know... and he would put himself in their shoes and it was just, he did it for the right reason. But to emulate him and how much he cared, that, that I think was one of the biggest things I took away. Now, he was also a technically great surgeon. And so, you know, I picked up a lot of different things from him. He too, to the very end, was one of my mentors. Another one, like I said, I could just go on and on.

But Jack Myers, who was a pediatric cardiac surgeon, was one of the greatest. It's one of those things that is always better when you look back at it than as you're going through it. I was at Penn State, and it had a big cardiac surgery program. It was one of the top programs, Damiano and all, there was the artificial organs program. I think they were the number one funded surgery department for years from NIH. And it was just this very active, busy program. They had two fellows. Neither of the fellows were interested in pediatric cardiac surgery at the time. And so, as the third-year resident, I always went to the cardiac pediatric cards room, which... that's an intense place. And Jack Myers, who is a wonderfully gifted surgeon, you have to be gifted to be a cardiac surgeon... the intensity in that room was incredible. And it just seemed in the beginning, you just couldn't do anything right. And you're just trying to assist. And you have to be careful how this is transcribed, but there was constant yelling. But you understood he wasn't yelling at you. It was just... this had to be perfect. And one of the most memorable moments, and I've told him this, I keep in touch with this too, is that after all of that, and you wonder, you know, can I ever do this or whatever? Toward the end of my rotation, he handed me the Castros (Castroviejo delicate cardiovascular needle driver), and he gave them to me as a third-year resident to close the atrium of the heart. And I remember...you would have thought I had just won the Nobel prize. But I appreciated the Karate Kid "Wax On, Wax Off." You know, I did not deserve to hold the Castros until I passed that course. But the feeling that I hung in there and I had learned, and was prepared when he handed me the Castros, to be able to do it and do it, you know, perfectly. Picking up the tissue exactly right, not pulling too tight on the suture, making sure the stitches were exactly right. I mean, it was just closing an atrium, but it is closing a kid's atrium at that point.... the fact that he would let me hold the Castros.

JM: These are very important moment because they can separate one group of people from another regarding their further career interest. Medical students might experience a variety of different reactions to such scenes. They may come back and say, "Oh, those surgeons, this is how they behave." Whereas you, you looked at this very differently. You saw the potential.

CW: I don't know what it... that I could put myself in the shoes of an attending, and I think I often tried to do this and understand that residency is a temporary thing. It's easy for me to stand here and accept that this guy's making sure I don't mess anything up. But to think about it, here's this guy coming in and he's opening up this little kid's chest. The parents are sitting in the waiting room. They have all the expectations that this kid will hopefully live for 80 years, right? And it's in his hands. And I used to think like, well, you know, will I ever be able to do something like this? You know, to actually feel like, okay, I am ultimately responsible for this thing. And I actually understood the level of intensity, how there could be no mistakes. And I wanted to get myself into that position. So, I never took it [personally]. And actually, and I think you probably recognize this too, there are malignant people who just yell and make it a personal attack and they're malignant because they're just malicious or whatever, or they were abused. This was not like that at all. And I'll, you know, move on to Dr. J. You could tell that the criticism and giving directions and things like that was not because they didn't like you or not because they were trying to make you feel bad. It just had to be perfect. And I needed that because I'd never done this before, right? And so, if I don't get the constant feedback, I don't know I'm doing it right. So, I almost appreciated it. And you know, even though there was this silence, I felt proud. We would take the kid up to the intensive care unit after the heart operation and we would stand there and I would do the sign out, what we did. And he would stand there like that and quietly and just allow me to give the sign out. I felt proud because everybody's standing there looking at me thinking, "Now this guy was in the operating room with Jack Myers, and they just did this incredible operation on a kid." You know, I got the impression that maybe he didn't say it, but there was a little bit of "I think this kid will be okay," and [with] a little bit of a pride. You know, I have talked to him since in very different settings and Dr. Cilley, who was a mutual friend of ours, the one who was my other mentor who passed of pancreatic cancer, unfortunately it took that for me to reconnect with Jack Myers, but I can tell you after the fact that my impression of him was, he's a wonderful human being, a family man, somebody who really cares about patients. But that's what it took to take care of those patients and to train a generation of surgeons. And I would never trade that for the world.

JM: So, let's just take a slightly tangential move here. We've been talking a lot about your development, but now let's talk a little bit about your role as an educator. You're now in a very significant position. A lot of people look to you the way perhaps you at one time looked at Jack Myers or others. And so, if you have a student or a resident who has an encounter of the sort that you just described and they come to you with this, what kind of a conversation do you think you would have? How would you handle it? Do you think that people can't be talked into surgery?

CW: Yeah, it's gotta be, it's gotta be in them somehow. They've got to, they've got to really want to do it. If they want to, they're going to. And that's one way we could probably just bring it to an end. If someone comes to you and says, I don't think I could do this, et cetera, et cetera, maybe you're going to sit there and say, you're right. You can't do it. Yeah.

JM: Or you might say something different because you see potential in this person. How would you approach this?

CW: I would advise him that "you should think about, you know, what, what exactly is it that you want to do?" You want to be a Jack Myers one day and think about what, what that takes and think about holding a baby's life in your hands or even an adult surgeon and holding somebody's life in your hands: I mean, the amount of skill [it takes] to get to that. And, and there's only very few people who can teach you and separate a personal attack on, which is not right with, with intensity and embrace the opportunity that there's somebody there that's making you better. And I always use, I use examples, and I think it's a good examples of Navy SEALs, right? You know, the intensity of that in some, maybe mentally maybe not, maybe the same physically, maybe not so much. But if you want to be a Navy SEAL, it's not going to be easy. And you have to, as they say in the military, "embrace the suck," right? Because that's just what you have to, you have to do, because it's going to make you stronger, right? It's the same way here. It's not a personal attack. You have, you have to get to that next level to be a master surgeon and embrace that. It's not going to be easy. Education is never an easy thing. And you know, and, and just embrace that opportunity that you're standing across the table from Dr. J or Jack Myers who have, you know, just immense kind of knowledge. And you have the privilege of standing there and learning it and... just get it through your mind, it's not going to be easy because not everybody can do it. And what you have to sort out is if you can do it or not.

JM: And so along the lines of not everybody can do it, you're involved probably in the selection of residents for your program.

CW: Yes.

JM: What kind of qualities do you look for in people who want to be surgeons?

CW: I would probably never get into a surgical residency nowadays. I don't think we realize just how much we've done by the time we get there. I'll give you an example. We accept eight chief residents here and we get 1800 applications. So, I can tell you that, perhaps it's a little bit unfortunate, but from that group, we have to select the top academic candidates. But what separates number one from number 180, it's not much. What I look for are people who are in it for the right reason. And, you know, you can tell, by sometimes interviewing and personal statements and things like that, but truly, I think passion is the key word, what they're passionate about it. Yes, I will abide by the 80-h work week, [they'll say] but that's not all, I'm here to learn. Right. I want to hear, how we have all of these things in place. I want to hear: can I stand across the table from Bob Montgomery? Can I stand across the table from the giants and learn from the giants? How are you going to help me get better? And I think that it comes out in their passion: you can separate the ones who are passionate about what they do. The other thing is, I know it sounds a little, you know, maybe not relevant, but people who have excelled in something else, because

I think to become a master surgeon, you have to be able to sacrifice and excel. So somebody who is a concert pianist, somebody who's played sports on a team and excelled in sports, somebody who has done community service to a high level and done it for a genuine reason, and there's enough out there that those are the kinds of things that I think help [an applicant] rise to the top. You can see that they were passionate about something, overcame hardship, overcame adversity, and they made sacrifices to get to that; that there's really no level of entitlement. I think that it was one of those privileges of growing up on the farm. And you know, not everybody can grow up on a farm, but you can pick these kinds of things out. So as a farmer, this actually has a lot of relevance to what we do in surgery. You can be the best farmer, you can be the best surgeon, but at the end of the day, we're at the mercy of nature, right? And so, okay, the drought, the drought comes, or whatever, it's a bad, there's nobody [that can fix it], that's just the way it is. And you're either going to adapt to it and figure out how to survive, or you're not. Nobody, nobody owes you anything. And it's the same way in surgery, you know, you see where you rise to the occasion, I always say, you're going to sink to the level of your skill. You know, when you're out there and you have enough rope to hang yourself, you're not going to rise to the occasion.

JM: I really thought when you said, we're at the mercy, I thought you were going to say, at the mercy of God. It just felt like the next word, if I were ChatGPT, that's what I would have put in there.

CW: Yeah, I'm okay to talk about religion. I think I'm a spiritual person. I was raised a Lutheran and raised a Christian, but I don't see myself necessarily as a Christian. I think that I respect that very much. I respect all of the faiths, but I think that, you know, I'm more of a spiritual type of person. As you can see (pointing to his bookshelf), I have all of, I have my crucifix, I have the Virgin Mary, I have Buddha, I have everybody up there. And so, you know, I think many ways, and I think, so I guess in my sort of spirituality, you know, that nature is the, is, is, yeah.

JM: So, what about patients who have stayed with you? We've talked a lot about mentors and your experience. What about the people that you've helped who have been the recipients of your surgical care?

CW: Well, I can tell you there's nothing more rewarding. And this is one of the great things about getting older and having done it for a long time. I follow all my patients for life. And now having at least several clinics at which I see patients with pancreatic cancer that are 5 years out, 10 years out, all the stories start the same. Everybody comes with a death sentence. And to have those people who come to clinic... a lot of them will interact with me personally. A lot of them will send, "it's the anniversary of my operation." or "it's my birthday," and "I just went, you know, I'm 10 years out and I just went biking across Europe" or something like that. That's the most rewarding thing. And I think that is what keeps you going. Even though there are more failures than successes, there is the fact that we can have successes. What drives my research then is getting more people toward success.

JM: So, you mentioned that you follow all your patients.

CW: For life.

JM: How many do you think you've operated on in your lifetime?

CW: Well, operated on probably in the 2000s or so in terms of pancreatic operations I've gone over 2000.

JM: You follow all those patients?

CW: Yeah. I've got patients who, you know, can, who want to follow and continue to follow, but, but I probably have over a thousand patients that I see. And of course, you know, a lot of them, 80% of them have passed from pancreas cancer and I follow them until, and even often am actively involved in a transition from aggressive to palliative care. A lot of them will be even admitted to my service and go through that transition.

JM: Will they be admitted to your service, and will they die on the service?

CW: Well, a lot of times it's either home hospice or, yes, a lot of them will die usually on inpatient hospice or similar things. You know, I try to... I'm an optimist and I'm aggressive, but in a smart kind of way, but also as a, what I tell patients directly is that there are worse things than death. They can sometimes happen because of what we do in the aggressive treatment that has no, you know, it just has no chance of helping you to keep swinging for the fence when it's time to say... again, getting back to nature. Nature. Some problems are not solvable with surgery or medicine. Because I have a relationship with these patients., you know, before the surgery that they go through, these resections: it's probably the highlight in their treatment. It gives them hope. Not false hope. We all know that we're in it for the long run, but then I feel that in a way I would be abandoning them if I were not there also when they have to go through the other transition. And that's usually not a surgical transition. That's something else... When you get to that stage and I don't know where this came from, but I think that John Cameron is the same way: I believe that he follows a lot of his patients where it's feasible. And you know, you're just... you're their physician. I mean, you stop happening to be a surgeon at some point. It can be a little bit annoying, but it's also rewarding. I have a lot of patients out there from whom I'll get an email, perhaps a couple of years out from removal: "Hey, my doctor wants to start me on a...," you know, "they want to give me an injection for my bone density. Do you think that's okay?" Yeah, I think that's okay. They see you as their physician, where they want to run things by you, or "I want you to know I was admitted to the hospital with the flu and had pneumonia" and stuff. Okay [I'll respond], thanks for letting me know.

JM: Do you think that's unusual for someone in your role to follow patients like that? Or do you think it's more commonly done than is generally appreciated?

CW: I think it's more commonly done than generally appreciated. I think that in our small world of pancreatic surgeons we are very involved. Obviously, it's the patient who has to go through things, but if you think about it, they have a very lethal disease. We're about to subject them to a huge operation that carries mortality and certainly a long recovery and morbidity. I think there's a little bit of a mindset that, you know, I'm going to put you through this for your own sake. I mean, it's the best for you, but we're in it together. And if things work out, we're going to celebrate together. And if it doesn't work out, I'm there for you, whatever I can do.

JM: Have you had the chance or been ever at the deathbed of one of your patients? CW:

Yeah, yeah, absolutely.

JM: What do you remember? What was that like?

CW: The circumstances are always different, but I can generalize a little bit. Often the worst period is not at the time of passing. It's prior to the time of passing, of us making that decision that we're not going to fix this. You're going to die of pancreas cancer. You're going to die of this. Switching gears and transitioning from "we're being aggressive" to understanding that "you are not going to be cured" to transitioning to things for comfort. I think once that decision is made, there's almost, it's almost peace. And no matter what religion or background, I think that once the patient is okay letting go and the family is okay, and often it's the patient being okay letting go, but they do it for the family. But once everybody's in agreement, it's time to go. I think that, you know, it usually is just, there's sort of passages of life. There's birth and there's marriage and then there's...and we ultimately are all going to suffer from the same fate. It's just, when the acceptance is there for most people, that it just becomes another transition. It's never easy, but it's also a part of life. And again, I find it a privilege to be at, with the family at that time. There are other times when it's gut wrenching. And you know, because it quite literally is something that you've done as a surgeon. That is one of the things: none of us are perfect. We come in, you know, patient comes in and is walking and talking. And you know, even if you did nothing, they are going to be around for a while, but then you have a case that doesn't go well, and you have a complication. And there is a certain mortality with pancreatic cancer, and it's amazing to me how understanding the family is. It requires a lot of discussion and preparation up front and getting to know them. But when things don't go well, even though the family is forgiving about it... actually it could be the most gut-wrenching thing about how understanding they are, how understanding the patient is when things don't go as planned.

JM: Have you ever attended any of the funerals of your patients?

CW: Yeah, I have.

JM: What's that been like?

CW: For me, it was healing. This is actually one that sticks out in my mind. She was a patient from the Midwest I took care of early on, a young, healthy woman. And she was just loved. She was a high school principal. She was loved by her community. And she had a Whipple, and she did great and then had a recurrence. And obviously we couldn't do anything for that, and she passed. Through my whole time of caring for her, I could understand how special she was because of the outpouring of... and you know, you feel terrible, although that wasn't a direct result of the operation. We gave her a chance, but it feels a little bit like a failure or something. It was healing for me to go to the funeral and have everybody I had known as I had taken care of her. Everybody came up and thanked me for taking care of her and for the time I had given her and the family being very appreciative. Although you know, the aspect sticks with my science of this: why we fail. We need to fix it. It was heartwarming to actually see that it made an impact. And you know, and it's just...it sticks with me. There's a quotation and I won't say it exactly as it is. I have to look up the quote, but there's a quote by Leriche, who was a surgeon... "There's a graveyard that all surgeons go to at night and visit." (the full quotation from Rene Leriche: "Every surgeons carries within himself a small cemetery, where from time to time he goes to pray—a place of bitterness and regret where he must look for an explanation for his failures") and I can tell you that every early mortality or every significant complication, I mean, I could go and list off, you know, those names. It actually lives with you. I think it makes you a stronger person. Again, it just reminds you of the impact of what we do. But those kinds of things, and I don't think it's a negative. I think you have to learn to live with it if you're in that field. But what also has an impact is the understanding that you have the potential to make things better, but you also have the potential to make things worse. It gets back to the training. And I think you don't quite understand that when you're a resident, the impact of what you do, even on the negative side. Because as a resident, you see things going positive all of the time, all of the time. Negative impact is something that thankfully is rare, but it always has to be here. It always has to be that place that you visit at night. And it may be an uncomfortable thing, but it's just something that you can never lose.

JM: There's a movement to try and make medicine more human. And yet, as I listen to you speak, and so many of the scenes are so familiar, and I can picture you in them, I don't know how much more human it could be. The application of skill and scientific work to the care of people, trying to do the best you can, recognizing the importance of their lives. To my mind, and I also consider myself a spiritual and a humanistically oriented person, I love the arts, and I also have a doctorate in sciences. So, you know, I'm not a stranger to either one. I love both worlds and to me they are inseparable. They eventually return us to the kind of work that we do day to day when we're doing it.

But now that I've stepped away from it, I miss what you talk about, that day to day contact with people, the intensity, the urgency, the importance to people. I am now seeing it in a broader context, with perhaps more clarity. But in contrast to some others who might say, well, we need to put more humanity into medical education, into humanities, etc., it creates a difficult situation, because they mean well, and their arguments are well made and intentioned, and yet, it's not like some fresh suit of clothes you're going to put on. It's either in your heart or it isn't. That's how I see it. And it's manifested through the work.

Do you think that surgery, the way it's going now, is as human a discipline as it can be? Would you want to make changes to the way patients are cared for? What about the overall environment, the sort of superstructure of surgery, its training, its practices, its administration, all those sorts of things that form a global enterprise? Right now, you're focused on really important matters close at hand, but if you were to think more broadly about what your daily work is, what would you say?

CW: I think that surgery now is a bit of a better field than what it was before, and I have a lot of hope for the future. I think that people who go into surgery, it's never... no medicine is easy..., and I think that most people go into it for the right reason. And so, I think it's important to talk about humanism, but I think that it's something that in a different form we learned maybe in a different way all along. I mean, first we were driven to that by just wanting to take care of people, but then I think it comes from—I don't think I've ever had a class on humanism, but I watch people like Dr. Cilley, I watch people like Dr. Cameron, and it's just that this is the way that we need to be. You emulate because at the end of the day, you know, they uphold that [way of] doing the right thing for the patient so highly. I think where things are going a little bit awry has nothing to do with the type of people we are or how we train. It's just where medicine is heading in general. I still say I love my job, it's the best job in the world, but in order for me to do the things that I love, I would say 80% of my time is spent on things I don't love. Billing.

JM: Well, I've noticed that your phone has gone off a dozen times since we've been in conversation.

CW: Even that. If it's for the right reason, but if it's a phone call because I haven't filled out my query related to my billing, which is most likely what it is because I went through my emails this morning and very few of the emails were directly related to patient care, they were about open encounters, they were about billing queries, they were about one thing or another. We now, although I find the electronic medical record somewhat useful, we now have a computer between us and the patient. There's just something about writing notes. The other thing is, I understand that "no money, no mission," and there has to be a financial aspect to it. As a leader, I'm constantly getting reports on our volumes and our numbers of clinic visits. That's where I think things start to go awry. Now, it's easy for me to say, I'm almost 60 years old and I carry enough, how do you say, weight or something where I can say, "I'm not going to do that." But somebody starting out, if they get that query, they say, "You need to see more patients," or "You need to..." They're at the mercy of the finances of the institution, of the documentation, of the rules that we give them. I'll give you an example. From the perspective of a patient, I see patients with pancreatic cancer all the time, it's nothing new to me, but that patient is diagnosed for the first time. Sometimes I catch myself thinking, "How many times must I go through this?" But it's the first time for this person. If it takes 20 min, then it takes 20 min. If it takes 45 min, it takes 45 min. Everybody is a little bit different. Some people are like, "Okay, just tell me the facts. I trust you 100 percent." Other people, "I want to know the facts." Other people, it's like, "We don't understand it," and so it takes whatever. But at the end of the day, I have a metric. I've got to get through so many patients in clinic, so now how do we do those two things? It sort of balances it, and it's balanced often at the end of the productivity and things like that. It's like, "Okay, we're going to have to cut this off here." There is something that goes beyond practical, but I'm not even talking about that. It's just really giving the time due to a patient.

JM: I think these are rumblings that you can hear in many places. I've had similar conversations with others, and I'm sure you have as well. I don't know. This is work in progress, shall we say. It does sort of knock on our door every single day, and it interferes with what obviously matters to you. You did say one thing at the beginning of this, which was people go into medicine for the right reasons, or many of them do. What are those reasons?

CW: I think because... Caring for people is certainly one thing, but I think there are other important aspects of why you go into medicine, and that is because you're intellectually driven to solve problems. Solving problems on behalf of your fellow human, I think that's what takes people into medicine. It's not just about caring, because let's face it, if you care but you're not competent, that's not helpful. Just like I said, I wanted to be a football player, but I'm never going to be one. There are some people who may want to be a physician, but they just don't have the... I'm sure they're good at something else, but don't have that tech. It's the combination of having the skill and the talent, but then also being engaged in the intellectual aspects enough to do things to care for people. It has to be...

JM: What can you do, or what kind of an educational environment do you think is most conducive to facilitating that? Is it what we have now, or do you think that there are some changes that you would like to see?

CW: No, I think it is... Things have improved in that regard. We're limiting the work hour to 80 h a week. Think about that for a second, how crazy that is. Limiting to 80 h a week.

JM: You mentioned that. I also remember you mentioning the snowstorms and pediatric surgery and being there 24 h on and then another 14 h to follow. You didn't say anything bad about that. In fact, from what you told me, it sounds like that was a seminal event in your life.

CW: It was, but I was... Like I said, I have maybe in some regard lived a privileged childhood because I have such a strong family. My wife is my strength. My kids are my strength, both my son and my daughter. I've had that. I can tell you, when I'm at my worst, and believe me, there's times when I'm not the nicest person, it is when I don't have balance in my own life. I'm strung out to the point where I can't do it anymore. Then I'm of no use to anybody. I'm not helping my patients. I'm maybe even just going through the motions and just getting stuff done. I think that the changing of the... It's not the hours, but it's the mindset that there has to be wellness of yourself first and then everything else comes because if you're not well, you can't really help anybody.

JM: It's like the oxygen mask on the airplane. Before you put it on the child's face, put it on yours.

CW: That's exactly right. Yeah. Now, for me, like I said, it's not the hours. You and I work those hours or whatever, and for us, maybe it was a selection process. There might have been surgeons who came up the process when we trained who would have been outstanding surgeons but they just... they didn't handle... I think we did. I think this is just keeping people who are talented and allowing them to focus on their family and focus on themselves so they can actually be better. I don't regret the time I trained or the number of hours I put in, but I look back and think, "I might have been a better person too, had I been trained in a little bit of a different system." I think these changes are good. If we can't train a surgeon in 80 h a week, then it's on us. Again, not the hours but just the realization that there has to be balance. God bless our spouses. Again, I have a... It was a privilege to have a wonderful wife. She's a scientist. She's a PhD. I think we shared the passion for science and things like that. We have a great relationship, and she was very understanding. As I also said, I'm not going to win any "Father of the Year" awards. Had I not had somebody like that who was able to raise the kids, and raise two wonderful kids, and have kids who are understanding... I was lucky maybe in a way.

JM: You have a daughter who followed you in the operating theater, literally, with smaller creatures, but God's creatures, nonetheless. It couldn't have been that bad.

CW: I think that it makes it more... I think we all have those examples of people who survive the whole ordeal. I always say, "One of two things are going to happen after surgical training to the way you used to be. You either become a stronger person or it breaks you." Broken doesn't mean you can't practice. They're just broken beyond repair. I think that we have less broken people. I think that ultimately that is going to be... I think it's better for surgery as a field. I see people coming through now who... It's not work ethic or anything like that. They would not have had surgery as an opportunity had training continued into same way because they are great parents, and they do the right thing for their family. We're better off as a field, having them in the field because they are outstanding people, but [in the old days] they would have made the choice. That's not the most important thing. I think we actually are becoming stronger because of that.

JM: I wanted these interviews with real surgeons who do real surgical work. I share many of the beliefs that you do. I have come to accept the idea that the knowing is in the doing. It's not what you say, it's really what you do and how you do it. That's what people see. That's what they remember and that's what affects them. You see people at work, and you say, "Ah." You can't even put a word on it. That's the thing you can't put a name on. Somehow those things have a way of filtering into literature and the arts. But in the moment, in the moment and the action that is taking place, and surgery is a world of action, what you encounter just speaks to you. It doesn't require language, but it speaks to you in some sort of way. I was tempted to say at the end of your last comments that surgery is medicine's best kept secret. Maybe we should keep it that way.

CW: Exactly.

JM: We don't want to let the strays in. We want to be inviting, but at the same time...

CW: That's right. I still think that, and I adore my medical oncology colleagues, my internal medicine, but at the end of the day to survive even a surgical residency now, there's a certain DNA of people who go into surgery. You've got to want to do it. It's a calling. You have to want to do it. There's no question about it.

JM: I think you would miss it even more than me if you left the OR. You would miss it, until you got to the stage where you couldn't do it anymore.

CW: I would miss parts of it, but I enjoy... My kids are older now, and I enjoy it even more, my kids and my grandkids and things. I have my hobbies. I have so many things. There'd be an aspect I'd miss, but even now I'm happy to have the guys come back and talk about the big cases that they did and stuff, and I'm proud of them. I'm glad I didn't have to stay there.

JM: I could tell you what happened to me, but you'll know for yourself when the time comes. You're not at that stage where you need to step down yet, though sooner or later it comes to all of us. Then you'll be doing what I'm doing now, walking around with a tape recorder.

CW: I might be on my tractor.

1 "Every surgeon carries within himself a small cemetery, where from time to time he goes to pray-a place of bitterness and regret, where he must look for an explanation for his failures."

Chapter 9
To Be or Not to Be

Margarida Lobo Antunes

The humanities are the hormones which do for society at large what the thyroid gland does for the individual.

—Sir William Osler [1]

9.1 Education and Future Doctors

The education of children and young adults has been a basic cornerstone of political and social agendas for many years now. The changes in educational structures, as well as in more recent years, the effects of the COVID-19 pandemic, have both had a devastating impact on educational standards worldwide. Younger children who began their primary education during the lockdown are not only frequently ill prepared regarding basic numerical and literacy skills but are also more naïve in social settings. The overall tendency to provide education for a greater number of people, in many circumstances, led to the establishment of an easier curriculum. Considering that an easy school does not prepare us for a difficult life, what are we offering our children in terms of their future? On a broader scope, what types of literacy skills should we be providing?

Regarding the topic of "literacy" in this "Brave New World" of ours, George Steiner proposed that we consider the existence of a "third culture" [2] which is that of computer literacy. Modern computers, the internet, artificial intelligence and the possibility of unlimited data storage have revolutionized the way people think, study and work. "No previous artefact or invention, certainly since man's domestication of fire, will have exercised the shaping impact on everyday human pursuits brought about by the pc and the laptop, by mobile texting and the internet" [2]. Computers have become crucial elements in our daily lives, both at home and in the

M. L. Antunes (✉)
Lusiadas Hospital, Lisbon, Portugal
e-mail: margarida.lobo.antunes@lusiadas.pt

J. McFarland et al. (eds.), *Humanism in Surgery*, New Paradigms in Healthcare,
https://doi.org/10.1007/978-3-031-86018-8_9

private domain and throughout the workplace, in business, finance, government, media and medicine. The vast knowledge readily offered by computers encompasses humanities and sciences alike, but there is a price to be paid. Can artificial intelligence and computers substitute all human activities and provide the type of "literacy" that humankind needs? Steiner proposes that a "fundamental literacy" should include "the ability to engage with, to respond to, what is more challenging and creative in our societies" [2]. Designing a curriculum driven by curiosity and imagination, which responds to the ever-changing needs of fast-paced, impatient and restless societies, is not an easy task.

In the realm of higher education, standards, prerequisites and norms also vary in many world-class institutions. Nurturing intelligent, imaginative, critical thinkers that yearn to pursue further knowledge should be the basic philosophy of colleges and universities that aim for excellence and embrace change. The process of education that begins in the home and often culminates in higher education calls for reflection regarding the paths that have recently been defined. Healthcare and the medical profession are a critical part of our societies, and therefore, the education and preparation of future doctors should also be a vital concern. The optimal medical curriculum has long been a challenge for medical schools, and there is a need to rethink what should be taught to future doctors. Medical education can be defined "as an art with scientific principle" [3] and is singular in that it is an area that deals with human health and well-being, calling for unique knowledge, skills and behaviour.

Physicians hold a privileged place in most societies because their "art" dwells in dealing with the human condition and human suffering on a daily basis. The ideal physician must practice patient-centred care, rapidly preventing, diagnosing and treating all illnesses, while working long hours, frequently fraught with moral and ethical issues, swamped in pointless bureaucracy and hoping to escape burnout at all costs. This ideal physician should also possess certain behavioural attributes such as being "confident, empathetic, humane, personal, forthright, respectful and thorough" [4]. Atul Gawande questions even further the notion of the ideal physician, "We've been wrong about what our job is in medicine. We think our job is to ensure health and survival. But really it is larger than that. It is to enable well-being. And well-being is about the reasons one wishes to be alive. Those reasons matter not just at the end of life, or when debility comes, but all along the way" [5]. Ideally practising physicians who yearn to offer adequate care must know not only the scientific basis of disease but also the personal aspects of illness deliberately engaging with their patients and appreciating their experiences holistically.

Medical education has evolved immensely since the era of the Greeks, Persians and Romans. Originally, the teaching process was based on models of apprenticeship and future doctors would shadow their mentors in order to learn and perfect the skills of the trade. In the nineteenth century, when the first advances were made to identify the causes of diseases, such as the identification of bacteria by Louis Pasteur, medicine began "to turn into a science" [3]. In the twentieth century, medical education leaned more towards the basic sciences, aiming to provide medical students with the foremost scientific information and skills required to best treat their patients. However, the swift and extraordinary advances in science and technology eventually managed to push the humanities out of the curriculum. Currently, despite decades of literature sustaining the significance of humanities in medical practice, there is still no consensus as to the standard inclusion of the humanities, for example, Narrative Medicine, bioethics, medical history, medical social sciences and the arts, in the medical curriculum. In most medical schools, the existing curriculum is already extremely overwhelming, leaving a very small margin to pursue other subjects beyond the more scientific and technological realm.

In 1969, the creation of the Society for Health and Human Values, under the orientation of Edmund Pellegrino, emerged as one of the dynamic forces for reintegrating the humanities back into medical education [6]. Edmund Pellegrino was a physician, scholar and distinguished bioethicist, who not only promoted the humanities as being vital to medical practise, he considered that medicine was a skill, an art and above all, a moral enterprise. Towards the end of the twentieth century, it became clear that it was time to return to the valuable teachings of the father of modern medicine, Sir William Osler. Osler claimed that the physician–patient relationship could thrive if the physician had a proper background in the humanities. For Sir William Osler, educating medical students required the combination of medical knowledge and the humanities.

9.2 Medical Humanities

Various studies have supported the benefits of including art and humanities as a part of the curriculum for future physicians, producing positive outcomes in terms of cognitive, affective and creative functioning. The incorporation of the humanities in medical education is based on the premise that the practice of medicine is not only technical and scientific but also humanistic and moral [6]. Art, literature, music and drama, in their multiple forms, are products of human creativity, and they can reflect various human emotions, joy, sadness, fear and anger. According to Jane Macnaughton, in her paper, *The Humanities in Medical Education: context, outcomes and structures*, "Part of what is to be a complete human being is to participate in some form of artistic activity, either as a spectator, reader or viewer. Understanding this will help doctors to remember the purpose of their own art: to enable people to participate fully in life unhampered as far as is possible by illness or disability" [7].

Medical humanities can be defined as "an interdisciplinary, and increasingly international endeavour that draws on the creative and intellectual strengths of diverse disciplines, including literature, art, creative writing, drama, film, music, philosophy, ethical decision making, anthropology, and history, in pursuit of medical educational goals" [8]. The inclusion of the humanities in medical education and clinical practice can be beneficial on two levels. Firstly, physicians exposed to and invested in humanistic studies become better clinicians. Studying the humanities enables physicians to better comprehend their patients within the context of their lives, fostering critical thinking and a more thorough approach. Secondly, the humanities can provide a supportive background to physicians as well as their patients, promoting resilience and comprehensive life balance. Various renowned medical professors and scholars propose "that humanistic interests such as literature, art and music are potent restorative resources for physicians that can help them to maintain their humanity and perspective through the stresses of medical training and practice" [6].

9.3 Narrative Medicine

By exposing physicians to training in the humanities, they can better "see" and value their patients as whole persons, comprehend their life stories and circumstances and sharpen their skills in listening and interpreting their patient's narrative. The term "Narrative Medicine" was coined in 2000 by Rita Charon, a general internist and literary scholar at Columbia University, when it became clear that literary and narrative work in clinical settings could be beneficial for both physicians and patients. Simple acts of reading and analysing literature have proven to promote the learning of narrative skills, beneficial to medical practice and nuturing critical thinking. Rita Charon and her colleague Peter Williams support the concept that the inclusion of humanities in clinical care provides physicians with the ability "to reach to the heart of human learning about meaning, life and death" [9]. When defining the various objectives of an ideal medical education, a physician should not only have the scientific capacity to treat the patient but also the ability to listen to the patient's story, to grasp and honour its meaning and to then act on the patient's behalf. "Narrative Competence", according to Rita Charon, allows the physician to "practice medicine with empathy, reflection, professionalism and trustworthiness" [10].

Lessons learned from the humanities and narrative knowledge allow the physician to recognize details about a patient's life that may seem irrelevant or tangential to their medical problems and treatment but are core to what they value about themselves. An appreciation of literature and stories affords basic skills of imagining and responding to worlds and realities vastly different from our own. Disciplined reading and cultural exposure can lead to a greater attentiveness to human behaviour. Relevantly, Rita Charon proposes that, "training in the humanities lets one see the suffering" [11].

Medical practice cannot be dissociated from narrative. Any narrative or story requires an interaction between people, the storyteller and the listener, as well as the disposition to hear and to understand that story. Rita Charon uses the expression "Shock of Attention" [10] to describe true engagement between physician and patient. In those circumstances, the level of attention is comparable to a reader's experience while reading a text. As Charon reinforces, "Like narrative, medical practice requires the engagement of one person with another and realizes that authentic engagement is transformative for all participants" [12]. Illness creates a state of chaos in the patient's life, and the basic act of the patient narrating their story is considered to be therapeutic, forcing them to put into words, their complaints and worries. Expressing the disease process through stories helps the patient and the physician to come to terms with the various dimensions of the illness. More importantly, it helps the patient better manage the impact of the illness on their life.

9.4 Literature

According to the writer Matt Haig, in order to travel in time, one can read and in order to feel time, one can write [13]. These incredibly simple propositions illustrate the importance of literature. Books and stories expand our horizons, humanize our views of life and those of others and heighten our awareness of the frailty of the human condition—all essential requisites in medical care. Brenda Walker, novelist and professor of literature, wrote the book *Reading by Moonlight: How Books Saved a Life* [14] to illustrate the importance of reading during her ordeal with breast cancer. Walker describes the five stages of her treatment—surgery, chemotherapy, radiation, reconstruction and survival. The story begins with the author trying to decide which book to take with her to the hospital. "The book will be the first thing I put my hand on when I arrive, when I'm taken to an empty room in an almost unimaginable place". From the outset, the book is a central element in her tale. Walker considers that a story is "a release into the account of another's life. A release in extended storytelling." Regarding the title of her book, she explains that "When I tell myself that books can save a life, I don't mean that books can postpone death. That is the job of medicine. I mean that certain books, by showing us the inner fullness of individual life, can rescue us from a limited view of ourselves and one another". Narrative Medicine proposes that books enrich the reader, allowing them to comprehend life and illness with a broader perspective and within a deeper context.

Walker defends that books are a source of empathy, "empathy the way that we can place ourselves, imaginatively, in the position of another person, is at the heart of what we do as readers, as people striving for a generous understanding of one another". Stories provide physicians with an escape from the toil of long hospital hours, treating and communicating with complex patients, as well as the bureaucracies of corporate medicine. Stories allow physicians to appreciate and value their patients, beyond the scientific foundations of disease and illness. Science and technology teach physicians how to diagnose and treat disease but not how to assist patients living with chronic, debilitating illness or more importantly how to face death. Physicians must recognize the necessity of treating their patients' spiritual, emotional and physical aspects. Stories help them to respond to the human needs of medical practice.

Brenda Walker's story is peppered with some of her favourite books, and each chapter makes a connection between literature and a specific moment of her illness. She cites the book, *The Hours* by Michael Cunningham [15] and the time when Clarissa tries to buy a book for her sick friend, "You want to give him the book of his own life, the book that will locate him, parent him, arm him for the changes". That special time taken to choose the right book is a true ritual, resembling the moment Walker experienced before leaving for the hospital. The notion that there is a perfect story for the different moments in our lives, and that a book can guide, fix and protect its reader is quite astounding. Brenda Walker states that as the reader, "I know that death can be a way of finishing a novel or beginning one; it can be central to the plot. But as a writer, I feel that storytelling is about staying alive. All narration holds the promise of further stories, and another dawn". This passage underscores how stories permit introspection and allow physicians to recover their balance and renew their sense of purpose and self.

The novel *Of Human Bondage* by William Somerset Maugham [16] illustrates the influence of art and literature on the life of the protagonist. Philip Carey, an orphan with a club foot, was raised by a rigid and pious uncle and a feeble-minded aunt. Philip's main hobby was reading from his uncle's vast collection of books, thus escaping the humdrum of his dreary life. His deformity caused him great distress as a schoolboy, being constantly mocked by his peers. The author notes that "Philip had few friends. His habit of reading isolated him". After boarding school, Philip went first to Germany and then off to Paris to study art. He constantly questioned the meaning of life. When Philip was asked about the meaning of life, he replied, "I suppose to do one's duty, and make the best possible use of one's faculties and avoid hurting other people". Philip soon realized that he was a mediocre artist and returned to England to study medicine. When asked what he had learned in Paris, Philip responds, "I learned to look at hands, which I'd never looked at before. And instead of just looking at houses and tress I learned to look at houses and tress against the sky. And I learned also that shadows are not black but colored".

Philip's "ideas of the life of medical students, like those of the public at large, were founded on the pictures which Charles Dickens drew in the middle of the nineteenth century". He had a series of romances, but his main obsession was with the selfish and cruel Mildred. His passion for Mildred trapped Philip in her bondage, a doomed relationship which served to enrich him and make him stronger. Philip's other main passions, art and literature, also prompted an interest "in the varied spectacle of life". His increased awareness of the vast complexity of human nature helped him become a better physician. Philip shared that "When I read a book, I seem to read it with my eyes only, but now and then I come across a passage, perhaps only a phrase, which has a meaning for me, and it becomes part of me". Philip's story superbly illustrates that which is proposed by a series of renowned medical professors and scholars, "that humanistic interests such as literature, art and music are potent restorative resources for physicians that can help them to maintain their humanity and perspective through the stresses of medical training and practice" [6].

In the article, *The role of poetry and prose in medical education: the pen as mighty as the scalpel?* [17], Frank J. Wolters and Marjo Wijnen-Meijer highlight the contribution of poetry and prose to the development of empathy in medical students. There is no consensus on how to teach empathy to anyone, much less to university students. However, studying humanities helps them acquire the three dimensions of empathy; first, the cognitive aspect—the ability to understand another person's thoughts; second, the affective component—concerning the emotional involvement; and third, the active component of acknowledging being heard and understood. A physician should not only have the scientific capacity to treat the patient but also the ability to listen to the patient's story, to grasp and honour its meaning and to then act on the patient's behalf.

According to Arthur W. Frank in *The Wounded Storyteller* [18], "stories have to repair the damage that illness has done to the ill person's sense of where she is in life, and where she may be going". Illness, especially serious illness, creates a state of chaos, where the ill person loses sense of time, priorities and direction in life. According to Frank, "whether ill people want to tell stories or not, illness calls for stories". Rita Charon defends that "the narrating of the patient's story is a therapeutically central act, because to find the words to contain the disorder and its attendant worries, gives shape to and control over the chaos of illness" [10]. Expressing the disease process through stories helps the patient and the physician to come to terms with the various dimensions of the illness. More importantly, it helps the patient better manage the impact of the illness on their life.

The classic novel by Leo Tolstoy, *The Death of Ivan Ilych* [19], is perhaps one of the most cited literary works in medical education. Ivan Ilych worked as a public prosecutor and his family life was "agreeable, easy and correct" until he began to experience a "sense of pressure in his side accompanied by ill humour". He became increasingly more irritable, and his marriage an absolute torment to the point that his wife began to wish he would die. Ivan Ilych would blame his testy nature on some illness and, following the suggestion of his wife, sought out an eminent doctor. After this visit, all worsened.

Ivan Ilych was observed by many doctors, but no one was capable of making a definitive diagnosis. Not only did he suffer from an illness without a name, but the treatments prescribed were useless, creating feelings of deception. "What tormented Ivan Ilych most was the deception, the lie, which for some reason they all accepted, that he was not dying but was simply ill". Ivan Ilych needed a more compassionate and humane approach; he wished "for someone to pity him as a sick child is pitied. He longed to be petted and comforted". The doctors were perplexed searching for the diagnosis and forgot to look and listen to the suffering man. As Rita Charon proposes, "A scientifically competent medicine alone cannot help a patient grapple with the loss of health and find meaning in suffering" [10]. Ivan Ilych's disease and death illustrate that the person is more important than their disease.

Physicians are trained to diagnose and treat their patients but have no expertise, nor any desire to experience disease themselves. A sick physician will feel diminished and disorientated, transitioning from physician to patient and from patient to person. The knowledge they possess is generally far superior to that of the common patient, and this often leads to further distress and despair. Paul Kalanithi a 36-year-old Stanford neurosurgical resident was diagnosed with advanced-stage lung cancer in May 2013. In January 2014, he wrote an opinion article in the New York Times, *How Long Have I Got Left* [20] that illustrates the difficult struggle of the ailing physician. "But now that I had traversed the line from doctor to patient, I had the same yearning for the numbers all patients ask for. I hoped she would see me as someone who both understood statistics and the medical reality of illness, that she would give me certainty, the straight dope. I could take it. She flatly refused: 'No. Absolutely not.' She knew very well I could — and did — look up all the research on the topic. But lung cancer wasn't my specialty, and she was a world expert. At each appointment, a wrestling match began, and she always avoided being pinned down to any sort of number".

As a patient, Paul Kalanithi began to comprehend the real needs of a patient, "What patients seek is not scientific knowledge doctors hide, but existential authenticity each must find on her own. Getting too deep into statistics is like trying to quench a thirst with salty water. The angst of facing mortality has no remedy in probability". In the 2 years following his diagnosis, Paul Kalanithi continued his medical training. His experiences as a patient influenced and enriched his medical practice. He wrote a beautiful memoir published posthumously, *When Breath Becomes Air* [21], describing his experiences facing mortality as a doctor and a patient. "Some days, this is how it felt when I was in the hospital: trapped in an endless jungle summer; wet with sweat, the rain of tears of the families of the dying pouring down". Since "words have a longevity, I do not", his memoir was an important legacy for his baby girl, a story for her to get to know and understand her father.

9.5 Art

There is an intimate connection between education, art and medicine, the most ancient being that of the field of anatomy. A thorough knowledge of the human body is at the core of the medical profession. The study of anatomy flourished with the dissection of corpses, first publicly disclosed in Italy by Mondino dei Luzzi in 1315 and cultivated throughout the Renaissance. It was during this period that Leonardo da Vinci masterfully produced many anatomical illustrations. Da Vinci's work rigorously depicted various parts of the human body, introducing multiple perspectives, angles and views. His approach was also a novelty in those functional aspects, especially the muscles and joints of the limbs were beautifully illustrated. However, one should dare to go beyond the obvious connections between art and medicine, such as anatomy, documenting diseases as well as surgical and medical practices through the ages and contemplate the benefits of art for the future physician.

In the book, *Art as Therapy*, Alain de Botton and John Armstrong [22] propose that art has various functions that can also be extrapolated as useful tools to further improve medical education. Their primary thesis is that "the main point of engaging with art is to help us lead better lives – to access better versions of ourselves". Many universities provide art programmes for medical students during their training. Future physicians visit museums, observe and analyse works of art, and this exposure can be beneficial in a multitude of ways. First, students that meaningfully look at artworks develop greater observational skills. The attention to details, subtleties and nuances in appearance, structure and form help promote diagnostic competency. Second, comparing and studying works of art from different periods and artists enhance cultural diversity and knowledge and stimulate critical thinking. Finally, contact with art in its many different forms has extraordinary restorative powers. Art can evoke a myriad of emotional responses in the observer, tranquillity by viewing the gardens of Giverny by Monet, sorrow by observing the Pietà by Michelangelo, disquiet by gazing Broadway Boogie Woogie by Piet Modrian and even grief by staring at Picasso's Guernica.

In *Art as Therapy*, art is described as having seven functions that can be applied to students, teachers, physicians and patients alike—remembering, hope, sorrow, rebalancing, self-understanding, growth and appreciation. Art aids in remembering, by documenting and recording moments, scenes and events. Art can serve as an aid to preserve our memory, in terms of facts and sensations. Art allows one to focus on meaningful aspects of our lives by decluttering less important themes. Art offers hope by providing beauty and illustrating the goodness in humanity. Hope is fundamental to find peace and to navigate throughout the obstacles of life. Art can be used to remind us that sorrow is a normal part of our existence, and that there is no need to flee and feel diminished by feelings of sorrow. The rebalancing capacity of art is useful in medical settings especially in the prevention of burnout, so frequent among healthcare workers. Art encourages self-understanding, providing insights and guidance to what is pivotal to our lives. Art promotes growth, enriching our souls as we embrace cultures, experiences and ideas foreign to our own. Finally, art brings appreciation, to "look at the old in new ways". These seven functions of art should be nourished in all students.

9.6 The Future

Albert Camus once wrote that "Real generosity towards the future lies in giving all to the present" [23]. Ours is an agitated present, where priorities in terms of optimal medical care are often shadowed by financial issues. Time is fleeting, but there really is no time like the present to promote a change in the medical curriculum. A high standard in medical education is key to provide future physicians with the tools required to practice their art in an increasingly complex world. Medical education must have a fresh approach, notwithstanding the importance of specific medical training but also embracing the broader perspective provided by the humanities. The existential question posed by Hamlet in the famous Shakespearean play of the same name, "to be or not to be", is no longer an issue when addressing the value of the humanities in medical education. Future physicians must strive to be curious and yearn to be educated. As the educational theorist RS Peters said, "to be educated is not to have arrived; it is to travel with a different view" [24].

References

1. Osler W. The old humanities and the new science. Boston: Houghton Miflin; 1920. p. 26–8.
2. Steiner G. My unwritten books. Weidenfeld & Nicolson; 2008. p. 138–9.
3. Ronaghy H. A brief history of medical education. J Fam Med Forecast. 2018;1(1):1007.
4. Bendapudi NM, Berry LL, Frey KA, Parish JT, Rayburn WL. Patients' perspectives on ideal physician behaviors. Mayo Clin Proc. 2006 Mar;81(3):338–44.
5. Gawande A. Being mortal: medicine and what matters in the end. Metropolitan Books; 2014. p. 238–49.
6. Horton MEK. The orphan child: humanities in modern medical education. Philos Ethics Humanit Med. 2019;14(1):1–6.
7. Macnaughton J. The humanities in medical education: context, outcomes and structures. Med Humanit. 2000;26(1):23–30.
8. Kirklin D. The Centre for Medical Humanities, Royal Free and University College Medical School, London, England. Acad Med. 2003;78(10):1048–53.
9. Charon R, Williams P. Introduction: the humanities and medical education. Acad Med. 1995;70(9):758–60.
10. Charon R. Narrative medicine: a model for empathy, reflection, profession, and trust. JAMA. 2001;286(15):1897–902.
11. Charon R. To see the suffering. Acad Med. 2017;92(12):1668.
12. Charon R. Narrative reciprocity. Hastings Cent Rep. 2014;44(s1):S21–4.
13. Haig M. How to stop time. New York: Penguin Books, an imprint of Penguin Random House LLC; 2019.
14. Walker B. Reading by moonlight: How books saved a life. Penguin Group; 2010. p. 3, 84, 123, 131, 173.
15. Cunningham M. The hours: a novel. Fourth Estate. 1999:21.
16. Maugham W. Somerset. Of human bondage. London: Penguin Books; 1992.
17. Wolters FJ, Wijnen-Meijer M. The role of poetry and prose in medical education: the pen as mighty as the scalpel? Perspect Med Educ. 2012;1(1):43–50.
18. Frank AW. The wounded storyteller: body, illness, and ethics. University of Chicago Press; 2013.
19. Tolstoy L. The death of Ivan Ilych. Prabhat Prakashan; 1973.
20. Kalanithi P. How long have I got left. New York Times. 2014;24
21. Kalanithi P. When breath becomes air. Random House; 2016.
22. Botton D. Alain, and John Armstrong. Art as therapy. London: Phaidon Press Limited; 2013.
23. Camus A. Notebooks, 1935–1942. Harcourt Brace Jovanovich; 1978.
24. Peters RS. The concept of education. London: Routledge and Kegan Paul; 1967. p. 8.

Chapter 10
Conversation with Surgeon 5—Jeff Wilkinson

René Génadry

Recorded online on 03/08/2024 by René Génadry.

Abbreviations that follow:

JW: Jeff Wilkinson
RG: René Génadry
UNC: University of North Carolina
IOFWD: International Organization for Women and Development
NGO: Non-governmental Organization

RG: Hello Jeff, you've had a fantastic journey that I've been following, and I'm interested in primarily listening to your perspectives, motivations, challenges. The idea is to relate the issues that result in such a decision to engage in humanitarian work, and in the process figure out how to transmit that message as to what is the character of a humanitarian person, what are the motivations and so on…

JW: Well pretty broad topic.

RG: I'll try to direct as we go along but this is the idea. when did you start?

JW: I guess in medical school; I knew I wanted to work with an underserved population.

RG: And why is that?

JW: I am not exactly 100% sure. It wasn't out of some foundational religious belief, or that at least in some part religion may have played a role, but I don't think that that was fundamental or any formative decision. I feel like if I were going into medicine, there is an opportunity to do something, and it wasn't an uncommon path, but it certainly wasn't the most common path. It seemed more interesting, and potentially fulfilling to consider some form of working

R. Génadry (✉)
Carver College of Medicine, University of Iowa, Iowa City, IA, USA

J. McFarland et al. (eds.), *Humanism in Surgery*, New Paradigms in Healthcare, https://doi.org/10.1007/978-3-031-86018-8_10

with the underserved; and certainly, in East Baltimore we had plenty of opportunity to see the impact you could make or the danger or the damage that could be done working in the setting like E Baltimore.

RG: So how did you make it happen?

JW: Actually, those days as you'll recall it was a bit simpler or a little bit simpler: you talk to somebody, and they say ohh why don't you walk across the street to the school public health and talk to this person, and that person says, so why don't you call Raj and Mabel Arole in India and see if you can go join them. And a few phone calls later, the rotation was set up. And in my second year, I was able to go over to India for a couple months, and spend a good amount of time there, and that's where my decision was solidified but also the decision to pursue Women's Health was also solidified. I think I had an interesting rotation in OBGYN: I had amazing mentors, but the practical day-to-day aspect of working on the service was decidedly mixed. I mean the intern that I was working with was so unhappy that the first speculum exam I did, that person said, with the patient obviously in the room, or while I was trying to do it: "are you an idiot? Have you learned anything?" and that just got worse from there. I think it just was emblematic of some of the teaching ethos at the time, especially for residents; they weren't happy, they were overworked; they were stressed out and tired, hungry and afraid. I guess at some level even though it was not particularly comfortable, I understood from whence that attitude and behavior arose because you could see it; and then there were others who were just so amazing. Of course, I had great mentorship with Doctor Ed Wallach and Dr. Jean Anderson. So, I didn't know that I would do Women's Health till I got to India where I really saw the impact that women had on communities; and a lot of people will talk about obstetrics and gynecology and the reasons I went into it were pretty much the standard: you could operate, you could do public health, you could just take care of people from birth to death, and you can deliver babies and do primary care; I mean everything was there, but I knew that, in anatomy class I had like eight thumbs, you know like I didn't feel like I could dissect anything, and then suddenly when it came to live patients, it felt a little different. And for some, for whatever reason, it seemed like there was some, a tiny amount of potential skill there, and I enjoyed it, and I enjoyed the immediate nature of it and sort of made the connection also of the ability to do and teach surgery in low resource settings would be a benefit that was immediate and didn't rely on months and months of medication or prolonged public health initiatives…

RG: So, after India you came back and completed your residency?

JW: Yeah, I came back and went to University of North Carolina (UNC) for residency and had a little bit of time during residency and spent some time in Santa Lucia, and did some other mostly social traveling, and maintained the interest in what I perceived to be my clear goals. I think it was helpful, (and this is a little bit uncomfortable) but at the time, my wife Sumera also was very aligned towards similar goals, and she was going into family medicine, and so it was mutually reinforcing and helpful that we both had similar goals for our careers. Then I had an opportunity to stay on as a fellow in urogynecology because she had an extra year in her family medicine training, and then had an extra year as a fellow herself as well, and I was offered the spot in one of the first spots in urogynecology fellowship there to continue the surgical theme. It seemed like a good opportunity to become a better surgeon in what I was going to do and then during fellowship, I went back to India a couple times; I was actually somewhat helpful at that point, because I had a handful of skills underneath my belt from residency and part of fellowship, and then after fellowship moved to the Navajo reservation for a couple of years; we didn't have a commitment to the public health service or the Indian health service, but we wanted to do something interesting and rewarding and it turned out to be very much so.

RG: So were you primarily doing OBGYN on the Navajo reservations.

JW: Yeah, we were in Chinle which is in the center, pretty much as remote as you can get from the most remote of the major hospitals on the Navajo reservation, and so general OBGYN and I also did a lot of urogynecology, just because it's a big problem amongst Navajo, and consulted some in Gallup and a few other places on a periodic basis; so at least I was able to keep my urogyne skills up.

RG: I'm sure you've learned a lot of lessons between India and the Navajo reservations by then.

JW: The Navajo reservation was the closest thing to a low resource setting in the States in the Continental 48. A good deal of our patients didn't speak English, over half didn't have electricity or running water, and they clearly were suffering from a number of different health and social ills, that were in some ways similar to the East Baltimore population, with the disempowerment of men in society, and lack of opportunities for both men and women, but you know it's a very matriarchal society with a lot, a lot of suffering to go around. I'm not sure that I made any significant changes there apart from trying to take good care of patients, but it definitely was interesting and informative in terms of what it might be like to live and work in a place that was very remote, and definitely solve the difference between where we had basically been up to that point, in the ivory towers of medicine, taking care of patients, and looking down on the last medical provider. I was just telling somebody the other day recounting an experience that we've been having the sickest preeclampsia patients on the reservation and we'd have to send them out to Phoenix or Albuquerque or Flagstaff sometimes, and a number of times you had to go through the intern in Phoenix to transfer a patient you know, and eventually it was flagged up to the attending and I remember just talking to someone that reminded me that preeclampsia was a combination of high blood pressure and proteinuria and at that point I was board certified, had come from a couple of pretty prestigious institutions. I hopefully didn't treat any of our referring physicians like that when I was an intern, I might have unknowingly. Arrogance is a dangerous thing, and most of the time you don't know when you're being arrogant, because either you haven't learned enough lessons or you're just completely oblivious to it. so, we don't care…

RG: Did practicing on the Navajo reservation prepare you for your subsequent journey overseas, was it a continuum?

JW: It is! we didn't learn anything about obstetric fistula in residency and medical school and fellowship even, we learned a little bit about post-surgical fistula and things like that, but I had no idea about the scale of suffering and what was really involved in the social and societal and all the different medical system factors that were related to a woman developing a fistula and how that was interrelated with the larger problem of maternal morbidity and mortality. It was a kind of a wakeup call to learn more about it.

RG: And how did you get exposed to the problem?

JW: It was I think just more by chance, reading up on it and you know finding that because there wasn't a host of people around, people like you. I do remember talking to Steve Arrowsmith a bit when he persuaded me to come out to one of the private hospitals in Gallup NM where he was working, and help him with a urogyne prolapse repair and he nearly got fired: I was supposed to just come and kind of look over his shoulder, because I wasn't licensed in New Mexico, there was no like formality to it, and I get there and he's doing what, at the time, we might have done in another country, and he said: OK sit! I was running a little bit late, and the patient was already asleep, and I got there, and he said sit. and I said OK. Well, I guess the ethical right thing to do is probably to do it, and he nearly got fired. In any case we had talked about fistula some. He obviously was already quite experienced and had done a fair amount already, and then also I talked to Tom Elkins, and I think his motivations were interesting and I think faith based but also very practical, just trying to figure out how I could get involved with obstetric fistula. It wasn't like they were opportunities abounding to go do it and then, I'm not exactly sure who introduced me to Barbara at IOFWD. Then that was the first real experience I had, going to Niger, and I guess that is where we met, if I recall correctly. I think I knew a lot about surgery, but I didn't know enough: I still could do simple repairs and some difficult dissections, but I still didn't know anything about it. And the whole environment there was so interesting and challenging and the weird interface between the NGO, with all of these relatively rich white people coming into a place like Niger and all of the different politics with the ministry, and I had zero idea about any of that, but I was thankful to have an opportunity to learn, and help out a little bit and gradually begin to cultivate more of a career; and after a few trips to Niger, I just realized I was never going to be a fistula surgeon unless I went and lived and worked overseas; and that's when I decided to go to Tanzania and help start up the maternal health program for Duke at the Kilimanjaro Christian Medical Center, and they started a fellowship, a global health fellowship and that's really where I think I learned how to do fistula surgery, and do it at least with some skill. I think that fistula surgery is an easy sell for anybody, anyone can see how much the women are suffering, you know this better or as well as anybody: if you don't have empathy for a fistula patient, you're probably not alive, and or you're a sociopath or something: I mean they clearly are the least represented, with the least agency of pretty much anyone that you meet others equally potentially equally horrible problems, although it's hard to imagine but they're always from the lower socioeconomic run, and it was very clear that the number of people doing this was minimal, and the number of people who actually dedicated significant time to it was few. I remember talking to Lewis Wall before I went to Tanzania and I said, you know we've done a few things together like wrote a couple of papers and a symposium, but when I first talked to him, I said Lewis, because he had some connection with Duke and he was a fellow there or something, of course I had read a bunch of this stuff, and I called him for advice and he said: forget it, you're never going to do it; he said just give it up now and walk away. I said OK, I appreciate that advice, but let's just assume that it's possible, what would you do? and then we had a civil discussion about it. But I think that ever the practical and ever the observant Lewis realized that most people who think they're going to do it don't do it, and most people who think they're going to go live or work overseas, life just gets in the way or something else gets in the way: you know you have a family, you have kids, you have your own parents, you have your spouse's parents, you have any number of things that will detract from it and so it has just been about balancing those things over time.

RG: Well, these are challenges that you've overcome very well.

JW: Well, at times…

RG: Well, it's interesting you mentioned the impact of your exposure to the fistula problem and what effect it had on you, and that it really reminds me of the same situation whereby I was talking to Dr. Cliff Wheeless and to the people at the school of public health and that's the reason why we put together that symposium about obstetric fistula at the time we met. It really was clear that no single person was going to solve the problem and that the only way it could be made to be dented a little bit was to get all the various players together and try to map out some way out of it and with the help of the USAID, UNFPA FIGO and so on we were able to try to get things on track that time.

JW: It's an interesting story on trying to know how much to engage and how much to not engage. We find that, to this day, we got a case every week probably that I've never seen something quite exactly like it before, the most heterogeneous condition in the world; and then if you apply surgery to that, and the surgical care is decidedly suboptimal, and we're still like wallowing in complete ignorance with fistula surgery on how to do it properly, and what works well and what not; as we've all said if it was a disease of upper middle class white men in Europe or America it would have been addressed by now, first of all it wouldn't have happened to begin with.

RG: Well, that's right I mean prevention is obviously key. It is clearly tied up to the maternal morbidity and mortality issues that you were talking about trying to solve in Tanzania. Tell me more about how this came about, challenges, difficulties, was it easy, was it well supported?

JW: The Duke Global Health Institute was forming around the same time, and Duke had very strong research focus. Fistula is very difficult to do research on, because it's surgical and it's a highly heterogeneous, and there's all kinds of issues with patient autonomy and central abuses of one's role as a researcher, but we had an opportunity to go there and help jumpstart their Women's Health Program under an existing adult HIV program. There's also a residency program there; we started a fellowship for US learners. We went to Tanzania on basically a fellow's salary and at that point I was 10 years out of fellowship, but it was clear that they weren't going to support it at a real level, but you know I was done paying off my loans by then, and I didn't have any significant major debt. And it's something we always wanted to do, and I always wanted to do, and I probably never would have gone to Africa, if it weren't for the problem of fistula: just because I speak Spanish and I think I probably would have gone to the Central America or South America to work, but the overriding factor was the ability to make an impact on obstetric fistula and safe motherhood. And so, we worked in Moshi for a couple of years ending up gaining up 40% salary support or something that wasn't quite enough. And Duke needed help back in the gynecology department and so I sort of negotiated to come back, but I knew after that I was sunk: I knew for sure that I wanted to pretty much dedicate what time I had left on this earth to trying to do something with fistula, and so I had the opportunity after a year back in the states, I called Andrew Browning. I was like do you know any anybody who's looking for a fistula surgeon? and coincidentally UNC wanted to start a Women's Health program in Malawi, and Freedom from Fistula Foundation wanted to start the fistula center in Lilongwe, and, by that time, I was at least skilled enough to reasonably care for most patients, and then and also more importantly know who I shouldn't operate on and save those patients for more experienced doctors to come; and then over the last 13 years, I've suddenly become one of those people who you'd wait for to come. So it is an evolution: I think the myth or the pervasive notion about people who work in Africa or wherever in any lower resource setting where you have to deal with some things you might not have to deal with otherwise, is that you're somehow making some sacrifice and I feel like that's at least in part true: I mean I figured I could have had a much larger retirement account right now, and not necessarily worried about how I'm going to pay for my older kids to go to medical school, but I don't really, I've never really perceived it as any sort of sacrifice. In my mind it was like why more people would not want to do this; the science and the clinical care is fascinating: I literally never have a dull day, I am never subsumed by medical records and medical legal concerns that I'm twisted in knots about that, I mean obviously we have many many other things.

RG: I feel like it's a privilege rather than a sacrifice Jeff at a certain level.

JW: I think a lot of people have written on that and come to that conclusion themselves. There's still this notion that people are giving up a whole lot, and in my mind, everybody who stays in the rat race in America or wherever Norway or the UK they're probably sacrificing a lot too, when they would have an opportunity to walk into the ward where there's a much higher percentage chance that you're either going to save a life or improve a life; whereas you know in the states there's 50 people who could replace me in a second, do urogynecology or whatever. I mean when I started urogynecology, it was still a bit new, it wasn't that new, but it was still a bit new and still there's such an abundance of urogynecologists.

RG: You get more out of what you give than what you would have in the States, there's no question about it. Jeff I'm sure there has been a lot of people along the way that have helped you and you had mentioned a few of them. Does anyone stand out as a mentor and how did that work in trying to steer you in the right direction?

JW: You know it's funny because I've thought about that at length, and you know being involved in education in some way shape or form from the beginning of my education, you try to parse that out a bit: for instance, I consider Doctor Droegemueller who was our chairman at UNC in residency and Ellen Wells, both great pelvic surgeons, but had little personal interest in global health; but their attention to detail and their dedication to patients was absolute. I mean you know Dr. Droegemueller, if somebody forgot to remove a staple on a patient, they called and they were like 6 h away, he would put the resident on the road the next morning to go out and take that staple out: "we're not making her drive back." I think that early sort of commitment to patient care and excellence is important. Even earlier than that, working with somebody like Jean Anderson who was so committed to patients with HIV, and just unwavering in her dedication to that, and also a fantastic surgeon just was great, along with doctor Wallach and then you know in residency and fellowship also someone like John Thorp in maternal fetal medicine who just was one of the people who were tirelessly dedicated to patients and patient care, yet were completely clueless about residents nearly dying from not sleeping. They still were in that sort of mold, that old school mold…It was a contradiction, but one that was understandable given their own training and suffering.

RG: So, the importance of role modeling and teaching by example essentially.

JW: Right, like Wade Bowes is the most skilled obstetrician I've ever seen and one of the smartest people in the world. He just talked about and demonstrated, more than talked about, how the equanimity and the capacity for cultivating that, when it is not an intrinsic gift that's given to you. I mean I can remember having deeper tachycardia, I can remember running into a room where there was an emergency going on, and just like not having the proper mindset to deal with it, and that is a detriment, and you see people who walk in the room and you know things are flying every which way, but they're walking through it like some sort of Buddha through the madness. Cultivating that calm approach during a storm is something that I think one can learn. I don't think that I've got it by any stretch, but it's something that can be taught, and more importantly modeled. And then of course, there are techniques you can use; but I think that for me, if I had to point to the 1st person who was a role model for me and a mentor, it was even before, when I was a kid, and just watching: I think this had maybe had a large part in making my decision to work with medically underrepresented community, but my best friend's father was one of the busiest substance abuse doctors in Baltimore and I mean he worked for years in the University of Maryland and then Maryland Medical Center, and just had a thriving but not necessarily well renumerated practice caring for people and he just was tireless in his dedication to it. It didn't matter that these were perceived by everybody else to be the lowest of the low in Baltimore let's just say, and that had parallels for working with fistula patients, not the whole thing about addiction, that people's judgment about it coming from their own weakness rather than an addiction or you know their life led them to that rather than something that they did causing it. I mean obviously it's a complicated set of things but anyway; to answer your original question, I think it was a such a hodgepodge of people and most of them weren't global health doctors.

RG: Right exactly that has nothing to do with it that comes afterwards. How do you impart that equanimity, that interest to the fellows that you're training. Is it something that's possible, or are you just relying on example and role modeling and have them take what they can out of it and learn by themselves: is it something that is teachable?

JW: I think aspects can be taught, and you clearly can bring in mindfulness-based techniques. One of the things that I would say the most to people is that when they come on the scene of blood hitting the wall, or baby stuck or whatever it is, first thing you do is take a deep breath and those 3 s or whatever it is are not going to make a difference between life, death to the mother and the baby but your mind is suddenly going to be sharper and focused, you're going to be present for it instead, like being a bystander to your own actions. I think that sort of mindfulness based approach to both stress reduction and to clinical care and teaching I've tried to bring in, but it's often difficult: I feel like the more I've done, the more I get pulled into things that end up not optimizing what I feel I was meant to do, because the longer you spend doing something the more you're called on to do everything else. For example, I started with a plan to do fistula, diversified very quickly into a lot of safe motherhood projects, to some extent to pay the bills, but also because you can't be in this setting without attending to safe motherhood. Starting a residency program for Malawians, starting a residency and the global health fellowship, residency track and so, to some extent I feel like that day-to-day clinical work suffers. Right now, for instance, I'll go in and I'll do 2 days official surgery a week and sometimes 2 1/2 or 3, but then the rest of the time mostly in meetings, and trying to figure out how to raise money and solve issues with the Ministry of Health, or solve issues with our own NGO here in Malawi, or try to figure out how we're going to pay for this or that. I'm even trying to figure out how to work back, to get rid of all those other responsibilities and work back to something and I'm sure as a chair of the department and leader of multiple programs you felt like it's an impossible job frankly.

RG: Well adaptability I guess you know is very important, flexibility obviously is very important too. Let me ask you Jeff, in your experience is it possible to identify the individuals that have that ability and those that don't? Obviously, you're dealing at this point with self-selected persons that are seeking to participate in some sort of global health, but from your experience beforehand do you think in medical school, one could you predict who was going to develop into a humanitarian and/or a humanistic physician in the future? any particular characteristics?

JW: I think you have to have just the right mix of humility to realize that you don't understand anything when you first arrive: if you can keep your mouth shut for the first few months, and not judge everything that you see around you, and feel like you have the answer to the issue when other people have been trying to solve it for years; but then balancing that with still remaining proactive, and not being desensitized, or not becoming totally numb to the death and dying around you. The one thing I try to instill in our learners is that everything they see and everything they experience is not about them. They come and they go back to their real life, and they're telling the story of how this person died, how this person was left dead and family members were devastated and they think woe is me that I had to go see that, or how amazing it was that I did this or did that… I feel so sad that all this happened, and I think that's a sort of a natural response to when you see the depravity of societies and the lack of care and attention and of governments without really understanding it in context: I think it's the person who can rapidly go through those stages and find the reality that's underneath that. They must understand that it's not about them. They're not coming for them, they're not coming to save people, per se, or as a big favor to humankind; they're coming to fulfill some need in themselves that either they haven't identified yet, or that they have identified but that just needs to be further explored. It's about telling yourself the truth because we all like go through most of our lives not really being truthful with ourselves about anything, and/or creating a narrative about something that ends up being a false narrative, or one that dispels the cognitive dissonance that arises when we see or do things that are not consistent with our values. I mean when you have to make impossible ethical choices in scenarios that you don't ever have to face in a high resource setting, and so you have to create an explanation in order to dispel the inner turmoil that's going on. So, you see people who have a more or less mature reaction, (and I by no means did when I first started, I had no clue) and being honest with yourself, not deceiving yourself that you're some saint. I guess that's why I've never really equated it at all with a religious belief or a religious tendency or whatever. I mean it's always just been about trying to do the next right thing, and that right thing arose from a humanitarian perspective and not a necessarily a religious perspective. For everybody it is different, right? It's great that some people do it because they feel like it's their God-given calling, maybe it is, but it's not entirely that for me. I may feel called by God to do something, but the overriding reason is because it is the right thing to do. The calling is a gift not a burden imposed.

RG: As you say, it is clearly a journey of self-discovery for the physicians or the people that get engaged in global health. How about your experience with patients? has there been any patient that really impressed you so much that would be worth relating? I'm looking for an example of a patient that has impressed you, in your experience working with the fistula patients, anybody whose either behavior or circumstances have really marked you and taught you a lesson.

JW: Well, I mean you could take virtually every fistula patient that you've ever had and look at them and see very clearly, if you're thinking straight, that they're absolutely the best. My worst day in my entire life, no matter what it was, is still better than their best day. They literally embody a patience and a resilience that is otherworldly, when you think about how the complaining and whining that I do, or we do as westerners. But I mean we have patients that have had 6–7 surgeries, that end up needing a diversion, and then a diversion reversal, and you know they don't have any IV's left and they're still leaking, and they come in and when they come into the fistula unit they are, especially at first, depressed, isolated and stigmatized and then you show them some kindness, and some care and attention and they blossom like it rained on some flower seeds. This is the story of fistula patients everywhere, and I think that's part of the appeal: there are so many, literally Rene, that I could point to. We have ones that stand out who have become outspoken leaders in their community, that end up going to run businesses, or go to teach other women about fistula, but unfortunately, some of the more like tragic stories stand out. I could tell you of a patient who has had five or six surgeries, had a nearly died a few times, had a urinary diversion 15 years ago, and is now in her home, running a business. For sure, she felt like she was never going to make it, but she's the ultimate in… you know she's always having a smile it's always genuine, it's never forced: no matter whether she was near death or whether she was home in the fields or at her business and she just embodied somebody who suffered immeasurably but dealt with it in sort of superhuman ways.

RG: Well Jeff I know time is passing and I could spend a few more hours talking about this with you, but I know you are busy and you have things to do, but if you were to describe yourself, your experience and all that, may I ask the question: who are you? how would you describe yourself?

JW: (Laugh) yeah, good question. (Pause) I think that the best I could say is that: eminently fallible yet tried to do the next right thing. And I made many, many mistakes but tried to learn from them and not repeat them; and also try to help a few people along the way.

RG: In summary, what lessons learned come immediately to mind?

JW: I think again what we kind of homed in on was just the fallacy of the so-called humanitarian being as making a sacrifice. I think people mean well whilst I can really pinpoint mentors along the way, I feel like as one would expect, rationally, that you take pieces of those mentors, and pieces of what they taught you, and you distill that into a whole for yourself: it's always the sum of parts and that those who tried to model themselves exactly after somebody who they admire and often idolized, they end up invariably being wrong or regretting it later, because you know that you are not them, and your values are different, your goals are different and it's just about being able to consciously process those things. Often it is unconscious, but if you can distill those things consciously that make that person so special to you then it helps.

RG: You must integrate it with your own philosophy of life.

JW: Yeah, and then also just like you said, self-discovery and being honest with yourself about what your motivations are, and what you truly are accomplishing and then being willing to change. No matter, even if you've dedicated your entire life to something, if it ends up being either proven wrong or you know it's wrong, don't be lulled into sticking with a wrong or bad idea. As physicians we're very subject to letting our ego and letting pride and arrogance rule what we do, and it's often unnoticed, and it's just always assessing yourself for that quality, to avoid it because it's the thing that poisons most people's lives and most people's careers.

RG: That's wonderful Jeff we finally got to the crux of it I think these last few words summarize it very well.

Chapter 11
Humanism and Medicine: Quo Vadis

Jacek Mostwin

11.1 Medicine Is the Study of the Person

When I entered the School of Medicine at the University of Maryland in 1971 over 50 years ago, my mother Danuta told me: "You will like the study of medicine, it is the study of man, the study of the person." Eighteen years earlier, newly arrived in America, she had presented her credentials to the same school to apply to continue her own medical studies that had begun during the German occupation of Warsaw during World War II and continued in Edinburgh after escaping from Communist Poland. When that school in Edinburgh closed and we came to America in 1952, she was given credit for the pre-clinical years, but no financial aid to enroll as a third-year student. Not much would have been required, for when I began my studies in that same medical school in 1971, the annual tuition for state residents was only six hundred dollars. And so, she turned to social work, supporting and then studying the Polish immigration while she continued to write about the lives of people caught up in war, uprooted and forced into immigration. She left a legacy of some 14 books published in Polish. Her focus was always on the person as affected by events and circumstances beyond their control, seen and presented through a humane, artistic eye. Her concern was always for the person who, as Martin Heidegger would say, has been "thrown into the world": *Geworfenheit*.

As a medical student, our first lessons involved cadaver dissection in a large anatomical laboratory. We would cross Greene Street to the Bressler prosectorium (the dissecting room), passing through the outdoor aroma of cloves and cinnamon

Adapted from a presentation entitled: Humanism and Medicine: Quo Vadis? at the 75th Conference of the Polish American Medical Society Chicago, IL, October 7, 2022.

J. Mostwin (✉)
Department of Urology, Johns Hopkins Medical Institutions, Baltimore, MD, USA

J. McFarland et al. (eds.), *Humanism in Surgery*, New Paradigms in Healthcare,
https://doi.org/10.1007/978-3-031-86018-8_11

drifting up from the McCormick spice factory by the Baltimore harbor before descending into a world soaked in formaldehyde, used to preserve the bodies of our subjects. After several months of working our way through the remnants of an old man whose body had been assigned to our group of students, I remember well the moment when my dissecting scalpel cut through the skin of his back to scrape against the metal of the table beneath. I found myself thinking, "I have gone through the body, but where was the person?" And I do believe the rest of my medical experience has been led by that question, where is the person?

11.2 What Is Humanism in Medicine?

"Where is the person" is a question that permeates our current interest in humanism in medicine but raises further questions of its own. Just what is humanism? How do we know it when we encounter it? Is that what we sense is missing in our medical world today? How do we integrate this perceived absence into what many consider an overly scientific view of the person? Should the human side of medicine be encouraged or suppressed to preserve what some call "clinical objectivity"? What shall we teach our students? How can we help them find their way? Can bringing the Humanities into the curriculum solve these problems?

There appears to be a resurgence of interest in humanizing or re-humanizing medicine, hence the appearance of many educational movements with the prefix "hum-": humanism, Humanities, humane, humanistic. Does the humanization of medicine seek to add something new (humanizing medicine), or rediscover something old that needs to be restored (re-humanization)? Do we wish to return to some golden age that has somehow been lost, presumably by the growth of "impersonal" science and "progress"?

Calls for patient-centered care abound in educational and clinical settings. Debates about whether the empirical sciences can help solve problems encountered by patients and doctors have recently led to demands that Medical Humanities form part of the basic preparation for medical careers. The AAMC (American Association of Medical Colleges) has launched its own initiative on restoring Humanities to Medical Education. Courses in Medical Humanities as areas of concentration for pre-medical students have been growing steadily throughout universities in the United States [1]. But there has been no real consensus within the academies about how to integrate or accept these many "hum-" disciplines into curricula for undergraduates, post-graduates, or continuing education. Most often they are relegated to special events or ceremonies such as presentations of white coats, graduation ceremonies, or memorial services held by medical students for the donors of bodies to their anatomical studies. These events, which follow a completely different set of ritual formalities than do scientific colloquia or presentations, and which nonetheless appear to draw something from assemblies that seem to want and warmly welcome them, resist easy definition or operationalization. They fall under that elusive category of "culture."

11.3 What Is a University For?

Regardless of their rank in the order of socially defined values, such events that recognize human experience and the arts eventually find their way to learned audiences who listen attentively. The following comments by Christopher Patten, former Chancellor of Oxford University, were presented at Wolfson College, Oxford on March 16, 2017 in response to the question "What is a University for?" addressing not only the value of the Humanities at a University but the criticisms they face for not offering practical preparation for careers.

> Why bother to study and research the Humanities? Why do I cherish for instance the fact that when at Oxford *Encaenia* a couple of weeks ago I asked the new Public Orator what he was woking on at the moment, he said he was principally concerned this term with studying Sanskrit musicology. Will that add life into the British capacity to innovate while matching productivity to GDP? Conceivably, research like that doesn't make us any richer. Yet we would be incomparably poorer if we weren't doing it. Above all we must support the Humanities because we are human, because the Humanities help us to answer the question why we need Universities at all, because they provide us with a fuller understanding of our world and of one another, because they enable us to think creatively and critically, because they inform our moral sense, because they teach us to love jazz and Beethoven, Rafael and Cézanne, a Shakespeare sonnet and a Flaubert novel, and because they teach us about life and beauty and love and death. To those who question a serious, generous and lasting commitment to teaching and researching the Humanities at our Universities, I offer this story of Samuel Johnson's refutation of Bishop Berkley. You may recall that his biographer Boswell suggested to Johnson that even if one did not accept the philosophical argument of Bishop Berkley that matter did not exist, that matter was only perception, it was impossible to refute it. Samuel Johnson reacted with alacrity. "With mighty force," Boswell wrote," he kicked against a large stone. 'I refute it thus.' "That is more or less how those of us who care about Universities should respond to mindless and meretricious criticisms of the Humanities: we refute it thus. [2]

The Humanities are in keeping with this desire to preserve something "human" to answer the questions, negotiate the demands, and calm the storms into which we have been thrown and for which empirical rationalism, machines, and technology seem to provide only partially satisfying solutions, let alone answers, guidance or reassurance, unless we wish to limit medical universities to the role of trade schools. Should we then focus Universities on preparing students for skilled trades or to be members of "the workforce" or "the health care team"? Should students be trained to be functionaries in a system over which they have no real influence, or should they instead be allowed to ask questions arising from human encounters as they grapple with the fundamental question of the machine age into which they have been thrown: "what does it mean to be human"? A prospective medical student might well wonder just how a medical school addresses this question: where is the person; what does it mean to be human, and to wonder whether such a question can be answered only in materialistic, reductionist terms.

11.4 The Cultures of the Academic World

These recent debates about the relative roles of science and the Humanities in education, human progress, and even in what might be called a *Weltanschauung* can be traced back to C.P Snow's 1959 Rede Lecture *The Two Cultures* [3] describing the rift in scholarly methods and communities that led to what he argued were two separate and distinct cultures in the academic world: one of the humanities which had dominated education until his own era, and the other of the more recently emerging sciences. Snow argued that humanists who had dominated the educational environment should become literate in the scientific disciplines, a view for which he was soundly criticized. But one could argue that he did not so much create this controversy as bring attention to it, stirring a debate that continues. More recently his ideas were revisited by Jerome Sagan, a developmental psychologist at Columbia University under the title: T*he Three Cultures: Natural Sciences, Social Science and the Humanities in the 21st Centuries* [4]. Kagan describes how a third culture of Social Sciences had emerged since Snow's 1959 presentation. Each culture, Kagan argued, has its own goals, its own language, its own forms of scholarship, research, and its own sources of data. The Humanities and Social Sciences, in particular, advance our understanding of human nature in ways that differ from the natural sciences. Whether they are complimentary or antagonistic is left to others to decide, but the lines of demarcation appear to have been drawn quite clearly. He argued that while scientific work supported by considerable funding progresses in Universities, the Humanities are mired in arguments about their roles and values, drawing much less funding and suffering from increasingly lower participation by students entering higher education, despite the respect they should be afforded judging from Lord Patten's comments at Wolfson in 2017.

11.5 Medical Curriculum Evolution

Over 100 years ago, in 1910, the Flexner report on medical education in America argued for the benefits of a heavily scientific curriculum for the preparation and education of medical students. The model was widely adopted throughout the United States. There would be no similar re-assessment of medical education until the more recent Carnegie report of 2010 [5, 6]. Although Osler, already at Hopkins when Flexner was preparing his report, had introduced the idea of bedside teaching of medicine and become recognized as an advocate for patient-centered and thoughtful medicine as expressed in his reflective essay, *Aequanimitas* [7], the basic sciences gradually took over the primary responsibility of pre-clinical physician education, especially given the growth in financial support for their departments by the National Institutes of Health, and eventually by the medical industries after World War II, a time when comparable support for the Humanities was minimal.

In 1999, Catherine DeAngelis, at that time a Professor of Pediatrics at Johns Hopkins and before she became editor of the Journal of the American Medical Association (JAMA), edited a publication entitled *The Johns Hopkins University School of Medicine Curriculum for the Twenty–first Century* [8], outlining the implementation of reforms that were felt to be needed by medical academic leaders. An earlier movement, the so-called New Pathway to be mentioned below, had already begun at the Harvard Medical School in 1982 under the direction of Daniel Tosteson, the Dean at that time [9].

In the Fifth Chapter of DeAngelis' *Curriculum for the 21st Century*, Leon Gordis and Henry Seidel, both of whom were distinguished senior academic physicians and members of the Hopkins Medical faculty, described the creation of a new course entitled "Physician and Society." In the Preface to the book, the Course was described as follows:

> A completely new four-year Physician and Society course that derived from two separate short courses in the history of medicine and bioethics, which had been taught in the first year. This course is the only one of its kind—a four-year coordinated course that is based in fundamentals of bioethics, and spans the fields of history, art, literature, economics, law and sociology.

The mention of history of medicine and bioethics as formative sources is noteworthy, as for the most part, these were the only established humanities disciplines that had been accepted as legitimate non-scientific disciplines within medical universities. History of Medicine had been a part of the Medical School for more than a century at Hopkins, and bioethics had grown as an independent discipline after its more recent emergence in the 1970s. No mention was made of The Department of Art as Applied to Medicine, as studio arts were generally considered of lesser rank than verbal disciplines. Also, as a visual rather than a verbal skill, they were not considered part of university programs in the same way that History of Art or Museum Studies might be. Medical Illustration was thought of as an applied art, an industrial art, but its role in advancing surgical education and progress was enormous, and its role has a fascinating history of its own.

11.6 Critical Incidents, Personal Experience and Reflection: Pathways to Learning

In a way similar to the Hopkins New Curriculum, but 20 years earlier in 1982, the Harvard Medical School had launched its own New Pathway in General Medical Education under the leadership of the dean, Daniel Tosteson [9]. One feature of this curriculum was the formation of a doctor-patient course which included reflective writing and discussion. The course was directed by two general internists, William Branch and Robert Lawrence. Branch had become familiar with focus groups to provide support for physicians created by Enid and Michael Balint, psychoanalysts who had created these groups so that psychodynamic features of general medical work could be discussed among working physicians. These groups were created to support actively practicing physicians who were already out of medical school and had acquired experience, in contrast to students who were just beginning their exposure to medical education. To provide starting points for discussion in these Balint-like groups for students, Lawrence adapted the critical incident report method initially applied by what would become the U. S. Air Force during WW II pilot training to successfully reduce crashes during the pilot training period. The method was later adapted to the field of anesthesiology to examine complications and difficulties experienced during work.

> "Critical-incident reports" are short narratives of events judged to be particularly meaningful by participants in the events … Our medical students wrote such reports at the beginning, in the middle, and in the latter part of their third year, while participating in a required course on the patient-doctor relationship. The students met weekly with faculty members in small groups … Assignments for critical-incident reports were open-ended; students were asked to pick an event they felt was important to their learning and to write a short account of it…..Investigation of critical incidents was first used in the 1940s by Flanagan… as a technique to improve safety and performance among military pilots. [10]

Lawrence and Branch adapted these methods to their course, and we, at Hopkins, later applied them to our own "Patient and Society" course. I became the director of that course in 2005, having previously facilitated comparable third-year classes based on critical incident reporting for many years. I came to appreciate the value of this kind of prompt to explore how students sought meaning from early clinical experiences.

Students, I found, as had many others, were able to express themselves in thoughtful and sometimes striking ways. I found that many of my faculty colleagues in other groups were unsure of how to proceed with student writing. Some would read fragments anonymously or abstract them by topics or themes to start the discussion. There seemed to be an excessive concern over privacy that appeared to reflect a fear of censure, reprisal, or even shame. The hidden message to students seemed to be that they were not entitled to express themselves about critical indents with complete freedom, as if their concerns were something to be concealed or even ashamed of. There appeared to be discomfort on the part of the faculty in allowing students to be recognized for owning their insights and writing, perhaps a symptom of the greater discomfort of medical education to discuss the very issues that critical incident reports were meant to reveal.

I approached it in a way modified from that described in the Harvard New Pathway course, asking students, if they agreed, to stand in class to read fragments or the entire content of their essays. This provided an opportunity for profession, stating what one believes before others and being respected for it. I recall one student in particular (and unfortunately, I can no longer find his name in any records to give him the credit he deserves) referring to his first encounters transitioning from pre-clinical studies to the hospitalized sick. I recall his exact words: "… then we cross the street to meet these strangers we call patients…" And as I write now, I see how closely these "strangers we call patients" recall my own experience in the dissecting room as a first-year student when I wondered "where is the person?" Maybe that is why I have remembered his words to this day.

Subjective experience is often dismissed as inferior in value or relegated to categories of similarly denigrated "qualitative research" that must compete with objectivity and data analytics for recognition in research. It is struggling to find its place in the medical academy.

Below is an example of an extract from a critical incident report as presented by Branch et al. in their paper "The road to professionalism: reflective practice and reflective learning:"

> When I was in the MICU, I was called by cross-cover to evaluate a patient for transfer. She had a slightly altered mental status and was hypotensive... We were giving her fluids, blood, pressors; it was around midnight. I got another admission and went to the ER to start seeing him. The first patient coded, and I went up to take care of her again. It was a terrible, endless, isolated night. I went back to the ER to see the new admission, and another code was called. I went to that. I was the only resident who responded. That patient died. I went back to the ER, but another code was called in the MICU... When I got to the MICU, my intern was running the code, and then we called, and the patient was dead...
>
> ... The next morning on rounds, my attending asked how many had survived. He said we didn't need to talk about any that had died... It was a hellish night of nearly unbearable stress and in the morning it was never acknowledged, as if it had never happened, as if (my patients) had never existed... What bothers me most about it, was that I felt completely flat. They were dead, and I didn't feel anything at all. [11]

11.7 The Natural Philosophy of Medical Students

In such studies of medical student and trainee writing about critical incidents reporting experiences with patients, Branch and colleagues found that medical students often expressed a "natural philosophy" of caring for the patients they encountered.

> The initial qualitative analysis of the critical incident reports concluded that students' acculturation into medicine was the theme that underlay the largest number of narratives [10]. A ubiquitous sub-theme was the powerful empathy that pervaded third year students' relationships with patients [12]. Medical students' empathic feelings clashed with the more dispassionate care displayed by the residents. Hence, the students resisted socialization when it seemed to demand relinquishing empathy. They often described wishing and sometimes struggling to comfort suffering and dying patients ...A separate analysis of critical incident reports applied the philosophy of caring to the third-year experiences [13]. This analysis concluded that caring was the natural philosophy of medical students as they ministered to patients. [11].

In sharing their experience in writing, students revealed something intrinsic to their work that ran counter to the behavior demonstrated by residents who might have been intended to serve as role models, but who were most likely to be the sources from whom "survival skills" needed for efficient clinical functioning had to be learned. The student experiences revealed by these studies could not have been predicted either by their scientific pre-clinical preparation, nor were they properly addressed by exposure to normative ethical paradigms that had grown out of the

Belmont report, even though the theory of care-based ethics based on the psychological studies of Carol Gilligan [14] as presented by Patricia Benner to the nursing profession [15], had been added from emerging feminist literature to the Belmont canon. To most medical students, however, the principles of medical ethics they "were taught" and that they would recall could be summarized as "autonomy, nonmaleficence, and justice," a summary as simple as describing economics as the study of "supply and demand." But in their writing, the qualitative studies performed by Branch and his colleagues found that students were expressing their ethics, their "natural philosophy" in a different language revealed in the way they wrote about their experiences.

The qualitative research performed on this kind of reflective exploration by students supports the impressions of other educators who have performed similar work with students, a direction that could open further educational doors to better explore what really happens in medical formation. But even in recent years, Gordon Peacock Harper, a former professor of Psychiatry at Harvard, and co-editor of a compendium of student essays entitled *The Soul of a Doctor* [16] would openly comment at educational meetings that there was an "anti-reflective movement" in medicine. And qualitative research faces considerable challenges for acceptance in an evidence-based profession.

11.8 The Role of the Subjective, Qualitative, and Experiential in Learning

In 2016, an open letter to the British Medical Journal drew attention to this tendency. Trish Greenhalgh, a professor of primary care health sciences at Oxford University who had long advocated for "narrative medicine in an evidence-based world," wrote an "Open Letter to the BMJ on qualitative research" with a group of 75 senior academics [17]. Some of the text, (the sequence of sentences has been minimally re-arranged from its original presentation), follows:

> We are concerned that The BMJ seems to have developed a policy of rejecting qualitative research on the grounds that such studies are "low priority," "unlikely to be highly cited," "lacking practical value," or "not of interest to our readers" [Example follows:].
>
> Excerpt from rejection letter: "Thank you for sending us your paper. We read it with interest but I am sorry to say that qualitative studies are an extremely low priority for The BMJ. Our research shows that they are not as widely accessed, downloaded, or cited as other research."
>
> We argue that The BMJ should develop and publish a formal policy on qualitative and mixed method research and that this should include appropriate and explicit criteria for judging the relevance of submissions.

Yet paradoxically, "experiential learning" based on theories of education that can be found in current curricula arising from the work of John Dewey and David Kolb were themselves theories of how experience is transformed into knowledge

William James utilized subjective experience for preparing his Gifford lectures of 1901–1902, published as *The Varieties of Religious Experience* [18]. This is still a highly celebrated book that remains part of the psychological canon. The book has never been out of print. It may well be considered one of the first qualitative research projects of the century. In it, James deliberately stepped away from theology, theory, and abstraction as authoritative sources, choosing instead to observe the experience of individuals. He wrote:

> Religion, therefore, as I now ask you arbitrarily to take it, shall mean for us the feelings, acts, and experiences of individual men in their solitude, so far as they apprehend themselves to stand in relation to whatever they may consider the divine…In these lectures, it is the immediate personal experiences [that] will … fill our time.

James' work has endured and been applied in the second half of the twentieth century to at least some portions of medical education, notably *Medicine as a Human Experience* (1984) by David E. Reiser and David H. Rosen and in a second updated edition of that work (2017) published under the same title, edited by David Rosen and Even Huang [19, 20]. The reference to James' title *Varieties* should not go unnoticed, as there are important similarities to qualitative approaches that take seriously the value of experience.

11.9 Experience and Epiphany

How can our own experience in medicine help guide the cultivation of humanistic values that we hope will lead to a more humane medicine? These are not only questions in need of practical and operational answers, but also questions about a more general philosophy, or *Weltanschauung* of medicine. The question with which we began, *Quo Vadis*? Where are you going? Refers to the title of the novel by Henryk Sienkiewicz of 1895 recalling the legend of Saint Peter related by sources other than the synoptic gospels. There we learn of Peter's flight from Rome in search of his own protection to avoid the kind of crucifixion suffered by Christ. On the same road which he chose for what he thought would save him, he encounters a mystical vision of the risen Christ, now also traveling. Peter asks him: Quo Vadis, Domine, where are you going, Lord? It is a moment of epiphany, an important moment to understand because, although its roots may reside in our sense of the sacred, its broader meaning permeates the secular world as well.

Among the several definitions of *epiphany* found in the on-line Miriam-Webster dictionary, we find the following: (**a**) a usually sudden manifestation or perception of the essential nature or meaning of something. (**b**) an intuitive grasp of reality through something (such as an event) usually simple and striking. (**c**) an illuminating discovery, realization, or disclosure. (**d**) a revealing scene or moment.

An epiphany could certainly arise from a critical incident, but it implies the further transformation of experience into knowledge, providing insight: "the perception of an essential meaning" or "an intuitive grasp." It is a moment of clarity that transcends and transforms the experience "illuminating discovery, realization or disclosure". Epiphany is a cognitive manifestation of knowledge creation from a profound experience that goes beyond a simple descriptive reporting of that experience. It provides these insights in a form that may require individuals to go deeply within themselves to seek understanding by means that can be difficult to understand or operationalize and may be unique to each individual. If an epiphany is an educational experience, we have yet to learn more about how, as educators, we might facilitate it, or even deal with it.

Many of us have an intuitive grasp of what epiphany means and have probably experienced epiphanies of our own. The first of these came to me in the form of that question in the dissecting room: where was the person. Later, after completing medical school and residency in urology, now working full time on the medical school faculty, my road in medicine would bring me to deeper questions about suffering and death. One such case had a lasting effect: a thirty-one-year-old man, who looked more like a child, but twisted and deformed by complications of a spinal operation gone bad in the first years of life leading to stunted growth followed by disability from post-encephalitic brain damage. He was non-verbal when I met him, curled up and carried about in a stroller, an only child cared for lovingly by devoted working class parents. As it would turn out, what appeared at first to be simple hematuria (blood in the urine) that brought him to me would be due not to stone or infection but to a deeply invasive bladder cancer. Despite operations and treatments that he could not possibly begin to understand or say anything about, he died months later under my care, but not before his childish ways of expressing affection had penetrated my defenses and run away with me in a series of events for which nothing in my training or education had prepared me. I attended his funeral, deeply affected by the entire experience of his illness and death, but more importantly, by the mystery of his short, very unusual life, so important to the large community that he had created and that now gathered at his gravesite for a final farewell. There were no reflective sessions for faculty, no Balint groups at my medical school, and certainly none for surgeons. My feelings at the time could have been summarized by the comments of the medical student whose patient had died in the MICU: "… The next morning on rounds, my attending asked how many had survived. He said we didn't need to talk about any that had died… It was a hellish night of nearly unbearable stress and in the morning it was never acknowledged, as if it had never happened, as if (my patients) had never existed…"

At the time, I was no longer a student, and one would have thought I had advanced beyond this kind of vulnerable exposure, but I had not. After this experience, I did not stop to formulate questions or research projects, I just knew that I had been stopped in my tracks, or so it seemed, on the professional path upon which I thought I was traveling. Perhaps, like Peter, I had been struck down by something unexpected and now found myself asking of medicine: where are you going? I started then on a journey of my own to look more deeply into these experiences to which my path in medicine had brought me but for which it had not fully prepared me, drawing me into the final months and dying breath of this small person. I was now increasingly drawn to look for what else might matter to people and to me in this medical world of illness, deformity, hope, and death. I was to become the subject of my own educational research, but did not know it at the time The experience had first to be followed, to be endured, to be understood. It took me to religious shrines in pilgrimage with the sick, an activity that I remain involved in to this day. It awakened a powerful need to express what I saw arising from this complexity of human experience in medicine, using writing and still photographs, not just for reflection but for an expression that some might call a memoir, a confession, or a prayer. In so doing, I found myself saying, showing, and wanting to teach that the bodies of people, as we study and understand them in medicine, these human bodies, were inhabited. But before long, I realized I was only working from within a well-worn paradigm that separated mind from body, first advanced by Descartes in the early seventeenth century. It had successfully guided the empirical approach to human sciences for 300 years. It took Gilbert Ryle, the twentieth-century Oxford philosopher of Mind to identify the problem left by Descartes as that of "the ghost in the machine," the separated natures of the body as a machine, and controlling it, the ghost, another word for spirit, or, some might say, mind or soul [21]. That is how medicine views and teaches us about the body, separated from what we call the interiority of life, what philosophers might call the problem of consciousness, of sentience, or simply the fullness of life. In modern times, it is phenomenology, following the lead of the French philosopher Maurice Merleau-Ponty that has advanced a different concept of embodiment, the idea of the living organism which is "in the world" [22]. I stopped thinking of the bodies of my patients as being inhabited. I now saw and understood them, as well as myself, as spiritual beings, incarnations of word become flesh. This now became for me the real world of bedside and clinical medicine: encounters with incarnate human beings.

Was this an epiphany, a "critical incident"? It was hardly sudden. It seemed to have taken years to manifest itself. Yet that is how these things can be: years of preparation for a moment of insight. Albert Schweitzer, the great physician of Lambaréné in equatorial Africa, a late vocation to medicine, a medical missionary, Protestant minister, scholar of the life of Christ and the organ music of Johan Sebastian Bach, Albert Schweitzer for whom the furthest explorations of humanity and divinity would take place as a doctor among the natives of western Africa. It took him 20 years to arrive at the moment when he was watching a herd of hippopotamus bathing in the river as he motored along its shores at sunset, suddenly experiencing his own epiphany when the phrase "Reverence for Life" came to him [23]. Everything he had studied and searched for all his life finally made sense, he wrote: an integration of ethics, clinical work, spiritual studies, and a philosophical sense of existence. What Paul Tillich might call a response to ultimate questions he found in that phrase "reverence for life." It led to his receiving the Nobel Peace Prize in 1952, the year we came to America. When I ask medical students today if they have heard of Albert Schweitzer, only 10% raise their hands. Would Schweitzer mind? I can imagine he would be tolerant and forgiving, knowing that life alone will teach what it will, as it did him. Toward the latter years of his life, Schweitzer would say: "I have given up the ambition to be a great scholar… I want to be more simply a human…"

11.10 Humanism and Medicine: Quo Vadis?

And so we come round to the question with which we started: "humanism in medicine: where are you going? Quo Vadis?" Do we need to pack our medical school curricula with visits to museums, read stories by Anton Chekov, the poems of William Carlos Williams, the detailed, obsessive tomes of Oliver Sacks, or the thoughtful reflections of the surgeon Richard Selzer, all of whom were working physicians? Do we need to translate our patients' clinical histories into narratives as some have suggested, or would we be falling into the trap described by the disability advocate Tom Shakespeare when he wrote of Sacks, author of The Man Who Mistook His Wife for a Hat as "the doctor who mistook his patients for a literary career." [24]

Perhaps we should pay more attention to the activities of the Arnold P. Gold Foundation for Humanism in Medicine, or we might take sides in what sometimes seems a battle between empirical scientists and medical humanists now looking for new opportunities to join medical school faculties and curricula. More science? More Humanities? Arguments and proposals circle medical school board rooms and curriculum committees, task forces have been created, conferences held, speakers proclaim, and experts write in academic journals about what is needed, but there are unlikely to be many patients at these gatherings, nor are there likely to be any from among the vast majority of clinicians who care for them, going about their daily work. Should we demand more Humanities as requirements for admission to medical schools? Should we be looking for more "A"s in courses on Shakespeare or studies of Greek theater interspersed with organic chemistry and time spent grinding, binding, and performing Western blots from tissue cultures in someone else's laboratory?

Perhaps the answer is yes to all of the above, in suitable measure. And that is an essential part of the dialogue that we have undertaken in creating this publication.

I do not presume to know the answer to these many questions, but I do know one thing: that the humanism in medicine can be found in the humans in medicine, the persons we call patients, the sick, who year after year, precede us down the pathways of physical impairment and mortality and ourselves, the physicians, those who care for them, who stand by them, who lead them, and more often than we realize, are led by them. My own experience has supported this, as has the work of educators such as William Branch and others before him.

11.11 Helping Students to Makes Sense of Their Own Experience

There are several models for reflective practice that can be used by educators when seeking ways to help student make sense of their experience [11, 25–29]. Regardless of which approach is used, we should avoid overcorrecting a student's use or interpretation of their experience. Instead, we should be encouraging them to follow their own instincts even while they are instructed in the prevailing standards and practices of the profession. If we inadvertently obstruct a student's own ways of coming to understand the significance of his or her experiences, even if we do so with good intentions, we may be substituting our own interpretation for the student's own authentic interpretation, which has not yet found a satisfactory form of expression. This is a subtle quality of reflective practice that is not generally considered enough when applying such methods to student formation.

The learning process in medicine starts early and never ends. And it should not be confused with the other aspects of the medical world with which it overlaps but it does not control, such as licensure, regulation, credentials, degrees, and certification: all the things that are needed to permit and certify students of medicine to become practicing physicians. What's needed to pass the test or get the license is not necessarily the subject of greatest interest to a student of medicine, as legitimate as that interest may turn out to be. Though licensure, certification, and other credentials may be unavoidable requirements, they may not be the highest priority in that student's interests, and yet, that student in pursuing their own independent direction of thought can become a richer and better physician who understands the human condition that much more and can apply technical skills with greater refinement and understanding. Such a student may even create new ways of knowing that will help medicine reach new territory. While science may offer ways to explore some of these ways, the humanities have for centuries provided them. We should not restrict students to scientific research if research in humanities alongside skilled scholars can enrich the profession.

It is one thing to allow or even encourage students to pursue their own education, it's another thing to try to over-regulate it or worse, block it by mocking it, denouncing it or marginalizing it, or what may be the subtest form of censure, providing it with faint praise while at the same time lowering its value compared to practical skills and scientific progress. Perhaps we should respond by "refuting it thus" as Lord Patten suggested in his comments at Wolfson. But what we are after is not a curriculum war, but rather peace and reconciliation among these apparently conflicting dimensions of medicine. We are not out to create curriculum battles. Any such victory would be Pyrrhic, leaving the bloodied victor with little to show for conquering what would be left in a world that would soon start to mourn what was lost.

I share with others the belief that the experience of medicine remains its greatest teacher, and for the student, and by that I mean the lifelong student who grows never tired of learning more about the profession and for whom arts and sciences both contribute to a broad, well-seasoned maturity, for that person the experience of medicine initiates and sustains a series of reflections, investigations and a desire for expression that can occupy a lifetime. It may be that some of the best physicians are so busy doing their work, and so caught up and satisfied by it, that they never need to explore this other realm to share with the rest of the world about what they have seen and done for others. The wide range of approaches and diversity of our profession is one of its greatest resources.

Art and science travel side-by-side in our profession, and we should be glad that they do so. Scientific presentations also rely on aesthetic as well as intellectual forms. In my own lifetime, I know that I have benefited from them all, I have learned from them all their skills and their traditions, their specialized ways of seeing and doing. I know that this made me a better surgical anatomist, and that made me a better doctor and surgeon for my patients. This was true not only during the anatomical dissections that I performed for many years after my residency ended so that I could be a more exact and precise surgeon, but also later in photographing in the clinical world and the setting of religious pilgrimage of the sick, seeking personal expression for what I found in the process of doing those operations and caring for those patients. I'm convinced that this broad and somewhat peripatetic approach to my own personal education in medicine was all necessary in some way or another.

In my own lifetime, art and science intermingled to produce a kind of doctoring that I came to accept as my own, "writing my own book" to paraphrase Emerson, and I feel gratified to have done so, finding my own way of being in the profession. There was no one curriculum that could have planned or predicted this for me. I had to be left to my own resources, and I suspect that even if some students need more structured guidance and formation, others should be left to their own resources as well. After certification, licensure, and diplomas, there was still much to learn, much education to be had.

And so we should select intelligent, thoughtful students for the profession and believe that with our help, or in spite of it as the case may be, they will find their way toward being the kind of doctors they want to be, trusting to their "natural sympathy" as described by Branch, even if they cannot express in words what might be important to them in the earlier stages of their training.

Another supportive method that is not commonly used is to introduce students to the personal writings of other physicians and patients that can provide them not only with a treasury of the experience of others but also provide them with examples of how others write about their own critical conditions and experiences and what they learn from them. This exposure can encourage students and provide them with prompts and models from which to start their own explorations. In this regard, the Humanities, as curators of the literary and performing arts, have much to offer us from the world of collective experience and its various forms of expression. But rather than just bring in a library of well-known sources, specialists in the Humanities can also look into the original sources that come from the profession, primary sources from students and practitioners who are undergoing their own experiences, so important in understanding their formation in medicine.

As an educational enterprise, it is important to expose medical students and young practitioners to the world of the sick and provide them with the tools needed to solve the job to be done, if one is to apply a "problem-based" or "case-based" approach, whether those tools be technical, digital, anatomical, physiological, pharmacological, literary or poetic. These tools help us to meet people where they are in their moment of need, in the way they present themselves to us, helping them as best as we can, and then stepping back to learn from our experience, both the scientific and the emotional.

We have become very good at providing scientific and analytic tools to help understand disease, but how good have we become at helping students to understand what it means to be sick, what it means to be a physician, how to make sense of experiences, events, and situations that emerge before them? Here, the Humanities can greatly help, for these are the very questions that have concerned them for centuries.

Medical practice and medical education could better honor the experiences of people as recorded or expressed, learning from them what lessons are to be learned or simply bearing witness to them, acknowledging that we are, after all, only human. The treasury of human experience is far richer and more complex than either the data sets or the literature that arise from it. People's experience matters, the ways in which they express it matters, it is what makes us human, and it all takes place within the theater of our embodied existence in this world into which we have been thrown. We should do whatever it takes to look deeply into the lives of the patients that come to us, have been assigned to us, and even other patients we've never met. Understand what they are telling us, what they are showing us, and what they are asking of us in physical or spiritual terms, then go deeply into our own experience with them so that we can understand our work, our role in the world, and ultimately ourselves. As Theodore Woodward, the Chief of Medicine at my medical school told us upon graduation: "You cannot rush your maturity as a physician." But you can, as I have learned, ever be approaching its horizon and even envision reaching it.

11.12 The Humanism of Medicine Is in the Medicine

I think back again to that dissecting room in 1971, to that first epiphany and the question. "Where was the person?" Perhaps it was really him all along, that old man whose body we'd dissected, who was asking me, Quo Vadis; where are you going? That is how I see it now. He was always there and always following me, not haunting me, as some ghosts might, but encouraging me, as a wisdom figure from the past might do. At that time, I was still quite young, and just beginning those professional studies. I didn't even understand how to understand.

It is the same with humanism in medicine. The humanism in medicine is already in the medicine, intrinsic to its essence, present in the day's work, in the experience of people who live and die within its theater of events. It is a deep well from which we draw sustenance to preserve us, restore us, and refresh us. As Lord Patten reminded us, "Above all we must support the Humanities because we are human, because the Humanities help us to answer the question why we need Universities at all, because they provide us with a fuller understanding of our world and of one another…and because they teach us about life and beauty and love and death."

Throughout our lives in medicine, we should never forget that what really happens really matters. The recognition and creation of space for this deserves as much attention as all the sciences and the Humanities that can be loaded into an already overcrowded curriculum that students must endure to get to the place they have been seeking all along: a mature and seasoned participation in the life of the profession.

In his poem "Little Gidding" the last of "The Four Quartets" widely considered his most important work, T. S. Eliot concluded with words that may be familiar to some, expressing to me much of what I now see when I think back to those early moments in the dissecting room and the journey that followed [30]. He wrote:

We shall not cease from exploration
And the end of all our exploring
Will be to arrive where we started
And know the place for the first time.
Through the unknown, unremembered gate
When the last of earth left to discover
Is that which was the beginning;
At the source of the longest river
The voice of the hidden waterfall
And the children in the apple-tree

11.13 Summary

Medical educators wanting to "re-humanize" medical education and practice have been advocating for reform by turning to the Humanities, "bringing them in" to the medical curriculum. They might also consider looking within the profession itself at the intrinsic humanism to be found in the real-life experiences of its students and practitioners, "arriving where we started and know the place for the first time." Such humanism may be a form of professional behavior that displays what it knows in what it does, borrowing from the epistemologist Donald Schön [27]. Understanding how to transform this knowing into a form that facilitates further study, and development should be part of the work of educators applying a humanistic approach to education.

Practicing and future physicians are seeking ways to make sense of their experience and integrate it within the professional demands of their work and the human qualities of their patients. For at least 50 years, a small number of educators have been trying to do so by approaching medicine as a human experience. Various reflective and literary practices, humanistic by nature an in origin, have been introduced into medical education to both study and support trainees in their development [26–29, 31–33]. Despite initial enthusiasm, they do not survive, they do not "stick" to curricula in the way that the empirical sciences have.

Since the Renaissance, the Humanists, practitioners working in the various disciplines subsumed under the category of Humanities, have been the keepers of scholarly and artistic methods for exploring, cultivating, expressing, and curating such experiences. These disciplines have much to offer educational reform, as did the basic sciences at the dawn of the twentieth century, when Abraham Flexner urged incorporating them into medical education. But a reform that would re-humanize medicine is more complex: the goals are less clear and may seem vague or overwhelming. One cannot depend on the methods of the empirical disciplines that brought about so much progress in the twentieth century.

Educators today should not limit themselves to bringing in Humanities experts and courses to medical settings, indeed they may meet resistance from within the establishment or be forced to contend with an already overcrowded curriculum and overburdened students. Humanities experts may feel pressured to reduce the specialized methods by which they have traditionally pursued their activities. They run the risk of being set aside as a form of cultural ornamentation or enrichment, rather than being accepted as a valued educators within the professional canon.

One way to circumvent these potential obstacles would be to apply the methods of the Humanities to help students and practitioners find an authentic perspective within their own experience. In this way, they are following some of the management advice provided by the anthropologist and management consultant Barry Dornfeld, described in "Finding the Future Within" as the recognition and cultivation of desirable behaviors or projects already underway or emerging, but unrecognized [34].

One final aspect of medicine that has not been carefully reformed is the method by which we accept students for medical studies. Jim Collins, in studying the qualities that turned "good" corporations into "great" corporations developed the phrase "first who, then what," first find the right person, then let them do what they do best [35, 36]. Of course, this begs the question: who are these "right persons" and how do we identify and recruit them?

We might consider more seriously how such a simple phrase as "First who then what" might apply to medical school admissions. If medicine is to be a human discipline for people, who are the people applying to enter its gates? At present, we consider academic achievement in school and standardized tests to be, for the most part, the standard by which students are selected, even as we profess considering other activities such as research, social volunteering, and experiences in medicine. Personal letters of reference may reflect qualities of character that would seem desirable for future physicians but overall, the entire process, except for measurable test results and check lists of required activities, is mostly subjective. Are we as a profession and as a society satisfied that we are choosing people that will provide a humane medicine balanced with technical excellence and progress? And if we are, how do we preserve that humanity during the training period and professional lifespan? How do we select and sustain medical faculties dedicated to the humane qualities of medicine?

For the time being, exploring the intrinsic humanism of medicine to be found in the experiences of its students and practitioners offers a practical and immediately available method to contribute to the humanization of medical education and practice by expanding beyond empirical sciences as the only foundation of medicine. It cannot be over-regulated, but it must not be overlooked or ignored lest it be lost or inundated by a multitude of other demands.

The story of Peter asking his mystical vision *Quo Vadis* is framed in religious iconography and has become part of his hagiography. But even if we consider it in secular terms, we could imagine Peter projecting this question onto a vision of what he held to be most sacred, in the way that William James considered religion to be an encounter with whatever a person held to be most sacred. In that case, it would be tempting to re-interpret Peter's encounter as a projection, a question he wants to ask himself, but it does not appear on its own, but only when he believes he has encountered an external vision. Quo Vadis/ Where am *I* going/ Where should *I* be led? The answer comes to him though a melding of his innermost being with the external experiences and encounters he had shared with his image of Christ, present before him as a vision. We could ask ourselves in the same way: where are we going? That is the question medicine is asking now about humanism and the humanities. Perhaps it could start by looking at the innermost qualities of its practitioners as well as the external realities of our encounters with life. The experience itself will be our greatest guide.

Bibliography

1. AAMC AAoMC. The Fundamental Role of Arts and Humanities in Medical Education 2024. Available from: The Fundamental Role of Arts and Humanities in Medical Education | AAMC.
2. Patten C. What is the point of universities? [Internet]. Wolfson College, Oxford University; 2016. 15/08/2016. Podcast: 1:07:22. Available from: What is the point of universities? | University of Oxford Podcasts.
3. Snow CP. The Two Cultures and The Scientific Revolution. Cambridge: University Press; 1959.
4. Kagan J. The Three Cultures: Natural Sciences, Social Sciences, and the Humanities in the 21st century. Cambridge/New York: Cambridge University Press; 2009.
5. Cooke M, Irby DM, O'Brien BC. Carnegie foundation for the advancement of teaching. Educating physicians: a call for reform of medical school and residency. San Francisco: Jossey-Bass; 2010. Available from: Table of contents only http://www.loc.gov/catdir/enhancements/fy1508/2015299001-t.html. Publisher description http://www.loc.gov/catdir/enhancements/fy1508/2015299001-d.html. Contributor biographical information http://www.loc.gov/catdir/enhancements/fy1508/2015299001-b.html
6. Irby DM, Cooke M, O'Brien BC. Calls for reform of medical education by the Carnegie Foundation for the Advancement of Teaching: 1910 and 2010. Acad Med. 2010;85(2):220–7.
7. Osler W. Aequanimitas. London: H. K. Lewis; 1904.
8. DeAngelis C. The Johns Hopkins University School of Medicine Curriculum For the Twenty-first Century. Baltimore: Johns Hopkins University Press; 1999.
9. Tosteson DC, Adelstein SJ, Carver ST. New Pathways to Medical Education: Learning to Learn at Harvard Medical School. Cambridge: Harvard University Press; 1994.
10. Branch W, Pels RJ, Lawrence RS, Arky R. Becoming a doctor. Critical-incident reports from third-year medical students. N Engl J Med. 1993;329(15):1130–2.
11. Branch WT Jr. The road to professionalism: reflective practice and reflective learning. Patient Educ Couns. 2010;80(3):327–32.
12. Branch WT Jr, Pels RJ, Hafler JP. Medical students' empathic understanding of their patients. Acad Med. 1998;73(4):360–2.
13. Branch WT Jr. Professional and moral development in medical students: the ethics of caring for patients. Trans Am Clin Climatol Assoc. 1998;109:218–29. discussion 29–30

14. Gilligan C. In a Different Voice: Psychological Theory and Women's Development. Cambridge: Harvard University Press; 1982.
15. Benner PE, Wrubel J. The Primacy of Caring : Stress and Coping in Health and Illness. Menlo Park: Addison-Wesley Pub. Co.; 1989.
16. Pories S, Jain SH, Harper G. The Soul of a Doctor: Harvard Medical Students Face Life and Death. 1st ed. Chapel Hill: Algonquin Books of Chapel Hill; 2006.
17. Greenhalgh T, Annandale E, Ashcroft R, Barlow J, Black N, Bleakley A, et al. An open letter to the BMJ editors on qualitative research. BMJ. 2016;352:i563.
18. James W. The varieties of religious experience: a study in human nature, being the Gifford lectures on natural religion delivered at Edinburgh in 1901–1902. Dover thrift editions. ed, vol. x. 534 pages. Mineola/New York: Dover Publications, Inc; 2018.
19. Reiser DE, Rosen DH. Medicine as a Human Experience. Baltimore: University Park Press; 1984.
20. Rosen DH, Hoang UB, Reiser DE. Patient-Centered Medicine: a Human Experience. New York: Oxford University Press; 2017.
21. Ryle G. The Concept of Mind. London/New York: Hutchinson's University Library; 1949.
22. Merleau-Ponty M. Phenomenology of Perception.London/New York: Routledge; 1962.
23. Schweitzer A. Out of My Life and Thought, An Autobiography. New York: H. Holt; 1949.
24. Shakespeare T. Book review: an anthropologist on Mars. Disability and Society. 1996;11(1):137–42.
25. Progoff I. At a Journal Workshop : The Basic Text and Guide for Using the Intensive Journal. New York: Dialogue House Library; 1975.
26. Progoff I. The Practice of Process M editation : The Intensive Journal Way to Spiritual Experience. New York: Dialogue House Library; 1980.
27. Schön DA. The Reflective Practitioner: How Professionals Think In Action. New York: Basic Books; 1983.
28. Charon R. The patient-physician relationship. Narrative medicine: a model for empathy, reflection, profession, and trust. JAMA. 2001;286(15):1897–902.
29. Branch WT Jr. Use of critical incident reports in medical education. A perspective. J Gen Intern Med. 2005;20(11):1063–7.
30. Eliot TS. Four Quartets, vol. 5. New York: Harcourt; 1943.
31. Ellis A, Felder R, Levitsky A, Progoff I, Rogers CR, Rosen JN, et al. AAP research tape: six therapists [sound recording]. Orlando: American Academy of Psychotherapists.
32. Hendrix J. Nothing Never Happens: Experiential Learning and the Church. Macon: Smyth & Helwys; 2004.
33. Branch WT Jr, George M. Reflection-based learning for professional ethical formation. AMA J Ethics. 2017;19(4):349–56.
34. O'Connor M, Dornfeld B. The Moment You Can't Ignore : When Big Trouble Leads To a Great Future : How Culture Drives Strategic Change. New York: Public Affairs; 2014.
35. Collins JC. Good to Great: Why Some Companies Make the Leap—and Others Don't. 1st ed. New York: Harper Business; 2001.
36. Collins JC. Good to Great and the Social Sectors [Why Business Thinking is Not the Answer: A Monograph to Accompany Good to Great] New York: Harper Collins; 2006.

Chapter 12
Conversation with Surgeon 6—John Tarpley

Jacek Mostwin

April 2, 2024 at 7:41 PM
Conversation with John Tarpley in Lutherville, Maryland

JM: We'll transcribe this and in a moment we'll forget about [these recorders]. It'll just be a conversation.

JT: Right. And I think this is a very clever way to do it, as a matter of fact.

JM: No notes, no nothing. We're just face to face. If I had a big budget, I would have a sound guy come in and make sure all the levels are good. But we're not at that stage.

JT: Have you read the Book of Joy? The Book of Joy?

JM: I'm afraid I haven't.

JT: I'll send you a picture of it. It's one of the more important books I've read in the last 5 or 6 years.

JM: Is this the C.S. Lewis book on joy?

JT: This is actually, because they did exactly what you just said. Are you on a time crunch? You have something right after this?

JM: [No].

JT: So, this is the Dalai Lama [who] invited Tutu to come to his ashram. And Desmond Tutu had metastatic prostate cancer and did not have a lot of energy level. But he had enough energy. They had a week that they set aside. They videoed it. They audioed it. They had a Jewish moderator to keep things going and ask the questions and stuff. Then they would have an hour or two conversation for five mornings in a row about life and history and thoughts and perspective and differences. And they recorded all this with high-tech equipment and everything. And then they wrote a book which is a conversation between the Dalai Lama and Desmond Tutu.

J. Mostwin (✉)
Department of Urology, Johns Hopkins Medical Institutions, Baltimore, MD, USA

J. McFarland et al. (eds.), *Humanism in Surgery*, New Paradigms in Healthcare,
https://doi.org/10.1007/978-3-031-86018-8_12

JM: I'd like to see that.
JT: I've got a picture of it on my phone. I can just send you the picture of the book. It's one of the three or four most important books I've read in the last decade.
JM: I'm trying to think of the name of the moderator that might have been there. Because there was a fellow who went with my friend Marc Lieberman. Rodger Kamenetz, his name was. He wrote a book called "The Jew and the Lotus." But you'll tell me in a moment because I can see that you're looking it up. Marc was an ophthalmologist who had met the Dalai Lama and started a number of dialogues with Jewish leaders here in the States and with the Dalai Lama himself. He traveled and ran a traveling eye hospital, mostly for cataracts in upper altitudes.
JT: I'll be on top of this in just a second.
JM: And then Marc died of prostate cancer just a few years ago. I invited him to to speak about his experiences because whenever he took a job, he would have insisted on having 3 months free so he could travel …
JT: It was Douglas Abrams. Douglas Abrams. Fine.
JM: Well, I'm going to look for this.
JT: I'm just going to send it to you right now. I just took a picture of it.
JM: Thank you.
JT: I'll send this to you. We want to get it done. Let's do what we're here for. But I'll send that to you. That's a terrific read.
JM: So, when I met you, which was now 50 years ago at the…
JT: Are we on now?
JM: We're on now. When I met you 50 years ago at the Loch Raven VA, you had very red hair. And you had a poster of William Halsted on one side of your surgical desk and on the other side a poster or a photograph of Albert Schweitzer. And you had a mustache that matched both of them with the same flame red color that your hair was at that time. You had come up from Vanderbilt. You taught me the Vandy MS acronym for putting medical orders into the chart. I remember it so well. Please tell me a little bit about how this all started for you. Did you grow up in Tennessee originally?
JT: I was born in Nashville, Tennessee, but I was only there for 3 years. We moved to Kentucky for 2 years. My dad was a Baptist preacher. And then we moved to Knoxville for 2 years. And he got invited to come as the denominational missionary, if you will. It's like the program director for the pastors and the administrative person for the Baptist convention for the Hinds Madison County in Jackson, Mississippi. So, he was a person who counseled the young pastors, pastors who were having troubles and also looked about church plans, where to expand. And so, if he were a Methodist, he would be called like the district superintendent or something like that. So that's what he was. And so, I grew up third grade to twelfth grade in Jackson, Mississippi. And that's a very important part of my life. And then my grandfather, both my folks were from Middle Tennessee, one in Wilson County, just east of Nashville, one outside of Collinsville, just north of Nashville.

But I would play baseball June and July every summer. And August, I'd go work on a farm in middle Tennessee for a month every summer with my grandfather, he was very important to me. And actually, my middle name is his name. So, I learned a ton from him about life and about work and everything. So, I grew up in between Tennessee, but mostly Jackson, Mississippi, third grade to twelfth grade. And I applied to Vanderbilt early admission and got accepted there. And my dad made five thousand dollars a year and I was going to be going to Vanderbilt. So, I got a partial scholarship, partial loan. And so, I went to Vanderbilt 62–66. So that was undergraduate.

JM: When you went as an undergraduate, was it your intention to study medicine at that time or were you headed for the ministry?

JT: No, I probably wasn't headed for the ministry. I had I love basketball. I love sports. I tell people I may be short, but I sure am slow. So, I was like an assistant manager for the basketball team in high school. And our team went to the state. I think we came in number two in the state. And some of our people had SEC scholarships. And it was really a high-level basketball that I could not be competitive in, being a short guy who was slow and a little bit overweight. But I love basketball, being around basketball. And one of the main people in my life was a basketball coach. He was a high school chemistry teacher and a basketball coach. So, I went to Vanderbilt thinking maybe I would be pre-med. Maybe I would be a high school chemistry teacher and a basketball coach. And when I got to Vanderbilt, I was on the dorm, freshman dorm. There were three guys on my floor who were basketball players on scholarship. And the freshman coach back then, you didn't play varsity ball as a freshman. In 1962, you had a freshman team and you had to be there, get through your freshman year, and then you would be varsity. The freshman coach said, does anybody know anybody who might be freshman manager? And so, these guys said, yeah, we've got a guy on our hall who's a fanatic about basketball and he'd be great. And so, I became a manager and trainer for Vanderbilt basketball for 4 years. And that helped give me a partial scholarship.

And I also helped out with the football team and actually helped out with the baseball team. So, I was in the athletic department 3 or 4 h every day all the way through my undergraduate years. And so, my decision was either be a basketball coach or go pre-med. And I made the right decision.

So, I worked with a team trainer, and I worked with a team physician who was an orthopedic surgeon. And I was very, very interested in that and still am. So those are the two things. And then I gravitated over to medicine and was pre-med. I majored in chemistry. I started out minoring in mathematics, but I had a struggle with that because we were gone so much on road trips my second semester that I did not. And I had an elderly professor, and I basically got a D minus, minus, minus in that course. And I went and thanked him for the D minus because I deserved an F. And I had to keep my scholarship at a B level. So, it helped me not to get an F. But bottom line is, is that I gravitated toward pre-med and applied to basically three medical schools. And University of Mississippi Medical School accepted me, but I had to tell them within 3 weeks if I was going to accept or not. Well, I hadn't heard back from Vanderbilt and Baylor, which were the other two. And I took a gamble and I let the people at Vanderbilt know that that's really where I wanted to go. And the bottom line is, is that I can't remember if I turned down Mississippi or put them off or whatever. But anyway, I ended up interviewing at Vanderbilt and getting accepted at Vanderbilt pretty quickly, maybe ahead of the usual response time because of the pressure from Mississippi.

But I was interviewed by a guy named Brittingham, who is basically the William Osler of Vanderbilt, and by a guy named Virgil LaQuire, who was a pathologist whose son is a premier sculptor and did the Athena and also the Musica statues in Nashville, which are two of the most important things to see if you come to Nashville. So, I had got accepted to Vanderbilt Medical School and that's where I went for 4 years.

JM: So, when you were an undergraduate, I'm hearing only a few words about chemistry, but I'm hearing a lot about basketball and sports. And what that says to me is you like being around people. You like that. You like that energy and that contact that you had with people. And then you also mentioned that there was a trainer and an orthopedic surgeon that you had contact with. Do you remember any more details about your interactions with them? Is it a vague sort of memory or are there more specific things?

JT: No, no. The guy's name was Joe Ward, and they called him Joe Bird. And I knew the equipment manager for football. His name was Sarge Tregona. And these are as vivid to me as ever. And actually, our basketball team made it to the Elite Eight. We were as high as number two in the country. And then we got beat by one or two points at Virginia Tech. But we upset Duke when they were ranked. We upset North Carolina when they were ranked. And we got beat by Michigan in the Elite Eight in Lexington by one or two points when they said that our 180-pound guys were pushing their 240-pound guys around too much. We really got cooked because we would have made the Final Four. We got beat by two points at the Elite Eight my junior year. We couldn't go to the NCAAs. Back in those days, only one team per conference could go. They had 32 teams and only one team could go. In our senior year, we lost. Mississippi State ended up winning. And that's when their coach, McCarthy, snuck them out of Mississippi when the legislature in Mississippi decreed that they could not go and play in the NCAAs because they would be playing against the black athletes. And they did not want to allow that for a Mississippi school that was receiving taxpayers' money.

JM: How times have changed.

JT: So, he put them on a bus and stole them out of the state, and he went and competed. Bailey Howell ended up playing for the Boston Celtics. And they had—anyway, it's a different era.

JM: So, your contacts with orthopedics and with sports, etc., was that already planting a seed about surgery, or you weren't thinking about surgery at all when you first went to medical school?

JT: Well, after my first semester of medical school, I came home and told Maggie, I said, "Well, one thing I'm not going to be is a surgeon." And I'm not sure exactly why I said that and everything, but the bottom line is that my wife had polio when she was like a year and a half old, and she actually has a flail upper extremity and had some lower extremity issues, and she had heel cord lengthening and things like that. But I told people it was like our third date before I realized there was anything wrong with the left upper extremity, so I probably wasn't a diagnostician. But the bottom line is that I was interested in orthopedics because of sports medicine. And so, each summer I did 3 months of orthopedics during medical school. Each summer at Vanderbilt. Right, because back then we didn't go 11 months a year. We went nine and three. So, J. William Hillman, Jr., who was a Hopkins-trained orthopedic surgeon, gave me a summer job, and I did a month at the Children's Hospital, a month at the VA Hospital, a month at Vanderbilt Hospital, and I learned some of the most important lessons in my life. There was a guy named Art Brooks who was not an academic who wrote articles, but he was the guy that did the operations and taught the residents how to operate. And probably one of my favorite quotes in all of my career is from Art Brooks, and he said, "Boys," because there were no women orthopedic surgeons in those days, "there is no condition that can't be made worse with an operation." And I quote that to my students and my residents all the time.

And I have a group of things called "TARPisms" and quotes and stuff like that, but that's one of the most important quotes in my life is that: should we operate, we make recommendations, not decisions. The patients make the decisions.

JM: I'm hearing you say that you came back after your first year and said, "The last thing I want to do is be a surgeon."

JT: First semester.

JM: "The last thing I want to do is be a surgeon." And then to remember you with this poster of Halsted, who's like the godfather of surgery, at least one of them, certainly at Hopkins. I never would have put those two things together. What happened?

JT: I think it related to maybe I had neuroanatomy or something like that and all the spinal cord tracks and the rubrospinal track and all the minutia that was associated with that. And we had gross anatomy, and we had cadavers that were fouled with formaldehyde and everything like that. But I remember saying that to her. But the bottom line is that changed in the course of the—I mean, I pursued orthopedic surgery within the next semester, so I think that was related to sports medicine and different things like that terrible triad of O'Donoghue where you get your knee injured when you get clipped and different things like that. But, yeah, I spent a year—I spent 3 months at Vanderbilt. And then at the end of my second year, he sent me to the Children's Hospital in Boston, and I was there with a guy named Henry Green Sr., who was a premier old-school pediatric orthopedic surgeon. And in my third year, I got an American orthopedic scholarship to go to England, and I worked at the Royal National Orthopedic Hospital in Stanmore and Greater Portland Street with

Geoffrey Burwell. So, I had really 9 months of really intense orthopedic training at some major centers and everything, which turned out, in retrospect, to be really important because about half my practice in Nigeria was musculoskeletal orthopedic surgery. That was like a godsend in retrospect. We say we live life in prospect, and we interpret it in retrospect. And so, you know, this was preparing me because I was actually—when I got to Baltimore as an intern, my professor, Hillman, had an M.I. in his 40 s, like April of my senior year. He died my senior year. And I think if he had lived, I'd probably have been an orthopedic surgeon. But when I got to Baltimore, we were there during the Vietnam War, and everybody had the Berry Plan, or you had to have an Indian Health Service or something, or you were going to go into the military. So, Robbie Robinson called me up and said, "I have an orthopedic position for you, Tarpley." He said, "I need to recruit you here. Sight unseen." I was just in on his word. "We don't even have to interview you. I've got a position for you." And I said, "Well, because of the Berry Plan and concerns like that, I actually applied to the Public Health Service, and I was accepted to go to the NCI Surgery Branch." So, I did that in lieu of Vietnam. So, I told him to keep me in mind because I'm interested, but I'm not available for a year and a half, two years.

JM: So, from medical school, you went to NCI before coming to your residency?

JT: No. The way they did it then, you didn't—if you were going into urology, you had to go do 2 years of general surgery.

JM: That's right. I did that at Ann Arbor, and most people now would just do it at Hopkins.

JT: Yeah. So, in those days, everybody that was going into surgery usually had 2 years of what would be like an introduction to surgery. You'd get 24 months of surgery, neurosurgery. And when you went there, you didn't have a job. So, when I went to Hopkins, I had a job for that year with the option to renew, but they only took two chief residents out of 18 residents that were there. And so, people came in with what they were interested in, but it was really a crapshoot because they figured appropriately that you hadn't seen everything, and it was good for you to get this basic core. I'm a surgeon first, like a history and physical and pre-op and post-op care and some operative care, and then you had a chance to see the smorgasbord, and you could decide what you wanted to do with your life's work and everything. That's all been truncated and thrown out the door now, and everybody's kind of going straight through in their integrated residencies and everything like that. But anyway, when I went to Bethesda, one of the things I was interested in was osteosarcomas and different things like that. So see, that was oncology. It was still going to be orthopedics. But while I was there, I changed over to general surgery. I decided I wanted to be a general surgeon.

JM: What happened to facilitate that change?

JT: I think that part of the reason was that orthopedic surgery, I had been in an era of polio and some tuberculosis, and the children's work, my wife's history. But what had happened in orthopedics, it became joint replacement, piezoelectricity, coefficients of frictions of metals and metallurgy. So it had moved into physics and a lot of different changes as they were doing joint replacements instead of moving muscle groups for polio and things like that. Polio was on the wane because of all the immunizations and everything. And then the whole field of surgical oncology had opened up. And at that time, the medical oncologists weren't doing anything with breast [cancer]. But while I was at Bethesda, they were beginning to get interested with adjuvant therapy and neo- adjuvant therapy later and things like that. So it was a very, very exciting field. Orthopedic surgery had changed somewhat significantly. And I was doing immunology research. And I ran a head and neck clinic for 2 years and had 8 months of really intense clinical work. And then I had like 16 months of research with clinical work and different things like that. So I did things like T-lymphocytes and immunology and things like that.

JM: So, a much broader education than what most surgical trainees are exposed to these days.

JT: So then when I went to Hopkins, I didn't know if I was going to be invited back to be a chief resident or not, to be a categorical resident or not because you had [to do] something to earn that. So I got a phone call from Dr. Zuidema's office and said, "Would it be possible for you to visit Dr. Zuidema on such and such a day?" And I said, "Yes." … If we've got time, I'll tell you this…. So I came up and I went in to see Zuidema and I was sitting outside. And so I got finally called into his office. And he said, "You're probably wondering why I invited you back." And I said, "Well, I had some ideas." And he said, "Well, you used to tell me that you and your wife could go out to eat on Sunday and both of you could eat for less than $5. Where are those restaurants?" [Laughter] And I told him there were three. There was this Peter Pan, there was the White Rice Inn. Because we were very—I'm very, very tight. I'm very…

JM: Parsimonious.

JT: Yes, exactly. And then he said, "Oh, by the way, would you be interested in coming back to go through the residency program here?" And so he became one of the—probably two or more—one of the most important people, it turned out, in retrospect, in my life career-wise, along with Dick Kieffer, whom you've already mentioned. Because Kieffer wasn't my mentor. I mean, you're lucky if you even have one mentor. You have advisors, you have role models, you have coaches, but very few people have mentors because that means that [person] becomes your child. I mean, that's what a mentor did for Telemachus or whatever. And very few people are parents, but they can be advisors and role models. And so I really kind of imprinted a little bit on Dr. Kieffer. Talk to the patients, touch the patients, be in clinic, have high standards, not spend the government's money. Spend the government's money like it's your money.

JM: You sort of summarized Dr. Kieffer in a few sentences, a few phrases, really. But what was it about him? Because he certainly was a powerful presence. When I was there for those few months, I remember him as a very powerful, very serious, and a bit crusty guy. He did not suffer fools. He was very concerned that things went well. I'm curious how you… you worked intimately with him.

JT: He was the most important person at Hopkins for me. Going through Hopkins, if you say what happened subsequent to Hopkins for my academic career, such as it is, it'd be Zuidema and I'll come to that because that's a really important chapter in my life. But Kieffer used to say, he was very… he saved suture. He used the minimum amount of equipment and different things like that. You didn't tie a knot and throw it away. You use it, you use instrument ties and you got 15 things out of one suture kind of a thing. And he used to say, you know, he said, a grand piano could be a disposable grand piano. You could play it one time and throw it away. But I told people the reason I got in the Hopkins program was because the tape that they were buying from the drug companies and everything was very, very expensive. And I was getting freezer tape from Kmart or something. And I was using that to put on the wounds and stuff because it saved money and stuff. And Kieffer liked that. But yeah, he was my role model. But he set the bar high. He came to clinic. He knew the patients. He expected you to know the history and the physical. And you better tell him the truth because we had some people that occasionally did quote instant information and that, that did not fly with him. His bar was very high and he didn't care about national acclaim. He didn't write a lot of papers. And actually when he died, very few people outside of Baltimore even knew who he was. And I'll come to that before we finish as well.

JM: What was he like in the operating room?

JT: Persnickety, crusty. He, he would, he was very, very good. He was a professional first assistant, which is basically what I became in my career. I imprinted on him. So I said I would not do any case that I thought one of my residents or juniors could do at least part of that or all of that. Sometimes I needed to take over. But the bottom line is I became pretty much a professional first assistant, just like Kieffer. And it was kind of like granting graded autonomy as they earned it with supervision and asking them why they were doing this and what were the other options and what, what are the cost benefit ratios for this track instead of that track. But I would, there was a guy that followed him named Tom Gadacz. It was equally important to me and he was very important in my career. But I would often ask myself, even until I finished operating, what would Kieffer do? What would Gadacz do? And, you know, it was different eras and everything like that.

JM: Kieffer was from the era of Denton Cooley and Jack Handelsman. I think that was probably about the time when he trained.

JT: He finished in the 50 s and he went straight. He had been at Franklin and Marshall. He went to Hopkins Medical School. He was a Hopkins resident who made it through to the chief. And then he went to the Loch Raven [Veterans Administration] in '52 or so and actually helped design and build the building that was there. And he stayed at Loch Raven until his wife had health issues and his son had graduated from medical school and then he retired and they moved to Asheville, North Carolina.

JM: But I remember seeing him once again before he moved. He was living, I think, he may have been on the Eastern Shore at that time.

JT: He did. We visited him. He would, John Cameron and I, he invited Cameron and his wife, Doris, and Maggie and me over for a meal. And we got into an intense conversation about what was the best corn. Cameron had one opinion. Kieffer had another opinion. But yeah, he and his wife moved to like Oxford or right in that area there.

JM: That's right. That's what I remember seeing him. But in addition to Halstead, you also had Albert Schweitzer, I think, on your…So how did Schweitzer come into your life?

JT: Well, one, he OK, he's a pretty important player. And actually my goal with my wife is to go to Gunsbach, which is very, very hard to get to in Alsace Lorraine. It's in the Alsace part. And I've looked about two or three times because my son lives in Switzerland and we visit Switzerland. And my wife and I are just going to go there the next time. But it's very hard to get there because that's where he was pastor of a church and everything. But my dad was a Baptist pastor subsequently. So he was a denominational missionary to start with. And then they started a church in our home and he was invited to be pastor. So he was pastor there for about 15 or 20 years. And that's the church that I grew up in. And so we would have visiting missionaries that would come by from the Home Mission Board, the Farm Mission Board. Some of them were medical missionaries, not most of them, but some would come by and they would tell what they were doing in the Philippines or they were doing in Africa, different things like that. So the idea of having a career as a foreign missionary or as a Home Missionary or as a pastor, that was obviously on the plate as I was growing up and everything. Because I grew up in the church. There was something going on all the time, all day on Sunday and Wednesday night and lots of other times during the summers and summer camps and things like that. So that was a very important part of my upbringing and my life and everything. But I had heard about Schweitzer, what's not to like? I mean, the guy had three careers and he was terrific in all three. And he wrote some great books and he has some great quotes and he had a great mustache. He ended up going to French Equatorial Africa. I'm actually on my way to Gabon in 2 weeks and I'll go by Lambaréné on the way to where I'm going in Bangalore. But anyway, I read some of the stories about him and I'd seen the pictures and he had been in Life Magazine and Look Magazine and all this kind of stuff.

JM: So just coming into contact with Schweitzer, in order for him to have an effect on you, you had to be exposed to it in some way. You mentioned that there would be people who would be coming from various missions that would come and speak or visit your house and talk about their work.

JT: Schweitzer's name may or may not have come up in the process of doing that. Not so much because they were mostly talking about what they were doing and their work and everything. But he was just this heroic character who got the Nobel Peace Prize and talked about Satyagraha.

JM: So I'll tell you something interesting. I mean, when I lecture to the medical students, for example, a first year ethics introductory course, I'll ask the students, "Who heard of Albert Schweitzer before coming to medical school?" You know, it's only 10%.

JT: I'm not surprised.

JM: That's the reason I'm asking the questions because it's unusual. It seems natural to hear about Albert Schweitzer, perhaps because of that era when he was sort of a more prominent figure, as you say. The essays were there about him in Life magazine. He was featured in many places. He won the Nobel Peace Prize. Not medicine prize, but peace prize. We know this very well. We're both Schweitzer fans, but you took it to a much higher degree. But Schweitzer was probably better known then. But still, it's one thing to say, "What a nice guy." It's another thing to say, "Take his poster and put it right next to William Halstead in front of your desk."

JT: Well, I'm actually interested in the history of medicine, history of surgery, background material. I actually co-taught history of medicine at Vanderbilt for 20 years. I was on the ethics committee for 20 years. I have reviewed articles on ethics. My wife and I have written on ethics. We think surgical ethics, medical ethics are incredibly important. We're actually integrating that into our work in Africa. We actually presented at the College of Surgeons of East and Central Africa the need for ethics to be a part of the curriculum. They call it notes now, but the non-technical skills in surgeries like communication, professionalism, ethics, and things like that. Anyway, there's a lot of cognates that are there that have accrued over the years.

JM: When Douglas MacArthur became Superintendent at West Point, he believed that military officers needed more exposure to sociology, economics, and shall we say the social sciences and social graces, so he introduced education to support that.

JT: Humanities.

JM: Humanities, exactly, which is exactly what you're talking about. This is a little bit of a deviation from your own history. It's more now about ideas. With reference to medical ethics, Schweitzer had this idea of reverence for life, which became for him a summative ethical principle. A term that got hidden in the Belmont principles under beneficence, non-maleficence, care, what have you. You don't hear about Schweitzer and you don't hear about reverence for life anymore, even though I think that's still a very relevant concept. I just wonder if you have any thoughts about Schweitzer's ideas on reverence for life.

JT: Yeah, you know, he didn't even want to step on a bug. I mean, it was like all life was very important to him. And I've read a lot of his stuff. And yes, I think things come in and out of the vocabulary. Here's one of the things I'm actually just writing up, an abstract for the Society of Black Academic Surgeons, of which I'm a member. I'm also a member of the Association of Women Surgeons, which I'm proud of. I thought about having that on my tombstone, but I'm not going to do it. But who is this weird bird? The bottom line is that Dr. H. William Scott Jr. was chair at Vanderbilt from '53 to '83. He was president of everything. If you talk to the residents right now, they don't even know who H. William Scott Jr. is. I mean, the shelf life for memory for most of these people is a decade or two. That's what's happening, especially nowadays. Now, they can tell you everything that's on TV and Twitter and all this other kind of stuff, X. But they don't know who Sabiston is. I mean, a decade with Dave, that quote means nothing nowadays.

JM: Pat Walsh would say he went from "who's who" to "who's he."

JT: That's exactly right. That's exactly right. And that's true for all of us.

JM: I'm afraid so. But that wasn't the way it was with Schweitzer for you. And I'm pursuing this because it will lead us eventually to talk about your work in Africa.

JT: That's right. So anyway, he could have done anything in philosophy and music and medicine and elected to go to French Equatorial Africa and create things there. It was interesting that he got criticized because of the crudeness of his hospital, but he tried to make it like a village so that the people were comfortable there because the people's family would come and make their own food. They would have to take care of them. It wasn't a palatial kind of a place. It was more of a village structure. He did do his proper training and actually got a degree in tropical medicine. He didn't do a surgical residency, but back in those days in the rural USA and in the smaller towns and everything, GPs were doing cholecystectomies and other procedures and things like that. So he was a person of his era, and I think that's what people don't appreciate when they're critical of some of this vocabulary nowadays and the language that was used. I mean, you have to judge people according—I mean, there are some terrific basketball players from the '60 s who couldn't start right now because they weren't doing year-long training. But there were some great NBA ballplayers in the '50 s and '60 s who nowadays—nobody knows their names anymore, but they were the people in their era, and Schweitzer was the person in his era.

And now they're talking about movie stars and professional sports. I mean, I think America's folk religion is entertainment, whether it's the movies or music. I mean, just look [at rock stars] right now—billions and billions of dollars, you know. It's $1000 a ticket to go to a concert.

JM: So however he came into your life, he came there and he was there with Halsted, and at some point you must have started thinking—either related to Schweitzer or not—you must have started thinking about this move towards missionary work.

JT: Well, I can tell you pretty much how that happened. During my senior year in medical school, the New England Journal of Medicine made [it] available, essentially free. I mean, it was like $15 or $20, and you got a magazine every week. [Phone rings] Quite all right. Let me just make sure this is—my wife's traveling, so let me make sure. [brief interruption] This is just a text from her real quick. [silence] She's on her way to Dar es Salaam for a women's global surgery Africa meeting.

So when I was in my fourth year of medical school, I got the New England Journal of Medicine, and this was the time of the Vietnam War. And there was a letter to the editor that basically said, "I'm the only physician in this part of Nigeria. My son has got X, Y, and Z disease. I'm going to have to return back to the States to take care of my son. How about some of you bleeding-heart liberals who are protesting and marching against the war on Saturday and going to your country club buffets on Sunday, kicking off your butts and coming over here and helping some of these sick folks?" Full stop. I cut that out, put it in my back pocket, went off to Baltimore to become a star. My goal was actually to go back to the University of Mississippi Medical Center and try to improve the health care for the blacks and the poor whites in the state of Mississippi, because it's not just the blacks. There's two groups down there. I was from Jackson. I'd done research 1 year at the University of Mississippi Medical Center, and I thought that that would be something to think about. That was really one of the things I was thinking about with my medical career. I didn't know if I'd be an academic surgeon or not.

I went to Vanderbilt, and my wife and I saw an advertisement that basically said, "Consider coming to the Christian Medical Society... We're going to have a meeting, one-hour meeting on Tuesday nights. Consider coming." We went to this starting from our first year of medical school. There were like 12 people in the group. One had spent some time in what was then Zaire, and one of the missionary surgeons there had been killed during some of the internecine warfare that was going on there. Another guy was getting ready to go in pulmonary medicine to Nigeria, and another lady who was a third-year medical student was planning to be a career missionary and go wherever God called her, and she ended up going to Bangalore, India for 30-something years. She came back and was at Parkland and won the Educator of the Year Award for the Association of Surgical Education.

Three people that I knew were considering doing something different than community practice, academics, research, or government medicine. You could also be thinking about doing international or global or mission medicine. That was introduced the first week of medical school, so that was actually an important event. Then in the Africa piece was this guy from Nigeria writing this. When we were in Bethesda for 2 years, we went to a Baptist church, Chevy Chase Baptist Church on the Circle, and Leland Albright, who's a pediatric neurosurgeon of note that we had met in Nashville in '69, he had gone there ahead of us, and so we went to church with him, joined that church. Long story short, he got up and complained at a church business meeting that they didn't have adequate enough education for the children in the church, the students, and they said, "You're right, Albright, so you take the senior high students, and Tarpley, you take the junior high students." I had 12 junior high school students, and in that group were three young women from Kenya. Ernest Lang'at was the number two ambassador from Kenya, and his wife, they had three daughters that were in my class, and I got to know the Lang'ats. At a picnic one day, I said, "Isn't the day of the white missionary in Africa over?" I said,

"I was in Baltimore. We had the Martin Luther King riots. They had the white riots, the black-white animosity, that kind of stuff." He said, "It all depends on you." He said, "We're really far behind. If you're going to be a colonialist and come over here and boss us around and tell us what to do, stay at home, but we really need help. If you will come and work along beside us, then I invite you to come. I'd love for you to come to Kenya." That was like a personal invitation from the number two ambassador from Kenya, and so that would have been 1974. That was really an important conversation for me and for us.

When we got into our residency and stuff, Dr. Zuidema was recruiting me to stay back at Hopkins along with Brooks Baker. In Bethesda, I had done good research. I'd gotten some papers out in major journals. Then I had gone to England to do thoracic oncology with [Ronald] Belsey, who was one of the premier thoracic surgeons in England. I had worked with Brooks Baker, and actually Dr. Kieffer was a TB-era thoracic surgeon. That was his main identity personally. He was a thoracic surgeon, and he was terrific. I learned from Kieffer. I had done some basic science, some translational work. It wasn't basic science, but translational kind of stuff, immunology research, and some clinical outcomes. We had done neo-adjuvant therapy for head and neck squamous cell carcinoma. This had not been introduced yet for lung cancer, esophageal cancer, and it was just being introduced for breast cancer. I was recruited back to thoracic oncology with Brooks Baker: "Let's think about moving this forward. We know what operation a lung needs. There's operation plus something else, whether it's radiation or chemotherapy. How will this help?" I basically interviewed with all the people, and it was all set up, and I was supposed to join. They actually took me out to the golf club and out to dinner and all. It looked like we were probably going to go that way. In the back of my mind, I kept thinking about this guy in Nigeria, and I looked around Baltimore.

JM: Nigeria or Kenya, because you had mentioned—.

JT: No, no. I remember that note. Bishop: The ambassador from Kenya, but the letter came from Nigeria. Brooks: The letter from Nigeria. We had thought about Africa, because the observation is… [phone interruption]—let me just deal with Maggie for a second, because she's going to bed, and she's in Amsterdam right this minute.

JM: We can take a break for a moment if you want.

JT: No, I'm fine. Okay. Okay, that last one was not from Maggie. That was about a baseball game, so I don't think it will go off again. Let me just turn it off now that she's gone to bed.

JM: So you're flying from both coasts of Africa. You got the letter from Nigeria in the New England Journal. You had the personal conversation because of the contact with the daughters of the Kenyan ambassador.

JT: Yeah, well, if you talk to me and you talk to Maggie, you get two different stories, okay. If you talk to me, I basically said—I looked around Baltimore, and there were really, really good surgeons, and many of them standing in line to do minor surgery. There's no minor surgery. There are minor surgeons, but I'm just saying they're doing lumps and bumps. They're not doing esophagectomies. They're not doing this. They've got plenty of horsepower in Baltimore. It's not like Baltimore needs more surgeons. They've got University of Maryland. We've got hospitals galore, and we've got Hopkins and all, Baltimore City, as it was called then. And I just said, "What if we go—let's consider going to Africa, and they would want us to sign on for life, but even if we just went for three years, that way we will have tried our career, and if it works and we stay, that's great. If it doesn't work and we come back, we've tried our careers, and then we can go to the country club buffet and not feel guilty." Now, that was my answer.

Maggie's answer was "he didn't want the responsibility of buying a house and settling down." We were looking at houses in Rodgers Forge and places like that, and the last thing I wanted to do was be a homeowner and be tied down to something. I wanted the freedom to be able to do other things. We discussed it, and she agreed to "at least let's talk to the Foreign Mission Board," which is based in Richmond, at the Baptist Convention, and consider it. She said, "Okay, I'm willing to consider it." So we wrote them, and we went down there and visited. I talked to the guy who was in charge of East Africa, and I said, "Y'all have just recruited—one of your missionaries, you just put on faculty at the University of Nairobi. That's what I would like to do. I think I'm an academic surgeon. I want to train surgeons. I want to do capacity building," though we didn't use that term at the time, "but increase the workforce. We would like to consider going to Kenya and being assigned to the hospital in Nairobi." He said, "Well, that's an experiment. We're not going to do that anymore, and I'm not very interested yet in committing any more personnel to that experiment, but why don't you walk across the hall and talk to the people in West Africa?" So we walked across the hall and talked to the guy that was in West Africa.

When I mentioned that I was a surgeon and we were considering God's call to Africa, he said, "Come on over into Ghana." They had a hospital in the northernmost part of Ghana. He said, "It wasn't the end of the earth, but you could see it from there." He needed a surgeon. He didn't need an academic surgeon. He needed a surgeon. I said, "No, my goal is not to go do operations. My goal is to go to train young Africans to do quality, safe surgery." So we got to talking. He said, "We actually have a program in Ogbomosho, Nigeria, where we have four, I would call them PGY1s, interns. That is a possibility, and that would work." My wife was a librarian. They would need her at the seminary that they had there and different things like that. So he was very interested in us coming to Nigeria. So we went back and talked about it. Subsequently, that was just a visit that we made on our own to the people in Richmond. They sent one of their regional people to come and interview with us, and he came to our apartment in the compound, and he talked to me for about 5 min, but he spent about 30 or 40 min basically telling Maggie that this is all his idea. You're not interested in this. He was correct, and basically, he verbally abused her. I mean, he was basically trying to make sure that she was called to do this, and it wasn't just me and that she wasn't going just because

I had a strong personality and was making her go. But it really offended Maggie, and we had actually had an appointment to go and be interviewed to see if we were going to be acceptable for the people in Richmond, and Maggie said, "To hell with that son of a bitch. Cancel our appointment." So we canceled our appointment, and I was not happy about that. Now we're kind of moping around a little bit, but then she was playing tennis, and we were having a dinner party that night a week or two later, and she basically hurt her ankle playing tennis with some of her women colleagues there before the dinner party such that a couple of her colleagues helped put on the dinner party, and she was upstairs in bed with her ankle elevated and ice on it, and for 2 weeks she was in bed, and different orthopedic surgeons were coming by once or twice a day to check on her, and I think she had a God event, which we've never discussed in detail, but she basically said, "I've got a trivial sports injury, and I've got surgeons galore in my bedroom." And she said, "There are other people over there who've got kids that are dying, and there's nobody to take care of them." Now that's my take, but we've never discussed it. So then she said, "I think we ought to go to Richmond and talk to them." I said, "Okay, I'll call them and tell them we're coming." So I called them, and they said, "I'm sorry. That spot's been taken. You can't come." I said, "Listen, you don't understand. We're coming. We'll see you. We'll be there." So we went there, and they did not ask her a single question. They asked a lot of other people a lot of questions. They interviewed probably three couples at a time, and they got one woman about her dad who was an alcoholic. They said stuff they shouldn't have. It was inappropriate. They had a psychiatrist see us and all this kind of stuff, but the bottom line is that they asked me a lot of questions, and I'm a bleeding-heart liberal to the left of Hubert Humphrey, but nobody knows who that is. So now I have to say to the left of Bernie. But I was not necessarily a good fit. I was a beer-drinking Baptist with a lowercase "b." I was too liberal for them and probably had habits that they didn't like, which we didn't bring up. We had to sign this faith statement document thing, and the guy that I was talking to knew where we were from, but he thought that we would be good missionaries for them and everything. And so we basically ended up saying we agree with it in principle sort of, a kind of statement at the end. But we signed it, but we added some wordage ahead of it and everything. But the bottom line is they accepted us, and so that's what we ended up doing.

So I told Maggie. She had the Security Council UN veto privileges. If it wasn't working out, we'd come back home. She says, "I don't want to teach the kids, and we've got to have running water." When we got there, some people told them if you're on the mission field, you'd have water, you'd have a cook, you'd have a gardener. It's actually a sweet life that you almost have to be a millionaire to have the equivalent in the States and everything. And there's a guy named Goodgame who just died recently, Rick Goodgame. I can send you an article about him. He's important. But anyway, bottom line is one of her friends in the compound who had been raised in the mission field said it was wonderful. It was great for your kids. It's the best thing you could do for your kids. We had two kids, and that was a big deal for Maggie, that that would be a positive instead of a negative. So the bottom line is we came back, thought about it, prayed about it, discussed it, and we went with the proviso that if she said, "We're going home," I said, "We're going home." And I said, "Let's try to make it the first three years, and if we don't, that's okay. If we do, then we can extend or not." And I went there, I thought it would be that 30 years, and we ended up just 15 years.

JM: So when you went there, were you the only Western trained surgeon in Nigeria at your medical center?

JT: No, there was one other guy there that had trained at—he was from Texas, and he had trained at UTMB in Galveston. And I learned a lot from him because he had been there for 10 years. It turned out to be that we were surgeons who confined our practice to the skin and its contents because orthopedics was like 40 or 50% of my practice, and I did a lot of urology. I did prostatectomies every week. We wrote papers on prostatectomy and the Malament technique, where you didn't do continuous irrigation if you did a transvesical prostatectomy, but that you would put a Malament suture around to kind of keep the hematoma—I remember very well: we've written papers on that, and I get letters today, emails today from people who say, "We use that technique." A guy from Kerrville, Texas—I'll send you an article that I wrote that related to the value of a 2-week volunteer, but there was a guy in Kerrville, Texas that came out, and he came and he showed us a better way. We invited him to help us improve our cystoscopy and urethroscopy. He came, he brought some scopes, he saw what we were doing, and he made some suggestions. And so we started doing DVIUs, direct vision internal urethrotomies, and he taught us how to do the Malament, and he actually fixed our autoclave. I mean, he came back for a second visit, and he really changed the way we did urology practice. And so Myer and I wanted to—Don Myer, my partner, joined me in '82, and he was from UT Southwestern. He was an academic surgeon. He had gotten fed up with going to parties in Parkland, and the only conversation was about how do you keep the algae out of the swimming pool? He said he'd been a student volunteer in Gaza at an Episcopal hospital on his way up, and he and his wife were active in the church and everything. Bottom line is that we—this guy, Toler, who's now deceased, but he taught me a lot of things, some of which were good, some of which were less than ideal....

JM: What about language with the patients themselves? How did that take place?

JT: Well, when we took this job, it was an English language assignment because really I was working with the resident physicians. They had four there, and we got a fifth one while I was there. We got it as high as 18, as a matter of fact. Actually, Myer and I, between us, established a residency training program in general medical practice. We didn't have all the bells and whistles to have a surgery program, but we looked into it. But we basically ended up producing more general medical practitioners than anybody in the country when they started that discipline in the '80 s, and Myer was the one that drove that. I didn't drive that, but I assisted on that. And they are still there, but what they would do is they'd do a PGY1 year. They would actually owe the government for a year, so that was a National Youth Service Corps year, and we would then recruit some of them to be in our residency if they were some of the really good ones. And then they would do 2 years with us, and they had to take exams and take some tests, and then they could come and back and do another 3 years where they would do general stuff but pick one area to emphasize and write their dissertation or their paper on.

So some would do—one did community medicine, a lot would do internal medicine or pediatrics, but several liked the [operating] theater, so we trained really four or five surgeons that did mostly surgery during their [time].

JM: And they remained in Nigeria?

JT: Yeah, and actually many of them remained at that hospital such that one just died. One of them just died of an ovarian cancer 2 days ago. Another one was actually—became a missionary, the one that did public medicine, community health. He went to Mozambique and worked there with World Vision for 10 or 15 years and came back. He was CEO. A guy that was really kind of my closest friend, Akin Ola O'Loran, he went to Vanderbilt for a year, Parkland for a year, and decided that he'd rather be back in Nigeria. And he ended up being head of surgery there, and now he's the CEO of the hospital. And I got an email from him just saying that Nneke Adenoran had just died, and then I got a letter—note yesterday from Bro Olapona that basically sent me a picture of Nneke Adenoran, whom I knew when she was a medical student and all the way through a residency program, and she stayed on with us and everything.

JM: What about individual patients that you encountered when you were there in your early years? What languages did you use to communicate with them? Was it English or did you need translators?

JT: I needed translators.

JM: What was the relationship like between you and the patients?

JT: I will give you my perspective. First off, Nigeria has 250 different languages, and even the Yoruba language has several different "dialects." So even some Yorubas have trouble speaking with some other Yorubas. But in our town, we had probably 40 languages, three or four major ones. So I mostly did my work in English. I had two interpreters who knew me and my language very well, and they knew their language very well, but we had interpreters, basically. I could tell them to stick out their tongue, drop their drawers, go to the blood bank, go to the theater, and things like that, but I could not carry on a decent conversation, history and physical-wise. But these people became integral to me and my practice there because they were with me in all my clinics.

JM: Translators.

JT: Yeah, translators. And we had translators in the OR, and I had a nurse supervisor who was incredible, and she and I really worked well together. When we were talking about mastectomies, especially, she and I would sit with the patient and the family for an hour, sometimes answering all the questions between us and everything because that was really a big deal. But she was a really important translator for me. But then my physicians, my co-residents that were there, and not all of them spoke Yoruba because English is the language after elementary school. Everything beyond elementary school was done in English across the country. And so all of my residents and all my trainees and everything and then my future partners that were there because we went from having—there was one surgeon there when I got there, then I was the second surgeon, and then Myer came in '82, and we had three. But what would happen is that we were on like 4-year rotation, so we would work for 3 years there, then go back to the States for a year. And so when Myer and I were there as the only two surgeons, we would have two fat years and two lean years because he'd be gone 1 year and I'd be solo, and then I'd be gone for one year and he'd be solo. But by that time we had trained residents, and so they became junior faculty, junior attendings, if you will. So there was a guy named Obi Amediego, for example, who operated on me, and Akinola Lawrence operated on me. And so these guys would be with us, not 24/7, but we were like together all the time, and we worked very, very closely together, and they taught me stuff and I taught them stuff. And so they—like, Amediego was Ibo, and Yoruba wasn't his national language.

JM: So you mentioned your—every fourth year you would come back—you would take turns coming back to the States.

JT: Right.

JM: I remember in the beginning when you started your travels that you would come back and you maintained a position at the VA in Loch Raven on the Hopkins faculty, and then at some point you moved as well to Vanderbilt. I recall that perhaps it was personal issues that drove you back there, but in the beginning you were—you would come back for a full year to Hopkins to work there?

JT: Yeah, so this is where Zuidema was so important. Dr. Zuidema made my career academically, whatever career I've got right now, which is actually really—we've been really blessed, Maggie and me, quite frankly. But so I was supposed to stay at Hopkins. After we did this visit with the Farm Mission Board, they came to our house, we went back and had the interview, we got accepted, Maggie and I discussed it, and we accepted that, and I had to tell Zuidema that I wasn't coming to Hopkins. And at that time he was still smoking his pipe. So I set up a conference with Dr. Zuidema, and so I went in. I said, "Dr. Zuidema, this is going to be a tough conversation for me." And he was sitting there puffing on his pipe. And so I told him our story. I told him about the article in the New England Journal. I told him about the people that I knew from the embassy, Ernest Lanyard. I told him about X, Y, and Z, and that we had decided that for now—I had planned originally to go back to Mississippi, but then I had supplanted Mississippi with saying maybe we'd stay at Hopkins because this was a golden opportunity to do neo-adjuvant therapy and to work with Kieffer and Brooks and stay in Baltimore, which I knew. But I said that I didn't have peace about it. And so Maggie and I were planning to go to Nigeria for probably a minimum of 3 years. But, you know, we might make a career of it and everything. Well, he was sympathetic to that.

He went to Hope College. He was from a Reformed tradition in Michigan. And he was very active in his church. I think his wife taught Sunday school. He sang in a choir. I mean, he was what I call a serious believer, a practicing Christian. And so he smoked on his pipe three or four times, and he said, "Well," he looked up at the ceiling, he said, "If I'm going to be out-recruited, I'd rather be out-recruited by God than anybody." And then he said—and this changed my life—he said, "This doesn't always work out." I know one surgeon who went over there, and he ended up getting drowned. People get meningitis. They have other issues. They have civil wars. They have illnesses. He said, "As long as I'm chair, you will always have a job here." And then he said, "You'll have to come back for your home leave." And that's usually every 3 or 4 years. He said, "As long as I'm chair, I will always have a position for you here. You have to contact me a year ahead of time and say, 'Do you want to be at Baltimore City or at Hopkins or at the VA?'" And I said, "Well, I obviously want to be at the VA because that's America's experiment with socialized medicine. I don't have a fiduciary relationship with the patients. It's a team approach for us taking care of these patients and everything." And I said, "That is incredible, and thank you very much." And I'm still grateful to him to this day.

So we parted very positively with the thought that I would have a position. So I would go off-salary when I came back every fourth year. So I didn't get a salary from the mission board, and I'd get a VA salary. And so I did that. So I did it, bing, bing, bing. So I did 3-1, 3-1, 3-1.

And then Maggie and I were not a good fit for the Southern Baptist Convention. They had changed some of the ground rules. They had decided that—a whole lot of noise that I don't want to go into. But the bottom line is I was not truth-in-advertising to be a Southern Baptist missionary. They knew that, and I knew that. And my mother had dementia. My dad was going blind. Maggie's an only child. Her father had died our freshman year in medical school. Her mother was in her mid-60 s, getting older. And so we had some conversations and different things. And so we basically said, "Let's go back to the States for a year or two, maybe come back with a different sending agency or something like that. We need to go take care of our parents, X, Y, and Z." And so the reason I went to Vanderbilt is because Barbara Mikulski, your …{Senator] and all of Maryland had been upset because Hopkins had what is now, you know, Bayview or whatever you want to call it, Francis Scott Key. Somebody once asked me, "Why did they name a hospital for a bridge?" But that's another story. So Hopkins had the VA, and they had the city-county hospital. And Maryland said, "That's not fair," and that we needed all the VA. And so Mikulski negotiated a contract that if they rebuilt a new VA, it would be all Maryland and it would be on Greene Street. And so fast forward, that's what happened. So the year I was going to come back, I would have had to change from a Hopkins affiliation and go through a whole appointment process. Loch Raven at that point became a chronic care facility when the VA moved downtown.

JM: So the job that you were going to come back to suddenly had been sold to other owners, if you will. -.

JT: Right, that's it. So I was going to either go back to Maryland and still be in Baltimore, or Maggie said—I was invited as a visiting professor to Vanderbilt. We were driving down 81, and I said, "Maggie, for the last half hour, I've been thinking, instead of returning to Baltimore and changing over to University of Maryland, why don't I ask Dr. Sawyers if there might be a place for me to come to Vanderbilt for a year?" Because we had not decided to leave yet, Nigeria. And she said, "I've been thinking the same thing." Because Maggie's mother lived 40 min from Nashville on a farm by herself. She was on a 200-acre farm by herself, running cattle, on the roof, climbing trees in her 60 s. And my folks were not as healthy as they had been for a variety of reasons, especially my mother, and my dad was deteriorating. So when I got there, I asked Dr. Sawyers, who had taken Dr. Scott's position and said, "Would there be any chance [to] come and work at the VA my next furlough year?" He said, "One year? No problem. If you want 20 years, that's a problem. One year? Not a problem." And I ended up 23 years there. So that's why we went back down there.

JM: So when you went to Africa for the first 3 years, you were returning to Hopkins, but then you said you went to Vanderbilt.

JT: No, I went 3 years Nigeria Hopkins. Three years Nigeria Hopkins. Three years Nigeria Hopkins.

JM: So this actually happened for a decade before Vanderbilt, because I remember you being back at Hopkins for quite a while.

JT: I was three different times. I was back at Hopkins, I was on faculty, and then instead of going back there the fourth time, we went to Nashville. And I went there with an idea of being there for a year, and so I was—Walter Merrill, it turned out, who had been a Hopkins resident and cardiac surgeon, had recently become head of the VA, so I wrote him, and they were ready to welcome me back and everything, and I had arranged that all ahead of time.

JM: Now, at some point, your work in Africa had become part of your academic work, your presence, if you will. You became known for this kind of work, and probably you were asked to speak about it, or you wrote about it, or both.

JT: Both, right.

JM: How did this evolve?

JT: This probably wasn't something that was deliberate, it just—my guess is it kind of happened because—I went there to do capacity building. I didn't go there to write articles and become necessarily an academic surgeon, but what I did do—and somebody recommended this to me—but they said, "Why don't you consider getting a faculty appointment at University College Hospital Ibadan, which was 90 kilometers away. It's about a two-hour car drive away." So I went down to see them—I wanted to collaborate, not compete, with the Ministry of Health and the Nigerian system. I went down and talked to the chair of surgery and said, "I'm in Abomasaw." I said, "I was going to be an academic surgeon in Hopkins. I came to Abomasaw instead to help improve the training of some of these residents and stuff that they have on their house staff there. Is there any chance that I could have an adjunct position or affiliate with University College Hospital-Ibadan?" He said, "Yes." He said, "I'm very interested in that. We can do that."

So I got a faculty appointment there. I would go down there one day a week for M&M [morbidity and mortality] and for Grand Rounds, like on Tuesday afternoon. Originally, it was on Saturday, and I would go down on Saturday when I wasn't on call. I dropped Maggie and the kids off at UI campus, which had a swimming pool and a zoo. I would go for 2 or 3 h, but basically 2 or 3 days a month, I would go to University College Hospital-Ibadan. I made relationships with all these people. I got to know them. I went to the West Africa College of Surgeons meeting in 1979, and the guy that was the secretary general was my thoracic surgery colleague there. He asked me to join WACS, which is the West Africa College of Surgeons. I filled out all the paperwork. I'm a member of WACS since 1981, and I'm a life member of WACS. I try to go to most of the meetings, and I've gone to the last two meetings post-COVID. I went to all the meetings when I was in Nigeria before that time, to five or six different countries. I integrated myself into the University Teaching Hospital from the get-go, from the first year.

Then Jack Toler was not interested in academics at all, but Don Meyer got there, and that catalyzed us. Don Meyers, one of the guys that he worked with, put out the selected readings in general surgery. He basically got to know Meyer really well, respected what Meyer was doing. He was a believer. He basically gave us money to afford one of our nurse graduates, because we started a nursing school while we were there, to basically be our person. We had a research nurse who also worked with us. Our goal was to do a research project every year, present it at the West Africa College of Surgeons, and write it up and get it published. We did that. We kidded ourselves and said, "We need to do one publication a year to get our union card as academic surgeons revalidated." We did that every year, and so we became known.

JM: The way I hear you tell it, you became a role model for global medicine before there was global medicine.

JT: There was a guy named Larry Den Besten, whom you've probably never heard of, and about whom I hope to write a paper someday. We met him when we went to an association of academic surgeons meeting in Florida. He had been in Nigeria for 5 or 10 years, and had asked to be head of the University of Benin Teaching Hospital. He ended up considering it seriously, but he turned it down, and he went back to UCLA. He was vice chair at UCLA for 10 years, and Henry Pitt worked for him. Henry Pitt got all of his prairie dog stuff and all that kind of his research comes from Larry Den Besten, who had been a missionary surgeon in Africa for 5 or 10 years. Then Den Besten, in the latter part of his career, became the president of a major seminary in Los Angeles, because he was an evangelical Protestant. So, Den Besten was really important. He's deceased now. Pitt knows him well, and he trained a lot of other people at UCLA, because Pitt and (Michael) Zinner were both at UCLA at the same time. They both came back to Baltimore at the same time. Cameron recruited them both back from UCLA at the same time. But the bottom line is, Den Besten was out there, but he was not known as a global surgeon so much. Some people would basically say, “I was the first person that did this model.” Five people that I know of actually followed up on this VA thing that I’ve done, including one of the persons that came to Maryland, and other people that went to UCSD. Meyer did it at Parkland, and there’s another one or two.

People will say that I’m one of the first people who did academic global surgery, doing it with feet on the ground. Now they have something called academic global surgery, which is where you go a month, a year, or you set up a lab, or you do twinning, or things like that. But the thing that gave me credibility was that Maggie and I had feet on the ground over time.

JM: You’re probably familiar with Paul Farmer’s initiative he started about global surgery, describing it as the orphan of international health, along with the president of the World Bank.

JT: His roommate at school, yeah, that’s right. So Farmer and I became friends. I met Farmer, I got back in ‘93, and we had a global health day at Vanderbilt, starting in the mid-90 s. And Farmer was one of our first speakers, he came a couple of different times, and we got to know each other. And what most people don’t know is that Farmer was raised in a Catholic tradition, and he was a believer, and he actually delivered sermons.

He was not like orthodox, every Sunday go to Mass kind of a guy, or every Friday, Saturday, or Sunday go to mass kind of a guy. But he was actually a believer, but he didn’t wear it on his sleeve. But he and I communicated, and actually he was in Rwanda, and there was a guy named Robert Riviello who trained with him, who was my resident, a whole other story. A lot of things have happened. It’s just incredible. But Farmer and I knew each other, and we emailed with each other regularly, as a matter of fact. And obviously I read Mountains Beyond Mountains and all the rest.

But Riviello is very important to me, and he is now the poster child for global surgery, but he was a resident with me, and he ended up going to Angola for a year, and his wife went with him, and she’s an internist and a critical care physician, and she’s at Harvard, and he’s at Brigham and Women’s Harvard, and he’s got a chair at Harvard, and he took over John Mira’s program. There are two or three different global surgery programs here, but he was one of Paul Farmer’s people. And actually when I told Riviello, I said, “I need to get back in touch with Farmer. We hadn’t talked in a while.” And he said, “I mentioned that to Farmer, and he said that when he gets back, he wants you all to meet.” And then he had his M.I. [myocardial infarction] and died in February, 2 years ago, taking care of an HIV patient, as a matter of fact. And interestingly enough, the University of Global Health Equity, which he set up, which is in Butaro in the north, and so our group has been actively involved. I visited there 6 months ago, and they want to start a PAACS [Pan-African Association of Christian Surgeons] residency training program at Butaro, associated with a

Methodist hospital in the south of Rwanda. And so it's an active project with us right now.

But anyway, Farmer was very important to me, and he wore a badge when he was back. Because he took care of patients in Haiti with tuberculosis especially, and people criticized him for treating people with tuberculosis when they may not be able to get their drugs all the time, and different things like that, and was it sustainable, who's going to pay for it, and all this kind of stuff. And so he had a badge when he was back at the Brigham that said, "CBA = SFTP." And he wanted you to ask what that meant. Do you know what that means?

JM: What does it mean?

JT: "Cost-benefit analysis equals shit for the poor."

JM: Oh.

JT: Is that not a great quote?

JM: The subject of global medicine, the life of global medicine, is something that you have lived, and is itself a huge direction that we could go in and talk about for a long time. And this in itself is fascinating. There are a few other things that I would like to be able to speak about. One of them is your eventual educational role because not all your education was limited to the operating room, to building programs and capacity and the rest. You got involved in ethics, and you got involved in humanism, in medical education at Vanderbilt. So there were medical humanities in this as well. How did this come about? Did someone come knocking on your door? Did you feel the need for this?

JT: Part of the gig for being appointed the Southern Baptist missionary is that as a physician, I needed 10 h of seminary, and if I were a non-physician, I would need 20 h of seminary. So when I finished my residency at Hopkins, we loaded up a U- Haul and went to Louisville, Kentucky, and I did 6 months of seminary: Old Testament, New Testament, Book of John, world religions, and audit courses, and I was basically was a seminarian for 6 months, and that was important. Hiram Polk was chair in University of Louisville.

JM: Did you say Hiram Polk?

JT: Hiram Polk was from Jackson, Mississippi, went to Millsaps College. I was in Jackson, Mississippi. I did summer school at Millsaps College. So Hiram and I kind of connected with each other, and I would go to their Grand Rounds because I was getting ready to take my boards in December, helping me prepare for my general surgery boards, which I took in Louisville in December. I was in Louisville from the end of June till Christmas in 1977, after I finished my residency. I had an incredibly positive experience there, such that on my, much to Maggie's chagrin, on one of my times back in Baltimore, I went out to the Cathedral, the Catholic Church on Northern Parkway there.

JM: Cathedral of Mary Our Queen?

JT: Yeah. And I took New Testament Greek. I took Koine Greek. Carriage Return here.

JM: Oh, at the seminary there?

JT: Well, they held it in the church. I think they held it in the church, but it was seminary. But anyway, I took two semesters of Greek instead of taking care of the kids at home and giving Maggie some spare time. But she ended up working on an Ed.D. at Morgan State. So we both did stuff when we were back. So I think 1 year I did that and in 2 years she did working on an Ed.D., which has been very helpful for her. The bottom line is that it was important, it was interesting. I didn't have a TV in Nigeria. I did read a newspaper. We got a newspaper. But I've read all the time and I read a lot of books. I read a lot of Graham Greene. I read a lot of G.K. Chesterton. I read a lot of really important writers that were important to me. My wife was at the seminary. She was working as a librarian there. She helped put out an Obamacare Journal of Theology. She taught English and she did everything that needed to be done.

JM: Greene and Chesterton are both what you could consider spiritual writers, although as you would say, they don't wear it on their sleeve.

JT: That's exactly right. And there's another one that I'm blocking on right now, but I'll give you his name as well. But those were important writers for me and they brought up questions. So one of the things that I just sent you is something that's important to me right now. Right now, I tell people, and you're not supposed to be judgmental. I will tell you up front that I shouldn't say this, but I'm going to say it anyway. But I tell people the Christian right is neither. And I'm serious about that because they're telling God what God can do. OK, I mean, so William Sloan Coffin, he's one of my writers; he's written some great books, but The Passion for the Possible is a must read for me. He wrote another book called The Heart is a Little to the Left, which I think is a great title.

And so when they were having a rally, they didn't call it LGBTQ, but when they had a homosexual, I'm diverting, I know, but when they had a homosexual rally against homosexuality at a church, a Christian group and everything, he and some of his friends printed up these pamphlets. It said what Jesus had to say about homosexuality and had a front cover and a back cover. And they had five pages in between and they passed them out to 100 delegates and there were five blank pages. Right. And so there's not one word that Jesus said about it. There are a lot of words in the Bible about divorce, but nobody talks about divorce. Nobody talks about it's hard for a rich person to get into heaven, but everybody is hammering. So we all have our individual cannons. So one of the things is this targeting. And that's what I sent to you.

C.S. Lewis is a major writer for me, a really a major writer for me. So mere Christianity wasn't mere, meaning trivial, it was mere meaning the kernel, the heart of Christianity. So what's key, what's core as opposed to what's opinion and preference. And so what we do is we argue around a circumference over what's opinion and preference. Solzhenitsyn wrote a paper that said that the communist era in Russia was God's judgment on the Russian people because of the way the new believers treated the old believers. Now, most people don't have any idea what that means.

JM: Sounds like something that could be from the Psalms.

JT: Well, what it was, they had a new patriarch for the Orthodox Church in like the seventeenth or eighteenth century. And he decided to change and do church reform, X, Y, and Z, reform the clergy, reform the practice. And he dictated, dictated that when you cross yourself, you had to cross yourself with three fingers for the Trinity of Christ. The old believers said you cross yourself with two fingers because of God's, Jesus's physical and divine nature. And they cut out the old believers tongues and they killed them. And he said, that's crap.

JM: So when you preach, because you mentioned several times you preach and you speak. How does the medicine fit into this? Because now you've shifted to a different gear where you're talking very much about personal belief, dogma, spirituality. When you preach, how do you prepare? How does your medicine [fit in] or do you leave your medicine at the door?

JT: I give more grand rounds talks than I give sermons. If they invite me to preach, I'll preach, but I don't get invited to preach that much. I'm going to a Methodist church now because Maggie grew up cradle Methodist. I grew up cradle Baptist and she was a Baptist for 25 years. And so now we've been in Methodist church since 2002.

JM: When you go to these settings, when you go to a purely religious setting, do you leave part of yourself outside the door? How do you speak to an audience like that, given all the experiences you've had with medicine and surgery?

JT: I will tell you what I'm going to do when we finish is I've got a couple of talks that I've compressed that I can just send you. A lot of times at the end of the talks, I will basically bring up what you want written on your tombstone. "He took great vacations?

He had a terrific antique car collection? X, Y, and Z?" Or, "He washed people's feet. He took care of widows and orphans." And this comes up, this comes up with Kieffer. And it's an article that I presented when I was president of two different societies. And we combined it and wrote it up in The American Journal of Surgery. But when Kieffer, I stayed in touch with Kieffer and I would go by and visit Kieffer and his son, Bobby, who was living in Buncombe County in Western North Carolina. I stayed in touch with Kieffer. Bobby called me after he died because I would have gone to seen him. But he said, I just want you to know, Dad just died. So I called [John] Cameron to let him know that Kieffer died. I still call him Dr. Cameron, he doesn't like that. But I said, I just want you to let you know that Dr. Kieffer died. And there was a pause on the other end of the phone. And he said, "he taught us all how to operate." And I thought to myself, what an incredible epitaph for an academic surgeon.

So a lot of times I'll ask people, what do you want? And so [David] Brooks, who writes for The New York Times, he talks about, you know, the different types of resume virtues and academic virtues and things like that. Not how many papers and offices you held, but how did you treat your family and other people? And how do they speak about you after your demise and things like that? I was actually with Ken Sharp. You might remember Ken Sharp was a Hopkins guy. He's been at Vanderbilt for now for 30 years and he's president of the Southern Surgical this last year. But he, we, we, we talk about…and again … I lose my train of thought. I tell people my mind's not as good as it used to be. My mind's as good as it used to be. It just doesn't do same day delivery. It's true. I'm slipping and I know it.

JM: And to be fair, physically, we've been going on for a long time,

JT: … but no, that's not, that's not it. There was a train of thought I was trying to get to…I know what it was. So Claude H. Oregon, Jr., who is one of the premier African- American surgeons of the century, superstar. He was a serious, serious Catholic, by the way. He grew up in a rural town in Texas and he ended up becoming editor of the Archives of Surgery for 20 years. He was the second African-American president, American College of Surgeons. He started two residency programs. We've got one at Creighton, UC Davis, which became UCSF East Bay. He was a leader. He was a mentor. He was a gentleman. He was incredible. If you go to the note and I can send this to you, the reference to the November 2005 issue, the Archives of Surgery is testimonials to him and some of his major papers. And it's an incredible issue. This is an abstract that I've just been writing. I just sent in this last weekend.

JM: So this question of how you want to be remembered.

JT: Yeah. Which is a question. Live in the light of your own mortality. That's where we're going. Live in the light of your own mortality.

JM: That's like St. Jerome who had the skull on his desk.

JT: I can't go on Monday or Tuesday [to the Walters museum]. I come back to Baltimore once or twice a year to go to the art museum. And I go on the second floor to the study. Have you been in that room?

JM: Yes.

JT: And there are like three or four. It's not only Jerome. My favorite piece of art in the whole world is a fifteenth century boxwood portrait of the skeleton "as I am now, so you will be." That's my favorite. And like I would have it on my screensaver.

JM: I often think of Jerome as the as the unrecognized patron saint of surgery, because on the one hand, here he was a doctor of the church. On the other hand, here he turned away from his books and from his laws to take the thorn out of the lion's paw. It's a bit derived from Androcles. But it is…

JT: It's his hagiography.

JM: The message there is very interesting. Here's a person who is learned, erudite, scholarly, but at the same time can connect with a fellow living creature with whom he has no other language except to see that it's suffering and to remove that thorn from its paw, a creature who then remains his loyal companion for the rest of his life, and at his side while he's continuing to do his academic papers, etc., etc.

JT: So you've got this question of how do you want to be remembered? What's what's it all come down to?

JM: And then you've got medical students and residents who face the reality of career choices, the CVs that they have to produce, the fulfillment of requirements, etc.

These are your students. These are the people that sit in your classrooms and come into your life. You've reconciled this within yourself. You've done both, shall we say. But they come to you either not knowing that this is a question to ask or wondering if this is a question to ask. How do they handle this? How did you think about this? Have you had experience with the students?

JT: I do. And actually, I have a lot of feedback from my students. Even yesterday, I got something back. There's an article that was in the JAMA for Easter. I don't know if you saw it or not, but I'll send it to you. It's worth reading. My wife cruises the literature 5 days a week for 2 or 3 h, gets up 4:30, 6:30, 7:30. She sends out a newsletter 5 days a week; she finds articles everywhere and on the web and everywhere else. It was a great article about a program director who was treating his residents as if they were his parishioners. And he cared about them. And one of one of my residents who had gone through a divorce and that I supported and everything, she wrote back and she said, this is what you were for me. I got that within the last 4 days. And it was really a worthwhile article to read. JAMA put it out for Easter. It's basically ethics and humanities.

So I gave a talk at the Baltimore Academy of Surgery. And this was back in probably the late 80 s, early 90 s when I was back during one of my times here. And I was probably inappropriate. But I'm leading. This is this is what I tell the residents. When I say follow your own gut, follow your own gut, you know, follow your own gut. Not what everybody tells you. You probably saw the graduate where everybody said "plastics." Everybody's going to tell you what's hot and what you need to do now. OK. But at the end of the talk, I looked around and they were asking me some questions. Just that because my wife and I, we made twenty thousand dollars a year. We got the same salary as a guy that had a high school education. So we're like a priest. We just got support. We got our house. And so some question came up about, you know, remuneration or something like that from the crowd there. And I looked around and they were all white guys and they were all most of them were elderly, older. And I probably should not have said this, but I've said it ever since. I said, as I look around this room, I realize I am the best paid surgeon in this room. I just get paid in a different currency.

And so I finished my talks nowadays challenging people about what currency do you want to be paid with? Right now, that is very much a spiritual comment. It is not a medical one. And yet it shows that I have the ability to do as …

JM: I hear you.

JT: So I was asked. Sharp, Sharp, requested it because he was in the Southern Surgery. But every year they have a H. Oregon Junior Lectureship. And so Sharp asked me, would I be willing to give a talk about Levi [Watkins] as part of this lectureship? And it got accepted. So then COVID disrupted the year I was supposed to do it. But they let me do it. So I gave it when I got back from the national in '21 after five… Maggie gave me five. When we retired 2016, she gave me five more years back to Africa.

So I was in Kenya for a year. She got it. Well, Rwanda, for a year and 3 years in Botswana, where we have to start with our colleagues, a residency program. There's not a single residency program in general surgery in

Botswana. And now there is one that was 5 years on. But that was to give the person who followed me as program director space so that they weren't coming to me with questions and stuff. They would all go to her.

My dad was a Baptist preacher when he went back from the church at Ridgecrest. He was actually asked to kind of leave because he had voted for Mississippi College, a Baptist school. He was on the board to accept blacks. And so the congregants didn't like that. So they came and told him they didn't accept that. And so he became the associational missionary again after we came back that second time…I'm jumping around a little bit too much, but the bottom line is, is that I gave that talk and only that. And my experiences with Levi and lessons that I learned from Levi because Levi and I had been medical students together. We were residents together at Hopkins. We both entered as interns together as Hopkins. And there was a Jewish guy named Phil Rosenblum. So there's a picture of John Tarpley, white neck from Mississippi, Levi Watkins from Alabama and Phil Rosenblum, Jewish guy from Detroit. And so we all started the first day of our internship in July the first of 1970 and everything together. That's an interesting story. We stay in touch with Rosenblum. So bottom line, we came back and I gave that talk and I basically talked about what was Levi's… what was his epitaph? You know, he never married. He didn't have any kids. But when he started, Hopkins had like almost no blacks in their class. And when he left, they had 10 or 15% of blacks in their class. And what did he leave behind? Academic excellence, but also dealing with social issues of the day that are appropriate. And I didn't spell all this out because I had to. That had been in my whole talk about what he had done. So anyway, that's what I do nowadays.

So Bill Wood, who was chair of surgery at Emory for years in 2019 at the American Surgical Meeting in Phoenix, asked me, would I take over as academic dean for him? He had had a pancreatoduodenectomy and he couldn't make international trips anymore. And he was in his 80 s. And I said, I can't right now. I'm committed till August of 2021. Come back and ask me then if you still need somebody. I said, I'm interested. I certainly will consider it. So I've been academic dean for the Pan-African Academy of Christian Surgeons since September first of 2021. So I'm working. It's a halftime job, which means I work 40 h a week instead of 80 h a week. And I travel to Africa eight times a year. So I'm still pushing, pushing, pushing and writing papers and I'm giving talks. And I'm on mission, if you will, to try to encourage people to address what I think are ethical issues. And I can show you these slides. I want to show you. So Malawi's got 39 million people, same as New York State. New York State has 4400 surgeons and 4500 anesthesiologists. Malawi has got 70 surgeons and less than 10 anesthesiologists. If you look at the number of pediatric surgeons in Kenya and the number of pediatric surgeons in Nashville and Tennessee, there's 45 in one for six million people and two million kids. And there's like 15, most [of whom] we've trained, and one of our hospitals there for 30 million kids in Kenya. You do the numbers.

JM: Do you think we're over-training surgeons for the needs of the world?

JT: Not for the world, but maybe for the for the West. But right now, people complain they can't even get an appointment with an orthopedic surgeon. You know, I'm just saying we've got barriers. We have a non-system. We have a non-functional non-system in this country. The guy from Princeton is the one that said that. He wrote 20 papers about it. But what we have is bad and it's ethically not acceptable. So we have …

JM: We've been going on for a long time and there's just a very few more things I really would like to…

JT: You can get the pointed questions.

JM: I would like to just get to a few more things. One: is there came a time when you had to hang up your gloves. You had gotten to the point you said, this is it. I'm not going to operate anymore. I'm going to move in a different direction. Can you recall? You mentioned 2016.

JT: In 2016 I went and still took call and went to clinic. So I was there for 6 months from July till December. And then I was supposed to stay there for a year, but it's a long story. But I'd been requested to come and help in Rwanda and cover for Robert Riviello, who had adopted two African children. And it wasn't convenient for him to be going back and forth. So I was filling for him. I went to 7 months in Rwanda, then came back and went back to Kenya for another five. And I took call then and I had a bad experience or two. I didn't want to end with a bad experience, but I had a bad experience or two. And then I went back. After that, I went back to Rwanda. And when I went to… I didn't operate in Rwanda, except I would assist and I would help with anesthesia. I also have a secondary appointment at Vanderbilt in anesthesiology. So I was a professor of anesthesiology at Vanderbilt as well. I've done a thousand spinals. We did anesthesia as a whole other world part of my life. And it's a very important part of my life. And I'm a real advocate for anesthesia, because we can't do good surgery if we don't have good anesthesia.

But I did not take primary care. I was not the responsible surgeon for the patients in Rwanda. And when I went to Botswana, they recruited me there. I didn't want to go. I was planning to go back to Kajabi and basically just help with surgical education and research and stuff like that. And I asked them, "What do you want?" I said, "If you want somebody to come in and do a lot of cases, I'm not your person. If you want somebody to come in here and set up a research empire and philanthropy, I'm not your person. What do you want?" They said, "We want you to come and try to see if we can, if we should start a residency program, and we're interested in you as an educator." I said, "My wife and I are a team, and we can do that, and we'll give it a try." And they insisted on a 3-year contract, and I said, "No." I said, "You don't know who Walter Austin is, but he had 24 sequential one-year contracts with the Dodgers. I'll have a one-year contract that I'm willing to renew it for three years maximum." And I said, "I don't think in the 21st century you'd have a white guy from Mississippi as head of the Department of Surgery in the University of Botswana. You've got people that we can find … somebody here who's a local, who's at least an African that needs to be there. I don't need to be there." And they said, "Well, we have to have a three-year contract." I said, "Fine. I'm off to Kenya. You need a head of department? I don't need a job." They said, "Wait, wait, wait." So I did it one [year], one more that way, and it turned out to work very well. And when I left, I left a Botswanan who's in charge now, and the program's continuing. It's actually growing.

JM: That was the last of your time in the operating room?

JT: When I got there, my attendings operated once every 2 weeks because they only had 1 or 2 days a week for surgery, and there were no beds in the ICU. I mean, if I did a case, it meant that these guys who were in their 30 s and 40 s didn't do cases. And I was focusing on getting the residency started, and the medical students, because they kept increasing the size of the classes, but they didn't increase the size of the faculty. And they put a faculty-free zone, and people would leave and go into private practice. And so we had 50 or 60 students and only one or two people who were teaching them, and it was not acceptable. So I focused on medical student education and starting the residency system and visualizing and being active in morning reports. That's what I did. And I went to a gazillion meetings, and nobody—it was a very difficult time. It was a very wonderful time. But I didn't do any cases to speak of. I would come to the OR if they wanted my opinion, but I didn't do a single case from the time that I was released.

JM: For someone who has spent so much time devoted to technical surgery and acquired so much skill, plus all the anesthesia that you've done, it's really gratifying to hear that there's a kind of life after the OR.

JT: There is.

JM: And [to hear] how much—how connected you are with the world, the different groups that you speak to that want to hear your voice. What about writing? Have you had a chance to do very much writing? Do you want to do that, or do you prefer to be a person of action and speak when you can?

JT: I've had many, many people, even within the last 2 weeks, that say, "I need to write a book." There's a verse in John that says, "The number of books is innumerable," kind of a thing. I've elected not to because I think they're not read. Don Meyer, my partner, actually wrote an autobiography. I'm a significant part of that book, and that was enough for me. But I do write. I try to write an article every year, and I do more than that. I try not to be the first author. If it's anything related to things that are derived from Africa, I try to have an African in a major role.

JM: What are the things that you want to communicate to people in your writing?

JT: I think that this whole inequality of access—I mean, James talked about that: true religion is taking care of the widows and the orphans, basically the have-nots. Jesus, when he went to recruit his disciples, did not go to the Jerusalem seminary. He found workers, farmers, fishermen, a tax collector, people that were not considered the supreme elites of their day, and that's who he worked with. There's a great book called Master Plan of Evangelism that was written by a Methodist guy. He basically said, "Jesus intensely focused on these 12 guys, and even one of them didn't get it right." Actually, if you read the book of Mark, Mark basically says these guys were idiots. They didn't catch it almost all the time. He kept saying it to me. He talked about how simple they were and everything like that. Thomas is one of my favorite people because he wanted experiential knowledge instead of accepting the words of these people that he didn't necessarily trust. Then when Jesus showed up and said, "Touch me," it never said he touched him. He just said he fell on his knees, and he said, "My Lord and my God." I would say that the devil, anybody can say that he's my ethical teacher, but to say that he's the divine son of God, a Muslim can't say that. But even the devil can say he's God, but he's not my Lord. A Muslim can say he's number two. He's number two in Islam. That's another subject that I'd love to get on.

JM: I don't think we're going to have enough time for that today, but I would like ask your opinion on the relationship with Islam in Africa…

JT: …because that's a big emerging issue, particularly in the North. Islam is as varied as Christianity. It's like right now in Israel, so many of the people are not for all this stuff that's happening.

JM: But in Africa, are you on talking terms with these people? Do you have contact with them?

JT: Yes.

JM: What happens? Because I'm sure they have a presence as well.

JT: No, the Muslims would say that Nigeria is about 50–55% Muslim, but it's not. It's probably like 40–40-20. So ATR, everybody's an ATR under the surface: African Traditional Religion. And then there's a significant Christian presence, mostly in the South, but not exclusively in the South. And Muslim is statistically greater in the North, but really it's closer to probably a 45–40-15, as far as who identifies themselves.

JM: Is it like a divided neighborhood? I mean, do you share resources? Even within the same family.

JT: So the Shaun, who now just recently died, the Shaun of our town had four wives, but he had three Muslim wives. And his youngest wife, his social wife that he took to all the meetings, was his Christian wife. And some of the children were Christian, but from this one woman, some of their children are Christian and some of them are Muslim. And they live together in peace. And he's a Muslim, but he has a beer distributorship. So we have lived together well until about 20 years ago, and now we have Islamic fundamentalism. And you've got all the Boko Haram, what we have in Nigeria in the northeast corner. And that came about because of a group that feels like they weren't represented in the previous second class. But, you know, they didn't educate their kids except for how to read the Koran. They didn't have jobs. They weren't viable in a modern society. And so what they can do is, is that they can go on jihad. And if they're killed, they're immediately transported to heaven where there's voluptuous women everywhere. And they have signs all over the country that says Islam is peace. But the majority of the Muslims don't want Islamic fundamentals. That's what's happening in Pakistan right now. It's imploding.

JM: When you say Islam is peace, it reminds me of Orwell's three sayings from 1984. The various rules of English socialism, the first of which is that War is Peace.

JT: I read the book. We had to read it before we came to Vanderbilt in '62.

JM: So, you know, we could go on for days.

JT: You're one of the people that I really like talking to, by the way.

JM: I like listening to you. You have a lot to say. And you've got far more to say than we have in our time to begin to explore.

JT: I understand. That's fine. Better too much than not enough.

JM: One thing I do remember, I always have that images of you sitting at that desk, writing your notes, bearing down on those metal clad charts in the VA with, you know, Halsted on one side and Schweitzer on the other. One of the questions I had coming in to meeting you today was, how do those two meet or reconcile? And now I sort of see them as two sides of the same coin in a way. And I wonder how you see it. If you think back to those days or perhaps, that was something you did then.

JT: Well, you know, Halsted founded… I mean, and he was a complicated character. Carriage Return

JM: Of course.

JT: Like crazy, right?

JM: Of course.

JT: All right. So Halstead was incredible. But my favorite single paper, and I've got thousands of them, is the address he gave at Yale on the training of a surgeon. So he was called back on their 40th anniversary or something. And he gave a paper, the paper is like 25 pages long. It's incredible. And I can send that to you if you don't have it, but I'll send it to you. You may have to remind me. But so to my mind, he changed the way we did surgical education in the United States. I consider myself a surgical educator. That's really, I'm not the world's greatest surgeon. I mean, the Lucian Davises and the people like that, they're better technical surgeons than I was. I was OK, but I was not a superstar. You mentioned Hartzel Vernon Shaft. I mean, he's a superstar. Even the people at Mayo Clinic and the cardiac surgeons around the world say he's a superstar. He is out there. He's Michael Jordan.

JM: You didn't do the same things. He went his way. You went your way.

JT: I was safe. And appropriate. And really, decision making to me is just as important as the technical performance of the operation. You need both. If the world would like for many surgeons to be technicians and the administrators say stay in the OR and let the CNPs, the advanced clinical nurse practitioners do the patient clinic, you don't need [to], you're generating bucks. I mean, the surgical services fund the health care medical systems in these institutions, quite frankly, and they want you operating and billing. They don't want you talking to patients. That's a problem that I fight against because that's … I'm Oslerian in that regard.

JM: How do you fight against it?

JT: I basically… You know, they say professionalism is easier caught than taught. And I think this idea of talking to the patients…you know, Osler said that the care begins with the patient, centers on the patients and continues with the patients. And I think that how you practice is how the young people see the adults behave. So it's easier caught than taught. So that's been it. But I also try to articulate it. It's modeled. It's modeling, the role model. It's how you live. And this is why Kieffer was with me. He had high standards. He was a professional first assistant. He went to clinic. He stayed current.

JM: So interesting to hear you mention Osler, because when I was thinking of those two pictures, I was thinking that when Harvey Cushing came to Baltimore, he wanted to study with Halstead. But once he had the contact with Halstead, he ended up studying more with Osler. And then he wrote that famous biography as well.

JT: Which I read in Nigeria.

JM: You mentioned Osler as well. You had a number of these… what I would call the wisdom figures… in your life.

JT: He's very important to me. And I've read Aequanimitas. I've given many, many copies away. And he talked about the books you need to have by your bedside.

JM: And Osler was actually very closely related to surgery as well. He married Gross's widow.

JT: I gave her named lectureship at Jefferson.

JM: He and Cushing were good friends. They lived next door to each other. And the great architect who built the Hopkins Hospital, John Shaw Billings, who was both a physician and surgeon. It was Billings who personally went to Philadelphia to invite Osler to come to Hopkins. So there was a lot of surgery around Osler's life.

JT: And there really, even though we sub-specialized these different directions, whether it be medicine or surgery, I mean, it's really all, we're all in it in one big game, if you will.

JM: It's all related, but there's something very special about surgery in terms of the hands-on, the physical contact and the actual concrete doing of things for people. And yet there are the administrative things. There's the educational things that you talk about. Without that, the rest of it becomes purely technical. And I don't think either of us want to see it just be like that.

JT: So I asked third year medical students and I asked people when I'm giving grand rounds oftentimes, especially if they're younger residents, because when I go to do grand rounds, I basically say, I don't want to just come and have one dinner and give one talk and leave. If I'm going to come all the way out here and you're going to pay the travel and all that kind of stuff, let me meet with your students. Let me meet with your residents. So I'll ask them, how do you define a surgeon? I said, you can't be wrong because I said, how do you define a surgeon? And they often will include very heavily, you know, likes to operate, likes to cut, technical facility, X, Y, and Z and everything. And then I will tell them what my definition of a surgeon is, which is what you're alluding to. And I say that a surgeon is a physician who can operate when it's indicated and it's in the better interest of the patient, because we make recommendations, we educate and the patients have to make the decisions. And Ken Sharp told me this. He talked about the RANDO criteria. He said, we don't want to operate on somebody because of the RANDO criteria. What are the RANDO criteria? Resident ain't never done one. You don't want to do it to pay the rent. You don't want to do it to afford your boat. You don't want to do it to have a horse. But to my mind, that's what we are. We're physicians first. That's Oslerism. And this guy, Brittingham, I'll tell you my favorite Brittingham quote. He was the number one role model at Vanderbilt for my 4 years of medical school.

JM: Had he been an Osler resident?

JT: I think he was at Wayne, in Cleveland, at Case Western Reserve. Then he was at Washington University. Then he came to Vanderbilt. He was like he married wealthy and was independently wealthy. He drove an old Thunderbird with a very loud sound system. And he worked at the City County Hospital, but he was great. But he, he was kind of like a praying mantis. And he was a thin guy and he stuttered a little bit. He's a guy who interviewed me for medical school and asked me some really important questions. And so he … we loved the guy…so he asked our class president the week before we graduated. Is it OK if I address the class of 1970 at least one more time? He said, whatever you want, sir. For as long as you want. He's like… 5 min. And so we all gathered in the amphitheater at Vanderbilt and he said, class of 1970, I've really enjoyed you for these 4 years. He said, I want to apologize. He said, half of the stuff I've taught you is wrong. I just don't know which half. Is that not a great quote?

JM: That's great. We are in process. I think, you know, I'm going to leave the machines on. But we've gotten there. We covered a lot of material and… there's so much more I'd love to hear about. Everything you said opened up… like three different directions.

JT: Let's talk again.

JM: We can do that by Zoom. We don't have to be in person.

JT: I'm serious. And so, you know, I've enjoyed [this]…not everybody we speak… If I mention some names, you know who I'm talking about. A lot of times I mention names I got no clue about. Right. You do. So there's a book. I think you're from a Catholic background?

JM: Yes.

JT: So I don't know. Robert Ellsberg.

JM: I know Ellsberg.

JT: Yes. Do you know him personally?

JM: No, no. But I mean, I know who you're talking about.

JT: OK. Do you have his book, All Saints? No? I think I'll send you a picture of a couple of books that I think you ought to have in your library.

JM: Please do.

JT: So my wife and I were very involved in teaching in ethics. So we had the Catholic chaplain from St. Thomas Hospital, which is now Ascension West in

Nashville. But it's St. Thomas out of Ascension Health in St. Louis. Largest not-for-profit in the United States is Mary Lou O'Gorman. So she's a Catholic chaplain. Her husband is Robert O'Gorman, who is a Catholic theologian, taught at Loyola Chicago for 25 years. So she was there. I was there. Bonnie Miller was there, a Jewish lady who did a mitzvah at age 40. So we were the three main people with Maggie as our person who held us all together and everything like that. So Maggie and Mary Lou O'Gorman and I went to Denver for a spirituality and medicine conference because we had an elective called spirituality and medicine. And I gave talks at the…

JM: You had that elective at the Vanderbilt?

JT: Yeah. And so actually I gave talks at both the Brigham and at the Mass General on "Is there a role for spirituality and medicine in other places." That was one of my talks that I would update and everything. And I would say, is there a role? So there's a question mark. And so we would deal with that. So we were at a spirituality and medicine conference and we went to the Tattered Cover, which was a bookstore in Denver. And they had this book called All Saints by Ellsberg. I bought it. And not 100%, but probably 98% of every day since 1998. I've read the entry. That book is like hardwired into my brain because I read it.

JM: Well, I have to see it. I remember when you sent me a Carell's Voyage to Lourdes and how I read that.

JT: Oh, my gosh. He also wrote a book on prayer. I have all his books.

JM: I do, too.

JT: Yeah, I've got I've got all his, too, even though he's banned now because he was with the Vichy.

JM: You know, with the Vichy. There were streets named for him in Paris and they took those street names. And the medical school in Lyon was named after him.

JT: Yeah.

JM: You know, he learned to sew from… his father was a silk merchant … and so he learned to sew from the women who sewed silk with little tiny silver needles and Vaseline lubricated silk thread. That's how he did those non-clotting anastomoses.

JT: He did. He did a popliteal anastomosis on a 6 month old with old needles and no heparin. And it stayed open, no loops and no good light. Yeah, that's according to us right now.

JM: It's quite remarkable.

JT: It's incredible. So someday we'll have … and someday better come soon. All right. This is this. I'm going to send you a picture of this and of the other book that I mentioned. You probably have read The Long Walk to Freedom. I don't know if you have it. I've got Mandela, but that's another book. Well, I think it's really important.

JM: You must have a very interesting library.

JT: It's incredible. And my wife is a librarian. And the short answer is I read an hour every day at least. Yes. And that's part of my devotions. And yeah. Yeah.

JM: So Jeremiah Turcotte, when he was chief at Michigan before I left to come to Hopkins for urology, I went to see him to talk with him just to, you know, exchange parting words, etc. And I asked if he any words of advice to He said "read every day."

JT: Yeah.

JM: He said read every day. Of course, I thought he meant like, you know, Annals of Surgery, The New England Journal of Medicine. I didn't realize that the reading I'd be doing would be very different, but would be clearly related to our work.

JT: So here's what I tell people. This is one of the most important quotes in my life that I heard from a family practitioner when I was doing a CME course in Brackenhurst, Kenya, which is an hour north of Nairobi, where I go to every year. I mean, it's a CME course for missionaries to keep their state licenses. So we'd go for 10 days, 10 h a day for 10 days or 12 days. And so we keep our state licenses and not have to return to the states and things like that. This guy's from Zaire, he had almost died of an illness but he didn't die. He was really smart. His name was Farmer, David Farmer. And he said there's a Zairean proverb, now it's DRC, that says you have that degree of freedom to decide whose slave you're going to be. And then he quoted Paul, who said, I am doulos Christos. I am the slave of Christ. So one of the things I ask my people at the end of the day is whose slave are you going to be? Power, prestige, position, or "he washed feet and took care of the widows and orphans." I ask them that at the end of my talks, depending on the audience and depending on the setting. That's the message I'm trying to get to the young people as opposed to plastics, plastics, plastic.

JM: This issue of personal spirituality, spirituality with medicine, you know, what you're talking about, the courses that you've taught, etc. The conference is going to be in Indiana next week, the conference on medicine and religion that we've both been present at. This is a whole different dimension that I think is still very fragile in medical education. Fluid. But everything you've talked about, so many people that you've talked about, you talk about people who are believers, people who are practicing. You know, there's this undercurrent that this is kind of a network that links you to people throughout the world. And without saying anything specific, without doing anything that I would consider a proselytizing or preaching, you've addressed this undercurrent of connection, you know, perhaps in Catholic language, you would call this Holy Spirit. It is a connection that links people. And it is something that links us to other people as well. I think that some medical students are hungry for it, but others are not. It's very complicated.

JT: One other thing I need to ask, given your background. Does CAC mean anything to you?

JM: No.

JT: How about Father Richard Rohr? R-O-H-R?

JM: Sounds familiar.

JT: I read him every day, his group. He has something. It's like meditation. He's a Franciscan. He went to school in Spokane, undergraduate Gonzaga, and then he went to seminary in California, San Francisco. He's based in Albuquerque and he has a group. And some people have tried to say that he's a heretic and they need to send him to the Inquisition. But the bottom line, he's been vetted by his bishops and he's met the Pope and all that kind of stuff. But he's written a boatload of books, maybe 20 books. The most important book I've read in the last 8 years is by him: "The Universal Christ." He reads scripture. He brings out scriptures that I've read, but I've never seen them from his perspective. It's incredible. So I'm going to send you a list of some books…Rohr, he is incredible. He's ready to retire. He's 74. He lives with his dog. He is incredible. But he's recruited like four or five other different people. He's got a whole place. I'm actually thinking about going just to… He's in Albuquerque. He's not in Santa Fe. He's in Albuquerque. But he is incredible.

JM: A person you would enjoy meeting is my former patient, Bjarne Gabrielsen. He's gone public, so I'm not disclosing anything that's not known. BJ, as he likes to be known. He grew up as a Lutheran on Long Island. He was an immigrant child. He went to a Billy Graham crusade when he was 18. He came down to accept Jesus. And then after that, he never looked back. He became an evangelical Christian. He became an organic chemist, a church pianist, organist. He was involved in new drug development at NCI in Frederick. He developed prostate cancer. I operated on him 25 years ago. He eventually had a recurrence. We remained good friends. He's still living. But at some point, he would say, "God has plans for your prostate cancer." And he would go on with that and go on with that and go on with that. One day I gave him a book because I was interested in reading narratives by patients. This book was about a spiritual journey of a man with prostate cancer. I said, "BJ, read this book. Tell me what you think." He read it. He says, "Well, there's a lot in here about prostate cancer, but there's not much about spiritualism." I said, "Why don't you write your own book?" He said, "I'll have to think about that." He would think about it. Once a year, he would come back to get his PSA checked. He decided one day, he said, "I decided to have a website instead of a book." I said, "Okay." He started his website. He would come back. I said, "How many hits have you had on your website?" "750,000." I said, "I think it's time for us to go public with what you've done, and I'd like to present your story to this conference on medicine and religion. I'll introduce you the way we used to do at in conferences in Michigan. You tell your story, and then I'll draw a conclusion." It was very interesting. We went there. It was in Houston. On the morning of that presentation, the responsorial psalm at the Mass was the 40th psalm. "I have not hidden your name in the assembly, but I've given praise to you." I can't remember the exact words. I can find it quickly enough.

I have always been very careful in the realm of religion and spirituality, mindful that it can be very difficult in a secular environment. On the one hand, you're declaring yourself. On the one hand, you're alienating other people. It's very difficult. But B.J. had no trouble with this. He stood up and shamelessly, unapologetically, went on about witness, talking about how he was going to arrive in the next world in a new and perfect body, how this was all planned for him, how this is something of complete faith. It's the only thing that's pulled him through. In an open, completely unapologetic manner, quoting from Scripture, etc. I'm sitting there listening to this, wondering how this is going to go. At the end of the presentation, a woman in a hijab stands up. She says she's a physician. She's a Muslim. She's had breast cancer. The only way she was able to survive was through faith. She just wanted to connect and express her thanks to him for presenting this. I was really humbled by this connection that these two people had. I wouldn't have had the courage to speak like that in a public assembly, but he had no trouble at all. That's in the books, and that's on his website now, which is called Godandprostate.net. God bless him. We remain in contact. We talk every now and then. Godandprostate.net.

JT: Did you help write the book, or did he write the book?

JM: He wrote the whole thing. It's interesting. The abstract in the meeting says it all. He's a very articulate person. He says, "Because books have ending and my story is ongoing, I wanted it to be a website."

JT: That's very interesting.

JM: It was an interesting dialogue between us that led to this, but it was all his story.

JT: There's a lot of stuff you don't know about me. One of the things was in December 1, 2004, I had a prostatectomy at Vanderbilt for prostate cancer. Sam Chang. I don't know if you know him or not. Jay Smith and I worked together. We are starting a fellowship in urology in Kajabi, Kenya, my main hospital that I'm associated with right now. We've got two urologists on the ground that are Africans. Jay Smith is writing the curriculum. We've got a committee. We've got the funding, and we're fixing to start. Here's Kenya. They have 54 million citizens. There's a lot of prostate cancer, I'm sure. We've got 45 urologists, and they're all in the capital city and two other cities. 55 million people, 45 urologists. So Jay Smith and I meet regularly.

JM: Bjarne, if you have a chance ever to speak with him or meet with him, he's had a stroke. He stutters a bit in his speech now, and he's taking care of his wife, who has developed some cognitive impairments. But he's still very solid, a very interesting man. He's just one of thousands.

JT: That's right.

JM: That's the whole thing, is that he is one of thousands. You get to know these people.

JT: Yeah.

JM: I was reading about—I was talking to medical students, second-year medical students in Spain. These kids are 19 years old, about personal experiences in medicine, about patients' experience and practitioners' experience. But in the end, you know, it's one thing to read about it, but the real beauty is in living it and being there and being in contact with people and living the life. That's why people go into medicine. They want to live the life.

JT: There's a good quote that—I'll send you a couple of compressed slides, and you just kind of breeze through them. But at the end is where a lot of the stuff is, where I kind of finish up.

JM: This has been wonderful, absolutely wonderful. I'm going to turn the machines off now, although I think I could probably just leave one on you all the time because, you know, every word that comes out of you is worth hearing.

Chapter 13
The Word and the Hand

Manuel Pera and Jonathan McFarland

13.1 Introduction

> *The wounded surgeon plies the steel*
> *That questions the distempered part;*
> *Beneath the bleeding hands we feel*
> *The sharp compassion of the healer's art.*
> *Resolving the enigma of the fever chart.* (TS Eliot, East Coker, The Four Quartets)

The poet T.S. Eliot was born in the United States at the end of the nineteenth century, however, at the beginning of the twentieth century he moved first to Paris, where he attended lectures by Henri Bergson, finally settling in England in 1914. Eliot lived through the two most momentous and unsettling events of the twentieth century, the First World War and the Second World War, and both impacted his poetry since The Waste Land can be seen as a response to the First war, with The Four Quartets a response to the Second. The above poetic excerpt is taken from the latter poem, and specifically, East Coker, and we have used it as the starting point for our chapter on speech and touch, and their importance to, and, within surgery for the simple reason that it hints at many important themes that will thread through this chapter:

> the wounded surgeon (or healer), compassion, hands, feel (and feelings and emotions) and the healer's art.

This Chapter is dedicated to Professor Cristóbal Pera.

M. Pera (✉)
Faculty of Medicine, Pompeu Fabra University, Barcelona, Spain

J. McFarland
Faculty of Medicine, Pompeu Fabra University, Barcelona, Barcelona, Spain

Faculty of Medicine, Autonomous University of Madrid, Madrid, Spain

J. McFarland et al. (eds.), *Humanism in Surgery*, New Paradigms in Healthcare,
https://doi.org/10.1007/978-3-031-86018-8_13

The idea of the wounded surgeon seems paradoxical since it is the surgeon who wounds, or cuts into the patient, and not the other way round. However, although this is correct, surgeons, as Henry Marsh understood, suffer too and he cited René Leriche who noted.

"*we all carry cemeteries within ourselves*" [1]. Surgeons carry an enormous burden and responsibility; patients' lives depend on them and on the decisions, they make before, during, and after the operation. The idea of the wounded surgeon links well with that of the wounded healer.

Indeed, it was Carl Jung who coined the term "wounded healer" partly as a consequence of his childhood, and in reference to the fact that the analyst (or any healer) needs to treat others because he himself is wounded or has once been wounded [2]. For Jung, "*a good half of every treatment that probes at all deeply consists in the doctor's examining himself... it is his own hurt that gives a measure of his power to heal. This, and nothing else, is the meaning of the Greek myth of the wounded physician.*" [3]

In fact, the myth of Chiron, the wounded centaur and mentor and revered teacher to many, including Asclepius, the God of medicine and healing, links with compassion since those who have been wounded or ill can foster compassion for others through their empathy; an empathy arising from common suffering.

> Love and compassion are necessities, not luxuries. Without them, humanity cannot survive. [4]

Compassion is a crucial element in any healer-patient relationship, and we believe it is critical in the surgeon-patient relationship since it is very often transmitted through language, verbal and non-verbal, and touch in all its forms. This chapter will delve into this theme and highlight how the word of the surgeon and the hand of the surgeon are both indispensable to their work and relationship with their patient.

> As compassion is defined as a response to another's pain or suffering, it is implicit that human suffering is involved. Responding to that suffering is the essence of what it means to be human. If one lacks compassion, one is essentially lacking humanity [5]

Aristotle called the human hand "*the tool of tools*"; indeed, he drew an analogy between the soul and the hand, while in the words of the French poet, Paul Valery, the hand, "*strikes and blesses, gives and receives, feeds, takes an oath, measures, reads for the blind, speaks for the dumb, is extended to a friend, is raised against the adversary and becomes a hammer, a pair of pliers, an alphabet*" [6].

The true versatility and critical importance of the hand will be expanded in the second section of the chapter, where we will discuss, among other things, the different functions of the hand, technical, cognitive, or pathic, and also the importance of touch on its different levels.

> Touch is not just a sentimental human indulgence, it's a biological necessity [7]

When Eliot writes "*Beneath the bleeding hands we feel/ the sharp compassion of the healer's art*" incisively or intuitively he encompasses much of what we wish to convey in the chapter since we wish to explore not only how the surgeon when invading the interior of another person's body feels, that is touches, the organs of another human being but also the ***feelings*** that both surgeon and patient might have; their emotions, which even in modern twenty first century medicine and surgery have an integral role to play in healthcare since as Roger Kneebone writes,

> When we think of medicine, we think of it only in terms as a science; however, it is very much an intersection between science, craft, and performance [8]

We believe this is as true in surgery perhaps more so, since surgery has all the hallmarks of artistic performance.

13.2 The Word

> In the beginning was the Word, and the Word was with God, and the Word was God. [9]

This quotation at the beginning of the gospel according to John highlights the primordial importance of language. Rob Riemen in his book "Nobility of Spirit" comments, "Language is the essence of being human. We can think, thanks to language, for thought exists only by the grace of words. Our experiences and emotions are molded by language" [10]. This is no different in a medical context, and, although in surgery, the surgical act is often envisaged as the essence of the surgeon-patient relationship, that does not diminish how critical the words spoken between surgeon and patient are; we cannot deny that Rudyard Kipling's comments to the Royal College of Surgeons of London in 1926 were, and still are, of paramount importance in this relationship,

> Words are, of course, the most powerful drug known to humankind. [11]

One hundred years later, when medication and the technology available to both physicians and surgeons have been completely transformed, these words still emanate powerfully since words are never spoken in a vacuum and they must always be seen in their particular context. They have the power to build or break trust and establish or destroy confidence. In contrary to modern-day assumptions about surgery, the word and language are integral to the doctor-patient relationship, and, at heart, the surgeon must always be a good doctor to be a good surgeon.

> Seeing comes before words. [12]

Patients bring fear, anxiety, and self-pity into the consultation with their unique experiences (illness), and these feelings are often exacerbated when they are alone in the operating theater or in the surgical ward, naked apart from wearing a backless and flimsy hospital gown. The surgeon always has the responsibility to soothe their fears and provide hope when "the lights of health go down" [13].

The accomplished surgeon needs a proper bedside manner or bedside behavior that is humane and compassionate, and often it has been proposed that this ritual when developed with harmony and adequate time is responsible for establishing the formation of a surgeon-patient bond; "the beginning of a therapeutic partnership and the healing process" [14].

However, nowadays, there is growing concern that the essential components of the bedside manner skills are disappearing in our technology-focused practice of surgery, and the word and the language, that are principal components of the bedside manner are being lost. We are entering a language-free limbo.

What must the surgeon look for, or how must they regard their encounter with the patient? First, their look, and second, the spontaneous body expression and initial behavior. The Spanish physician, historian, and philosopher Laín Entralgo puts it well when he describes the instant when a doctor and a patient meet and look at each other. "For a moment, their eyes become the vector centers of their reciprocal communication. Later, perhaps after a brief fraction of a second, the oral expression—the word—will take over this central and organizing function of interpersonal communication; but, although in the background, the eyes will not cease to participate in it" [15]. The doctor's gaze—the doctor's expression through the vector center of his gaze—must above all provide a place of refuge for the suffering and needy existence of the person who asks for technical help [15].

After the first visual encounter comes the moment of the bidirectional narrative (conversation) between the patient, who narrates their personal experience, and the surgeon with the interpretation of the patient's story as "clinical history" [16]. In the words of Roger Kneebone, conversation, different from history-taking, is a deliberate process of construction that depends on giving as well as taking. It is the heart of clinical practice. It requires close listening and a generous-minded attention to what the patient is saying or not saying [17].

The word is the key to the contact established between those who need help and those who can help them. The word, in that first encounter, calls and names the patient and simply in the act of being called by name, the patient feels extracted from the mass, he finds himself, in the same way, personalized, liberated [16].The word asks questions and inquires about his ailments: it is an inquisitive word. But it is also a conductive word as far as it directs and modulates the patient's words: it stimulates them in their meaningful silences, and it reassures them in their excessive, verbose phases.The word of the physician or surgeon, finally, suggests or affirms the diagnosis, reassures the patient as to his prognosis, and proposes the treatment [16].

Silence is an integral part of language and in medicine even more so. Laín Entralgo discussed three kinds of silences: the pre-significant silence, the significant silence, and the trans-significant silence [15]. In the first, silence is like a background silence, similar in many ways to background music since it is the basis in which the words are formed. In the second, significant silence, something important is expressed and this can be through a look [a gaze], a gesture, or simply the act of not speaking. In the latter, trans-significant silence, the emphasis is on the silence in which the true meaning of the words is expressed. Good clinicians can read, or even see, the patient's silence in the same way as musicians know intuitively when silence is the key to the music.

We can envision four potential scenarios where the surgeon and the patient can have a clinical encounter (the preoperative visit, the operating theater, the postoperative period, and the aftermath/continuity of care).

The first is one of the most important because the surgeon and patient meet for the first time, two unknown human beings, one asking for help and the other with the capacity to provide a technical solution to their problem. The dramatic character of the relationship between the patient and the surgeon in their first encounter is the consequence that the surgical intervention they discuss is an aggressive act, with a curative or palliative intention. This aggression obliges that in the conversation between patient and surgeon in which the surgeon explains the benefits and risks of the proposed intervention and the patient his doubts and fears, the surgeon's language, that semantic air that comes out of the teeth in the words of the Spanish philosopher Emilio Lledó [18], transmits the appropriate security to the patient and at the same time, is humane and compassionate.

The language used by the surgeon when speaking to the patient is very different to that used by another medical specialist, such as an internist. This is because surgical language, per se is built predominantly around essential surgical words such as *operative field, excision, resection, ablation, radicality, reconstruction, hemorrhage*. These words by nature are aggressive since the surgical act is aggressive too.

The warlike metaphor of surgery is evident in the description of the surgical intervention, which takes place in an operating field, by means of a previously designed strategy (this is the technical option chosen a priori by the surgeon) and with the tactical variations that the operative findings and the development of the operation/combat make advisable.

In the patient/surgeon relationship, the aggressiveness of the surgical language must be tempered by the surgeon's own language: cultivated, sincere, compassionate, open, and reassuring. A language that allows the conversation between the two protagonists to conclude in a pact of trust that turns what is too often an aggressor/victim relationship into a healer/patient relationship. By doing that in an adequate manner, the patient invites the surgeon to access the interior of their corporal space rather than the surgeon invading or penetrating that space.

Frequently, during the surgeon-patient conversation prior to the operation, the surgeon draws a figurative explanation of the procedure that he will perform. So here, curiously enough the surgeon is using both the hand and the word to reassure the patient who is about to undergo the operation (Fig. 13.1).

The second encounter or scenario is in the operating theater; for most of the time the patient is anesthetized, asleep, and unconscious on the operating table if given general anesthesia. At this moment, the touch of the surgeon is key to the surgeon-patient relationship, however, the words that the surgeon says to the patient just before he falls asleep can be of the utmost importance since, they can reassure, comfort, and calm the patient. Nonetheless, there are other words being spoken in the operating theater since during the operation there are many more involved than just the surgeon and patient, and, once again, Roger Kneebone explains this beautifully [19],

> In the operating theatre, different voices are in play. At the center is the scrub team – those who operate on the body itself. Around them are other members of the group – equally important but differently so – and all have different voices. He continues to describe the different voices,

ABC

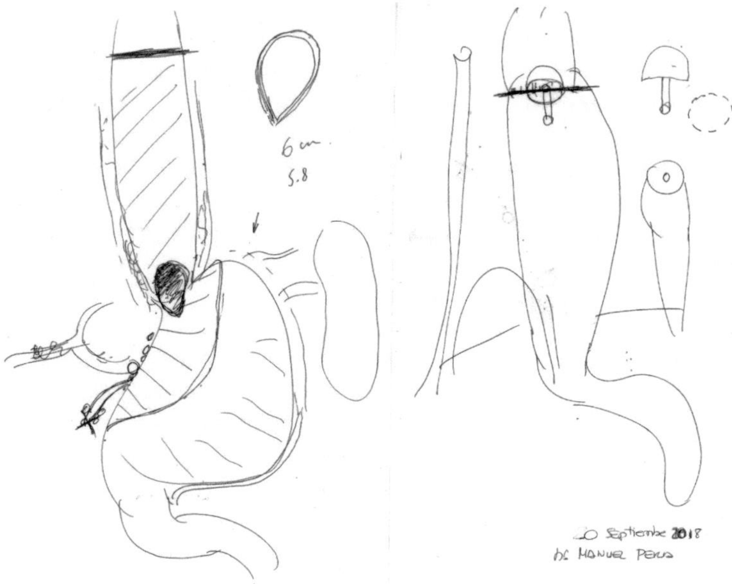

Fig. 13.1 Drawing of a total gastrectomy (Manuel Pera)

> The surgeon's voice is often muted, soft, muffled by a mask. Intended for the scrub team only, it may be inaudible beyond. Voices spread out in ripples from the scrub team: requests for instruments, instructions to others in the theatre.

However, what is fascinating in Kneebone's interpretation of the role of the word and voices in the operating theater is his insistence that often the most important voice is silence, and especially in critical and complicated moments,

> But if things are going badly, you sense the tension without even knowing how. The most eloquent voice of all is the voice of silence: the voice that says, 'we've got a problem here and we all need to focus on fixing it. [19]

After the operation, which hopefully has been successful, the job of the surgeon is by no means finished since he needs to be in the presence of the patient while he is recovering. In this moment, both the word and the touch of the surgeon can prove extremely beneficial for the recovery of the patient since compassionate care (involving both language and touch) "can improve patient outcomes, satisfaction, and loyalty as well as reduce stress and burnout for health care professionals." [20].

Of critical importance is to understand that the role of the surgeon continues; to some extent the operation is only the beginning of the journey that the surgeon and patient share. J.M Little describes this well in his editorial "Ethics in Surgery" [21], "surgical procedures leave scars, both on and in the body, and in the psyche. The last skin suture is not the end of the surgical story, nor does it end with discharge from hospital." Although supposedly cured, often patients undergoing a surgical procedure may remain with lifelong symptoms and sequalae that may even worsen their quality of life. Ellingsen S et al. [22] correctly noted that "health personnel must also become aware of their responsibilities to patients, understanding the need for critically ill patients to receive more complex and long-term follow-up." We agree. However, all patients need a long-term follow up, and again the presence of the surgeon plays a critical role in the journey with the patient since his words may even improve the outcome. Arthur Frank, in his book "The wounded storyteller" uses the term "remission society" to describe all those people who, like him, were effectively well but could never be considered cured. These people are all around, though often invisible [23]. In fact, in the end, everyone will be part of the remission society.

13.3 The Hand (Fig. 13.2)

> Colour is the keyboard, the eyes are the harmonies, the soul is the piano with many strings. The artist is the hand that plays, touching one key or another, to cause vibrations in the soul (Wassily Kandinsky) [24]

> We are animals, yet we behave like gods. Darwin riffed on *Hamlet* in 1871 in his second masterpiece, *The Descent of Man*, declaring that we have 'god-like intellect', yet we cannot deny that man – and woman – carries the 'indelible stamp of his lowly origin' [25]

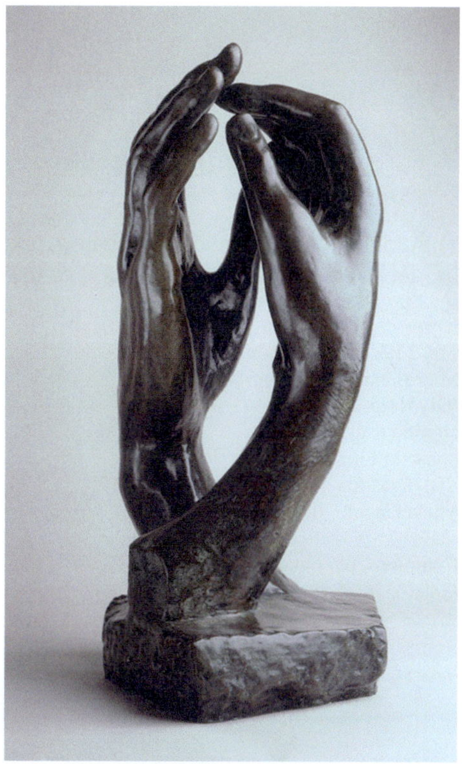

Fig. 13.2 The Cathedral, August Rodin, 1908 (https://commons.m.wikimedia.org/wiki/File:85_La_catedral.jpg#filehistory)

The hand is imbued with symbolism; it is all in the hand, and you only need to think of English expressions with the hand; "to lend a hand," "to give a hand," "to offer a hand," all of which are connected to helping another, person, sufferer, and soul. The hand symbolizes help, support, friendship, and love. The hand distinguishes us from all other animals on the planet and has been endlessly debated and discussed throughout history. The symbolism of the hand is infinite; indeed, William Blake wrote, "Hold infinity in the palm of your hand" [26].

The French poet, Paul Valery, spoke to the doctors and surgeons on the 17th of October 1938 in the amphitheater of the School of Medicine, just as the English poet, Rudyard Kipling had done little over a decade earlier to his English counterparts. Valery's speech "Discourse to surgeons" is a beautiful piece of poetry and philosophy, of its time as you can tell when he refers to gentleman· but as all great speeches or writings it is timeless in its beauty and its relevance [6]. He comments,

> If the surgeon is to be described as an artist, it is because his work is not reduced to the uniform execution of an impersonal programme of acts. An operating manual is not a surgeon. But there is, I think, more than one way of cutting and dispensing, and each one belongs to each one.

And once again we can see how the use of the hand is compared to that of an artist,

> Surgery, hand that operates, that works, hand of work, work of hand.

13.4 Touch (Fig. 13.3)

> Touch *comes before sight, before speech. It is our first language and the last, and it always tells the truth.* [27]

And then there is touch. The warm, assuring touch of mother's hand; the lingering feel of a lover's hand in yours; or the quick firm handshake of a colleague or

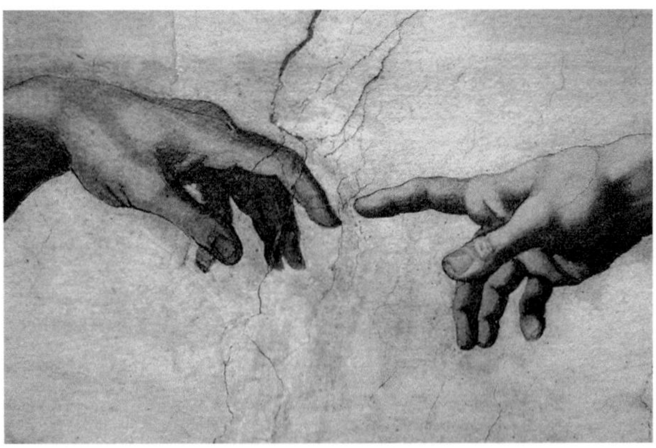

Fig. 13.3 The Creation Michelangelo, Vatican, Italy (https://commons.m.wikimedia.org/wiki/File:The_Creation_Michelangelo_Italy_Vatican_-_Creative_Commons_by_gnuckx_(3492637902).jpg)

acquaintance- in each instance, fingers against fingers, palm against palm, and yet a multitude of different emotions are conveyed [28]

These two quotations show how important touch is for human connection and communication; in the first, Atwood conveys how touch could be as important or more in communicating with another human, while Sternberg beautifully conveys the emotions behind touching. However, in recent years there has been a touch-skepticism mostly because of the touch prohibition during the COVID-19 pandemic that still lingers but also due to the #MeToo movement. The pandemic changed everyone's relationship with touch; it became taboo, like coughing or sneezing in public, and perhaps we now need a renaissance in touch and touching, especially in the healthcare context. The neuroscientist Laura Crucianelli wrote [29],

> What's unique about touch, when we set it against the other senses, is its mutuality. While we can look without being looked back at, we can't touch without being touched in return. (The need to touch)

Crucianelli highlights the mutuality of touch, and states, "*In a pandemic where touch is a proven vector, paradoxically it's also part of the cure,*" and this reminds me of the surgeon who needs to harm his patient by cutting through the skin to cure him [29]. The doctor and writer Abraham Verghese comments on how "*touch is so much more than touch,*" and in his article, A Touch of Sense, he laments how doctors touch their patients less and less, and, although it was written before the pandemic the trend was not initiated by it but has been steadily increasing due to the advent and rise of medical technology and especially imaging [30]. Young doctors use X-Rays, CT scans, and MRIs before human touch, and although this could in part be explained by defensive medicine (especially in the USA), this is not, I believe the principal reason. Verghese writes,

> *They find that the real action in the hospital revolves around the computer…* and continues that the illusion has been created that there is no other way to "see" the body.

"*The physical exam is really about one individual granting permission to another individual to touch his or her unclothed body, to probe their ticklish and private places.*" It is a privilege, a ritual concerning trust, which is the critical element to a good doctor-patient relationship, and it is worth remembering that one of the main complaints of patients about physicians is that "*they never touched me.*" This seems highly relevant and even more so in a technology-dependent twenty-first century.

Another physician who talks about touch as a language is Roger Kneebone [31], whose medical journey has been interesting, moving from trauma surgeon to GP to Professor of Academic Surgery, in discussing the importance of the physical examination adds,

"*What I didn't realize was that I was also learning a tactile language, a form of communication that worked in both directions. By constantly examining patients I was establishing a lexicon of touch that went far between distinguishing a lipoma from an epidermoid cyst.*" And interestingly he alludes to touch as vision and explains that clinicians often talk of teaching their fingers to see, which seems especially pertinent in surgery.

But before exploring the importance of touch and surgery more deeply, let us return to the roots and where the word comes from. Some words are beautiful and others not, and although beauty is in the "eye of the beholder" touch, for me, is a beautiful word, and like "hand," it has a diversity of meanings. Coming from the French word "touche" by the late fourteenth century it had come to be understood as "a *sense of touch, that sense by which pressure upon the surface of the body is perceived*" but also a "way *something feels*." In the arts it radiates meaning too; in music, the "*act or manner of handling the instrument to bring out its tones*," and in the visual arts the "*skill with the brush, pencil*." [32]

In this chapter section, we will cover all these meanings since they are all connected with surgery and the hand.

In a medical context, the hand and touch are critical for a surgeon as Cristobal Pera notes, "What *does the surgeon do with his hands? In the first place, he develops a technique in the operative field, a kind of know-how, in which* ***his hands are the instruments of instruments****: he cuts, he dissects, he binds together, he sutures. All these actions he accomplishes with a personal rhythm, which attempts to be, at one and the same time, energetic and caressing, marking the movements that strive to be beautiful through eurythmy*." [33] The bold letters are mine because they go back to Aristotle's—the tool of tools—which Pera highlights but he also emphasizes the "beauty" in the work of the surgeon, and its eurythmy, a Greek word meaning a system of harmonious body movements to the rhythm of music or the word. So, we return to the essence of this chapter—*the word and the touch*.

Escribano et al. [34] emphasize how the hand of the surgeon holds a weapon that wounds to heal; the surgical act balances between life and death. The technical (or instrumental) act handles this balance act.

Van Manen defines the noetic (or cognitive) hand as a "*data collecting instrument manipulated in a diagnostic manner*," explaining how,

"*The human hand is marvelously equipped to be receptive to different types of sensations. Medical and nursing handbooks provide a great deal of detail about the practice of palpation and a sensory discrimination detected through the use of the hand*." This coincides with the phenomenological vision proposed by both Husserl, emphasizing tactility and Merleau-Ponty who explores the critical role of the double-sided nature of touchant/touché since as Escribano [34] highlights, "*It is not possible to touch without acting on the object and without the object acting on oneself*" or Radman notes, "*the touching hand receives feedback from the touched object.*" [34].

This double-edged nature of touch is incredibly important in medicine in general, but surgery in particular for the surgeon in touching the patient, delving into the body of another person is being invited by that person to do so; it is a reciprocal action, which can also have spiritual connotations so deep is the bond between the toucher and the touched; the subject and the object, the surgeon and the patient.

The last kind of touch and perhaps that which embodies the humane act that the surgeon is doing in attempting to cure the patient, and in caring for that same person, is the affective hand. Curing for the patient is not always possible but caring for them, yes. Escribano [34] writes,

"The intention of the pathic touch is to provide support, comfort, company, reassurance, understanding, etc." Van Manen goes further when he says,

> This pathic quality may well constitute the core meaning of the healing act…If, as a patient, I trust this hand then it has the power to reunite me pathically with my body, reminds me that I am one with my body, and thus makes it possible for me to heal, to strengthen, to become whole. [34]

Touch is at the center of medicine but unfortunately, and, to the detriment of health care, nowadays it does not have this centrality either in medical education or clinical practice. Roger Kneebone starts his short essay "Getting back in touch" [31], "*Clinicians and patients are getting out of touch with one another.*" This is little short of tragic for, even though the advantages and benefits of advances in imaging techniques are indisputable, touch is far more than solely a physical action as Kneebone stresses, "Touch *is more like vision, where imperfect signals are processed into a rich and complex sensory experience. It is no accident that clinicians talk of teaching their fingers to see.*" Touch allows the clinician, in this case, the surgeon to see as well as feel the patient, and to communicate on many diverse levels.

But when we are talking about the surgical hand and its importance, what about robotic surgery? Robotic surgery has been around since the mid-1980s [35] but began to be used more frequently in the late 1990s when the Californian based da Vinci surgical system came into use. In some ways, the robotic arms of the machine can be seen as an extension of the surgeon's hands.

"He places his forearms on rests and uses hand controls to manipulate robotic arms fitted with surgical grabbers and clippers. Watching a high-resolution screen, Bathani, who is at St. Paul's Hospital in Saskatoon, Canada, guides the tools to perform minimally invasive surgery for prostate cancer" [36]. The surgeon, Bathani, says, "The visualization is incredible," and "That 3D view that you get makes surgery that much better, that much more precise." So, paradoxically the robotic hand can be seen as a more precise version of the human hand. However, there is still much debate over whether robotic surgery is better than traditional minimally invasive surgery since there are many drawbacks, including time and expense, and some surgeons doubt the benefit of this new technology,

"We still don't actually have a lot of proof that they're better than old-fashioned surgeons—at least old-fashioned surgeons doing minimally invasive surgery" [36], says Peter McCullough, Professor of Surgery at Oxford. So, the debate is open and presumably we will still be debating this in the coming future.

However, perhaps we are overly optimistic, but we believe if correctly used the new diagnostic and surgical "tools" will benefit the surgeon since they will ideally complement their touch. The critical importance of touch will not diminish, but, on the contrary, these new technologies will allow the surgeon to have more time to show their empathetic and compassionate side when treating the patient. J.M Little [21] underlines the critical value of "the patient's need for the surgeon's presence throughout the illness and beyond," [which] "will help us as surgeons to establish and maintain trust and a relationship of care with patients who are particularly vulnerable." The hand and touch elicit the trust that is central to the surgeon-patient relationship.

13.5 Conclusion

> Surgery is first and foremost a moral activity with a noble tradition of compassion, altruism, and public service. It is now time to reaffirm that tradition. High technology and humanity can coexist. [37]

Even though the University of Padua dates back to the thirteenth century and the first recorded autopsy was made by Pietro d'Abono (c.1250-c.1315) in the same century it was not until the sixteenth century when Andreas Vesalius, a Flemish anatomist, came to Padua in 1537 that dissections became an established part of medical education. Vesalius became Chair of Surgery and carried out regular dissections on criminals but also on dogs and monkeys. It was here in Padua that he worked on his masterpiece "De Humani Corporis Fabrica Libri Séptima" (On the fabric of the human body in seven books), which was based on his lectures in the Paduan amphitheater, and where he introduced the ***demonstrative method*** to medical education that implied an active involvement in studying anatomy, now based on the direct observation and verification of theories: henceforward, it became a habit for students not only to read books, but also to approach the subjects physically (Fig. 13.4).

It is interesting to note that the anatomy lessons were the only form of practical lessons in medical education with the theater enhancing the theatrical element of a real ceremony. Even more interesting is that it was also linked to the number seven, and its seven rings can be connected to the seven skies of Empireum, or the seven pits of Hell in Dante's Divine Comedy. So, the element of ritual is strong, and we believe that this component was crucial in those days: the touch of the surgeon-anatomist was critical in teaching new doctors as well as his word to explain what he was doing and why.

Thus, we hope that in this chapter we have emphasized the critical importance of the word (discourse) and the hand (touch) in twenty-first-century surgery and medicine in general, and although technology (with the continuous advancements in robotic surgery, AI, and other technologies) will play an increasingly crucial role, this is not the sole answer but what is of supreme importance is how future doctors and surgeons use language and words and the hand and touch to care for the patient. In the end, caring for the patient is more important than curing since we are not, and never will be, immortal.

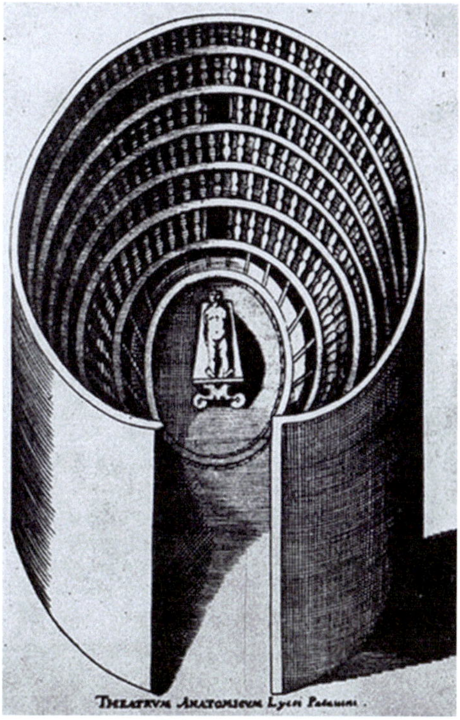

Fig. 13.4 Gravure représentant le théâtre anatomique de Padoue parue dans le *Gymnasium Patavium* de J. Ph. Tomasini paru à Udine en 1654 (https://en.m.wikipedia.org/wiki/File:Gravue-Gymnasium-Patavium.jpg)

> He *who works with his hands is a labourer. He who works with his hands and his head is a craftsman. He who works with his hands, his head, and his heart is an artist.* (St. Francis de Assisi)

13.6 Afterword

The aim of our chapter has been to defend the need for surgery to concentrate on the relationship between two persons: the surgeon and the patient. Unfortunately, in twenty-first-century medicine, healthcare systems around the world and the environment that they establish seem to construct barriers, leading to a complication in this relationship. Medical education, and thus clinical practice has been consistently evolving through an ever-stronger emphasis on the scientific side of medicine and so negating the humanistic, or compassionate, side of medicine.

Sir William Osler words [38],

> Care more for the individual patient than for the special features of the disease…. Put yourself in his place… The kindly word, the cheerful greeting, the sympathetic look—these the patient understands., are still relevant now.

References

1. Marsh H. Do no harm: stories of life, death and brain surgery. London: Hachette; 2014.
2. Dunne C. Carl Jung: wounded healer of the soul. Watkins Media Limited; 2015.
3. Stevens, Anthony. Jung/Anthony Stevens. Oxford: Oxford University Press, 1994. Print.
4. Dalai Lama XIV Dzin-rgya. The art of happiness. A handbook for living. Hodder and Stoughton; 1999.
5. Trzeciak S, Mazzarelli A. Compassionomics. The revolutionary scientific evidence that caring makes a difference: Huron Consulting Group Inc; 2019.
6. Valéry P. Discours aux chirurgiens. París: Gallimard; 1938.
7. McGlone F, Chatterjee R. Feel better, live more. Podcast, Episode 45. https://www.drchatterjee.com/touch-forgotten-sense-professor-francis-mcglone/; 2019.
8. Kneebone R, Kneebone D. The art of performing science. Utrecht University; 2019. https://www.eventbrite.com/e/tim-lecture-the-art-of-performing-science-roger-and-dusia-kneebone-tickets-60196933649?utm-medium=discovery&utm-campaign=social&utm-content=attendeeshare&aff=escb&utm-source=cp&utm-term=listing
9. John 1:1–5 King James Version (KJV).
10. Riemen R. Nobility of spirit. A forgotten ideal. Yale University Press; 2008.
11. Kipling R. "Surgeons and the soul," speech. London: Royal College of Surgeons; 1923.
12. Berger J. Ways of seeing. Penguin Books; 2008.
13. Woolf V. On being ill. Ashfield: Paris Press; 2012.
14. Verghese A, Brady E, Kapur CC, Horwitz RI. The bedside evaluation: ritual and reason. Ann Intern Med. 2011;155:550–3.
15. Pedro Laín Entralgo. La relación médico–enfermo: Historia y teoría. Madrid: Revista de Occidente; 1964.
16. Cristóbal Pera. La Mano y la Palabra. Archivos Españoles de Medicina Interna. N° 2 (March–April), 1968.
17. Kneebone R. The art of conversation. Lancet. 2018;391:731.
18. Lledó E. Palabra y Humanidad. KRK Ediciones; 2015.
19. Roger Kneebone. https://www.theguardian.com/science/blog/2013/nov/06/secret-language-surgery
20. Strange TJ, Castellanos MR. Medicine—both a science (care) and an art (CARE). JAMA. 2024;331(16):1357–8.
21. Little JM. Ethics in surgical practice. Br J Surg. 2001;88:769–70.
22. Ellingsen S, Moi AL, Gjengedal E, Flinterud SI, Natvik E, Raheim M, Sviland R, Sekse RJT. "Finding oneself after critical illness": voices from the remission society. Med Health Care Philos. 2021;24:35–44.
23. Frank A. The wounded storyteller. Body, illness and ethics. 2nd ed. Chicago/London: The University Chicago Press; 2013. p. 8–13.
24. https://www.cherylmachatdorskind.com/color-is-the-keyboard-the-eyes-are-the-hammers-and-the-soul-is-the-piano-with-many-strings-kandinsky/
25. https://www.theguardian.com/books/2018/sep/21/human-instinct-why-we-are-unique
26. Stevenson WH, editor. Blake: the complete poems. 3rd ed. Routledge; 2007. https://doi.org/10.4324/9781315761169.
27. Atwood M. The blind assassin. McClelland and Steward; 2000.
28. Esther M. Sternberg—the balance within: the science connecting health and emotions. St. Martin's Press; 2001. p. 140.
29. Laura C. https://aeon.co/essays/touch-is-a-language-we-cannot-afford-to-forget.
30. Verghese A. A touch of sense. Health Aff (Millwood). 2009;28:1177–82.
31. Kneebone R. Getting back in touch. Lancet. 2018;391:1348.
32. Merriam-Webster Dictionary. https://www.merriam-webster.com/
33. Pera C. El Cuerpo Herido. 1st ed. Barcelona: Acantilado; 2003.

34. Escribano X, Pérez-Bellmunt A. The therapeutic hand. In: Bertolaso M, Di Stefano N, editors. The hand: perception, cognition, action. Springer; 2017.
35. Kwoh YS, Hou J, Jonckheere EA, Hayati S. A robot with improved absolute positioning accuracy for CT guided stereotactic brain surgery. IEEE Trans Biomed Eng. 1988;35:153–60.
36. May M. The next generation of robotic surgery is emerging: but is it better than a human? Nat Med. 2024;30:2–5.
37. Organ BC, Claude H. Organ, Jr, MD: a son's tribute. Arch Surg. 2005;140(11):1052–4. https://doi.org/10.1001/archsurg.140.11.1052.
38. Osler W. Aequanimitas: with other addresses to medical students and practitioners of medicine. 2nd ed. Philadelphia: Blakiston's; 1925. p. 3–6.

Chapter 14
Conversation with Surgeon 7—James Handa

René Génadry

Recorded online on March 6, 2024, by René Génadry

Abbreviations

JH: James Handa
RG: René Génadry
CME: Continues Medical Education

RG: Good evening, Jim and thank you for making yourself available. I know that you've been working for a long time overseas, right?

JH: Yeah, I did, 27 years going to the Republic of Palau to do some mission work. It was mainly focused on diabetic retinopathy and it was a really interesting story: one of my colleagues was giving a CME course on diabetic retinopathy, and this was right at the time that Diode laser technology had been developed; all of the prior lasers were the size of a large closet, because it needed to be water cooled and Diode laser took away the water so the laser fits into a suitcase, and so his last slide was a picture of a suitcase with the laser- and his statement "I can go anywhere in the world…" And there happened to be an internist in the audience from Palau, he said "we have this explosion of diabetics," but nobody to look at their eyes! so we started going over and went 27 years in a row until COVID hit: we've been shut out since then but we're planning to go again next year; over time, that morphed into doing cataract surgery: this is an island nation on the equator, so the intense sun also brings out cataract formation, and so we did cataract surgery. From a surgical experience, the issues changed through the years, there's no question about it and that is germane to this topic.

R. Génadry (✉)
Carver College of Medicine, University of Iowa, Iowa City, IA, USA

J. McFarland et al. (eds.), *Humanism in Surgery*, New Paradigms in Healthcare,
https://doi.org/10.1007/978-3-031-86018-8_14

RG: That's fascinating. So, it was circumstantial basically, the exposure to that presentation that gave you the opportunity to get started, but what motivated you? Is it something that just happened, or is there something that created that desire to go ahead?

JH: Well, I think it's multifactorial. When you work at an academic institution, there's a lot of bureaucracy: the patient's clientele sometimes is different, so you tend to get a bit more litigious patients who come in with their lawyer to want to render your opinion to see if they should go forward with a lawsuit that the prior doctor had screwed up their eye or something like that; and I think cumulatively and as we've gone toward the electronic medical record where we spend more time with our back to our patients, you lose the essence of what it means to be a doctor, have that doctor patient relationship, and having the opportunity to step out of my comfort zone and go to a remote region of the world and really feel like I could make a difference on a small scale, but a clear difference to help people out, I think it was worth the risk. It also happened to be a beautiful region of the world and the opportunity to go with a really good friend from my residency who, when we work together we just kind of seamlessly work together, we just had this sort of telepathic ability to communicate to make the patient flow go well when we were residents, so it was an opportunity just to build the friendship there as well, and we both were scuba divers. That happens to be a great place to go scuba diving, so every aspect was a win-win, I think. But one of the things in terms of the doctor patient relationship was that through our 27 years of going there, you really do get at the essence of the doctor patient relationship where you really get to talk to the patients, they're extraordinarily appreciative of anything you do. There's this implicit trust that develops and that it really comes back to the roots of why we all become doctors. In addition, we learned the language and you get away from this litigious society: through the 27 years we had gone there, there had never been even the threat of a lawsuit anywhere in the medical system in Palau, just didn't exist. And that's a really refreshing environment to be in.

RG: Yeah, it's a humane relationship that really brings you back to what you went in the profession for; it's really a calling, and it's the expression of such calling as it should be basically.

JH: Yeah, and you can practice forward medicine instead of defensive medicine, right? How often do we get a test just to make sure we do it, so we cover ourselves as opposed to getting a test or planning something to look forward; so, I think there is a comfort in that, so removing yourself from defensive medicine is always nice as well.

RG: Jim, did you always go as a team with your colleague in residency?

JH: Yeah. When we first went there, we would see sort of 500 patients over the week and then we would sort of count up. We typically would do probably 50 or 100 laser treatments for diabetic retinopathy, and then we would do anywhere from 25 to 50 cataract operations. So, we would see patients all day and then we would do procedures or operate. They would feed us dinner at the hospital, and then we would go to the operating room until 9:00 or 10:00 at night; and at the end of it, each year we would tally up how many patients we would see and the procedures performed and then we would make a calculation of what it would cost to do those patient visits in the United States; and then we would add the cost of air flight to and back and hotel and the amount of money was in the millions of dollars that we would save them. So, the Minister of Health sat down and just said we would like you both to come back on a yearly basis and that's what we have done ever since: it's just a gentleman's handshake agreement and I think, so long as we provide the necessary care and the commitment and they're happy, then it continues. It was interesting that they had consultant doctors from different regions of Asia, and we saw some of the poor care that was provided, and they were aware of the poor outcomes, and we would educate them as to why. We also helped them identify places to go when we're not there; we always look to improve, so we did provide technology to them. For instance, we bought these simple retinal cameras to take pictures of the retina, and the idea is that they can take those photographs and use them as triage in their diabetic clinics, and they can send the images to us. We can analyze them: so, it's like a free visit 6 months before we go and so we can say here's what we want to see, here we don't want to see, and in that way when we go over, we'll see the patients who really need to be seen. Thus, our ability to help those in need increases, as opposed to those who are doing well, which is great, but that's not a wise use of our time when we're there for a limited period; so, each year we've improved the care. It's kind of funny in terms of the cataract surgery, at the beginning there were so many cataracts where they're completely white cataracts so people could only see movement in front of them, they couldn't recognize the face, or who the person was. So, pretty much whatever we did was fine. Obviously the cataract surgery is much more sophisticated than that, it became much more savvy and their standards rose and so it got to the point where we said you know we should really have a cataract surgeon: so, there is a Hawaiian eye foundation and a cataract surgeon who flies around that whole region of the world and we connected this person with Palau, and so that person goes over and does cataract surgery 6 months apart from when we go, so between that and our remote imaging now we've got three potential visits a year; so we're providing 3 typical care of what diabetics need in this country. Each year we've tried to improve the healthcare that we provide to the Islanders who are literally in the middle of nowhere.

RG: So how do you get to Palau.

JH: It's a 24-h flight. Either I would fly from Dallas to Hawaii to Guam and then into Palau or sometimes I'll fly from Dulles to Tokyo and to Palau. I have also flown to Seoul Korea and to Palau. There are several ways, but any way you look at it, it's a 24-h flight.

RG: I'm sure it's worth it because it sounds like you're running a very efficient organization there.

JH: Yeah, and you know we give lectures on different aspects of eye care that the emergency room docs can use. We learned the language so we can get through an eye examination in Palauan, and through the diving and the downtime we've kind of immersed ourselves in the community: that has been helpful in gaining trust among the people there.

RG: That's great. I'm sure you must have started out having a lot of challenges initially.

JH: Initially yeah: when we first got there people didn't know how to measure the vision, there certainly was reluctance to having dilating eye drops put in their eyes and saying that their vision goes blurry and their eyes are bright; those kind of things were obviously at the beginning but everybody spoke English, broken English but the language issues were always something; there were clearly words that don't translate or things that we would say had different connotation, those kind of things and then of course on the other side was the equipment or lack thereof. So, we would solicit different instrument companies to get donations so we bring a slit lamp, and we got an operating microscope and an autorefractor so people can get the right prescription for the glasses. Each time we would go over there we would try to bring some sort of infrastructure to build up which helped, but the weather is so harsh there with the humidity and the heat that the equipment just corrodes faster than it does here so that always requires updating. Those were kind of the big barriers but I think one funny story I remember having with the language issue: I remember I examined this elderly woman and the eyes were healthy, no diabetes changes and so there's this term that goes 'ungil amadam' which means 'healthy eyes,' your eyes are healthy but in a different context, if you were in the bar, it means you have beautiful eyes and the way she looked at me, and she looked at the translator, and they started talking for about 3 min and they started laughing and they started pointing out and told me what it was: it was kind of a funny circumstance, but I think that sort of highlights the kind of issues that you encounter.

RG: And it helps build trust I'm sure, and that's what you're trying to do in the beginning when they don't want to have their eyes dropped into, that kind of interaction, although funny in a way and risky in this country, can be useful over there.

JH: When I reflect on the years which have passed, it makes you forget about the troubles that we had, but really the acceptance by the people of what we were trying to do was seamless. And I think some of it is cultural, so the origins, these are fishermen and hunter gatherers by history, and there's this certain mental toughness that they have: when we would do the laser, sometimes the laser could be a little bit uncomfortable with the bright light you know, they wouldn't flinch at all, and they wouldn't admit if there was any discomfort or anything like that. So, I think that kind of overall cultural mentality probably made it easier. It certainly didn't scare anybody away, and I think as people saw improvement and success, word travels quickly.

RG: I'm sure it takes more than their toughness; it has to do with the provider. Jim, you know as I was trying to get your phone number and your contact online, I looked at your profile and I was very impressed by how you were perceived by your patients in the community, and so I'm sure that is what they perceive too over there and that is fantastic.

JH: I think it's important you try to treat people the way you want to be treated. Life is pretty simple. I think if you're straightforward and honest, I think people appreciate that, even if you must deliver bad news.

RG: True. Well, let me go back before I go forward, we talked about motivation and we talked about the initial time when you got started, is there anything in your background, in your childhood when you were growing up that had set you up on that path or is it all circumstantial?

JH: Well, it's very interesting: I'm Japanese and we're the very prototypical Japanese Americans in this country; my grandparents came over from Japan because, in the early 1900s, the economic climate was very tough, and they were given a new opportunity to come here. My dad grew up in a very financially troubling background of a farming community in California, and then he was drafted into World War 2 while my mom was interned during the war. So you know it's a troubled time but one of the things that my dad did and eventually after the war, (in the war he was made a medic) and that motivated him to go back to school and go to medical school and he became an anesthesiologist; and because he never had anything growing up, he always said to me that he wanted to give his kids everything that he didn't have; and so he just kind of projected that it's important to give back and to be generous, and I think maybe that had a big influence on how I look at the world. I come from privilege, but I don't feel like I need to have a lot of money to be happy, but I get a lot of enjoyment by giving back, and I think that probably has it, and you put that with the opportunity to be with a good friend and go scuba diving and that's win-win.

RG: Sure, you make the circumstances happen. Has there been any mentor that has played a role or is there anybody else besides your dad who obviously was the major influence there, any colleague as you were going through medical school and training and so on, anyone in that area that might have influenced you?

JH: Sure. During my residency there were several doctors who participated in this program called Orbis; Orbis is a nonprofit group that would take prominent ophthalmologists and fly them to impoverished regions in the world to provide eye care. I think that had an impact on me, because after my residency I thought about doing that for a year before doing a fellowship. Then when I thought about what they exactly were doing, I didn't agree with it: they would go to someplace in Africa for instance, they would do cataract surgery, help these people and then they leave. And there was nobody left qualified to take care of the patients or provide postoperative care; and it's something that my colleague Mark Wieland and I have discussed when we started doing this. The intent was really to help a few, we obviously weren't going to save the world, but we could have an impact in this particular location; and one of the big impacts was building on something going back year after year. And so, I think we learned from those colleagues, my mentors, I thought it was very altruistic, but it also forced us to analyze how it could be better. And so at least for what we do with the amount of time that we spend I think we've been very satisfied with the direction it is going.

RG: You were impressed positively and negatively, and you made the best of it.

JH: It is interesting, one of the people who I really admired who was doing that was my chairman and he happened to be an avid diver and when he learned that my friend Mark and I were going over, I saw him at a meeting and he said do you think I could go over with you, and I said, yeah you know you're 15th in line.

RG: That's right whatever the reason it works. How about medical students, Jim or residents has there been any interest in this professional circle that have been influenced, affected, interested in contributing?

JH: There's no question that there's interest, definitely. Medical students and residents have approached me but there just hasn't been capacity or an opportunity to do it. It is interesting this past fall there were two medical students from the University of Hawaii who called me because they had done a rotation on Tropical Medicine in Palau, and they we're interested in going into ophthalmology and when they found out about the program that Mark and I have been going over they got very excited and so they started resurrecting some of the programs and they've been looking to try to improve the infrastructure, organizing the diabetic clinics and reimplementing things that kind of stopped during COVID. So, the plan is theoretically they're going to help us when we go over in the fall; whether that actually happens I'm not sure because one thing we've learned is when you're dealing with a third world country the intention is always good, but the implementation can sometimes be challenging, whether it's lack of money or other things come up…

RG: Is it possible under the circumstances to train anybody local there or you know just primarily lectures that you provide them with and so on.

JH: In Palau, it's really very interesting what they did: they have the foundation of some outstanding doctors, so they have several internists who've been American or English trained, they have a surgeon who is US trained, they have a gynecologist who was UK trained and they had an expatriate pediatrician. And all of the Palauans who have been US trained were identified in the beginning of high school and they were then pushed and given scholarships to complete high school, college and medical school and residency in the United States with the intent of going back. So, the government actually funded their education; and as the Paluans say they want to return home, despite the greater financial opportunities in other regions of the world because they say when you live in paradise you have everything: you don't need a lot of money. I think it's true and so I think that's the foundation. The issue with ophthalmology is that the number of people with eye problems is not enough to keep a full-time ophthalmologist busy. And so there hasn't been enough motivation for that. What has actually happened through the years is that one of the internists has been interested and we have trained him, not only with the lectures but we've taught him to use a fundus camera that he can send us stuff when there's a problem and periodically e-mail us for getting advice; and he actually opened up a separate clinic to take care of simple things, and he's able to give glasses and simple things like that. There has been that aspect of it, but in terms of a surgeon, there's just not enough demand to do it.

RG: I'm sure you see a lot of pathology that is useful to bring back and use to teach medical students here.

JH: We haven't seen a lot of exotic diseases. It really is a lot of bread-and-butter complications from diabetes and cataract and it's interesting you know like myopia (near sightedness) is a rare event. There are a couple reasons: it turns out that sunlight exposure 60–90 min a day dramatically decreases the prevalence of myopia, and there's some science behind it, so obviously in a very sunny climate that's not a risk. The other thing we've sort of hypothesized is genetics: these are fishermen, that's a fishing culture and to see far on to the horizon, to see the little ripples in the water to see where the fish are as an advantage to survive and when we go fishing with the doctors they all see the ripples and we see it you know 100 yards later, because we're myopic, but the other thing is that they're hunter gatherers by nature, and so genetically they're like the Indians in the southwest: their tendency to gain weight is really easy, so metabolic syndrome, hypertension, obesity and then obviously diabetes is a real problem as they transition from a fish and Taro, which is like a low gut glycemic index potato, and fruit and vegetables diet to Budweiser, lays potato chip and spam that's really where the problem lies. That's the bulk of what we see. And like glaucoma, which is obviously very common, doesn't really exist on the island; the only glaucoma patients we see are those of mixed race that have Asian or other blood.

RG: Well, I'm sure you must have had a lot of fascinating experiences there Jim. Is there a patient or any circumstance or any event that has impressed you significantly there that is worth relating?

JH: There are a couple of experiences I think are really kind of unique: when we were sort of feeling our way around one of the things we were trying to do was get enough outreach, so we took one of our slit lamps and we put it on a boat, and we went to some of the remote islands. We would be on a boat for 2 h to get to the island, and probably 20–50 people live on it. We would go to the dispensary, and they would come to us, and these people are just dirt poor. We would evaluate them and assess their cataracts or their diabetes. And that was a very eye opening experience, because these are people who are suspicious of medical care, they don't feel like they need medical care, but one thing we did that I think helped was a simple gesture: we would bring over a bunch of reading glasses, and we would just predict based on their age what strength glass they need, and we would give them the glasses and at the end we would show them a document to read, and they would be astounded at how much clearer that was. I think to see that for the first time, to see how satisfied they were, was really amazing! I think some of the first cataract surgeries we had was really kind of funny: when we took it off of one patient and obviously this was a while ago, the patch goes off and the patient looks at me and says: "you're my doctor and you did the surgery?" and I say "yeah" and they go: "you look too young!" so that was really kind of funny. So the other kind of funny thing was they would, to give us a break when we'd be seeing patients, they would come in and they would have coconuts that they crack open and give us a straw and we would have coconut milk but I think those kind of stories the outreach and the glasses and then the realization after cataract surgery of restoring the vision: there definitely is the cultural norm for older people to go blind, and to have that restored was at the beginning really a powerful experience; and as more and more people got cataract surgery, then people started going off island when we weren't around and then the expectations rose and it got to the point where -Oh well we want cataract surgery and not need to have glasses afterwards-, and that's when it got a little bit out of our control. We didn't have the instruments to be able to calculate the right strength power lens implant into the eye…

RG: So, do you buy the lenses or are they given to you by charitable donations.

JH: All the sutures and all the supplies that we need were all through donations. The other interesting thing because they don't have much, they would ask us to bring over things: one of the things they absolutely cherish were the disposable little alcohol swabs, they loved having those swabs that we throw away or write notes on them. We would always bring stuff like that, or shoe covers, and they cherished them. It forces you to think about how we utilize our supplies, how we practice medicine; there's so much waste in what we do...

RG: Well was there any challenge in trying to get some time off to go? I'm thinking of a young physician who's interested in going there, any challenge in trying to make it happen at that time.

JH: No, it was really all in my own vacation time. The problem was really scheduling at a good time for Vicki and myself; and then early on, when the kids were young it was a big load on Vicky, so she was very tolerant of allowing me to go. That was really the bigger issue.

RG: I'm sure you must have seen things changing positively over time over there. You had the support of the Ministry of Health, obviously that makes it easier. Has there been any change in the physical environment over those 27 years or is it the same as when you first went there?

JH: It's pretty much the same. So, when we first went there, there was this old hospital and then it turns out that Palau was a UN trust territory which, following World War 2, the United States was assigned to manage, and so consequently US taxpayer dollars-built infrastructure. When we first went over, they had built a new hospital which still exists, and it's a beautiful hospital that has a lot of the typical amenities that you would have in any outpatient clinic: they have inpatients there and the OR's, no ICU per se, but they have got dialysis so they were able to administer dialysis and things like that, and that really hasn't changed all that much other than a CT scan came. They would get grants to make things more modern, but I think we took a lot of modern-day things for granted. When we first got there, water and power would shut off at 10:00 at night and go on at 6:00 in the morning. So, you had to adjust for that. You know improvements in the sanitation for water were made so you could drink water out of the tap if you want; these were really big things that were important for public health. I think they were very shrewd in emphasizing preventative care in public health, mainly out of necessity because preventative care was going to cut down the amount of dollars they needed to spend and so that's where most of their efforts have been such as simple things like controlling blood pressure, weight loss, and improving the diet. In the Town Center, they have this billboard where they would show how many patients were screened for diabetes, and how many people actually had diabetes, so they there was really a strong public health initiative to identify diabetics to make people aware. The other thing that was really interesting was when we first went there, there were no traffic lights and through the years as we went back, there was one, and learning about the public education needed just to have people obey the traffic light, learn the meaning of a red light was a significant undertaking …and then we would see two lights the next year, and then up to seven lights later, so it was interesting.

RG: Well Jim you are teaching and training students and residents, do you think the humanities have a role in the making of a humanitarian physician?

JH: I think it should. I think today's medical education is so focused on becoming competent in your specific field and I think in many ways rightfully so. Certainly when I look in ophthalmology when I look at the sophistication of how we examine or assess the patient, it's strikingly different even in the career that I've had, and so the amount of information that I think trainees need to know today is dramatically more than what I was expected to know; so I can appreciate that, but I always think there needs to be a time to pause to provide that humanitarian side to medicine. I don't know how you do that, but I do think that it really kind of gets back to reinforcing and emphasizing why people should be going into medicine. So, I certainly have let students know about my humanitarian trips to Palau, and I've given talks about going over and giving back and things like that, but I'll be honest with you, I get asked more to give talks about what it's like to be a clinician scientist than I would be asked to talk on how to be a humanitarian physician.

RG: I guess one can give back in so many ways and does not have to go far to do that. I mean there certainly are a lot of needy people in our own backyard that one can give back to. The question that I think is critical is: is it important and possible with all the material that medical students really must acquire to pause a bit and to use art, to use literature, to use movies to try to bring out that human dimension in interpersonal relationship between the physician and the patient. I don't know how you evaluate that which we now describe under the heading of professionalism, but that's industry getting into the picture, and I don't know how you identify that dimension of a physician except through seeing directly that interaction with the patient.

JH: Yeah as I think about it, we really look at endpoint metrics, so we look at patient satisfaction scores, are you a 4.5 or point 4.9 out of five, and you look at the comments that patients write about you, when we renew reappointments we look at professionalism or dress or getting appropriate consults or how we interact with staff which are all important but I think the reason I made that initial statement is I don't think that in medical school we actually teach how to treat people. I think in some ways it's a little bit like being successful in business, the bottom line is you want to get the right people on the bus and the wrong people off the bus, and then if you have the right people you don't need any rules because they'll just do the right thing and so by the same way, if we are selective in choosing people who have this, whether it's learned or natural tendency toward humanity, we're going to be better off. I don't know if that is circular reasoning or not, but I do think that you want to look for that potential when you're selecting students, and then I think the big gap is figuring out a way to embellish those skill sets. I do know that I still remember when I was in medical school, we started out very early where I went to do physical exam and diagnosis on patients and it was very much impressed upon us the importance of treating the patient with care and compassion, and part of that was learning how to make sure the stethoscope was warm before you put it on the person's chest, or whatever, little things like that. I think there was a lot of informal things that I took to heart. I remember when I was a resident one of my attendings said you know when we examined the eye looking in the retina we actually have to open the lid or touch the forehead, and the attending said how hard you press on the lid is an indication of how you're going to be as a surgeon: you want to be very gentle; it also portrays that you're very compassionate and a thoughtful person when you're examining, and don't turn the light on too strong, use the minimum amount of light so that you don't cause too much discomfort to the patient. So, I think those are the kind of things that we need to have. How do you formally integrate that into a medical school curriculum I don't know, but in today's world as we go toward the electronic medical record and things like that, I think it would be a welcome break to incorporate. I'm not all that much at the medical student level and I just don't know if that is in the curriculum, but I would highly endorse that, or even having it so that students get the opportunity to go away and to do a charity work would be a really valuable learning experience.

RG: Unfortunately, in a lot of studies done on medical students, their level of humanity seems to decrease progressively in favor of the technical and scientific aspect of medicine. And when you compare 1st and 2nd year students to preclinical students, as they move on to the third and 4th year of clinical work, the degree of empathy, the degree of interest in the whole patient seems to progressively decrease. I agree with you that selection is critical to make sure that the right people are in the profession but is there any place for a formal structured course in the humanistic care of the patient?

JH: Yeah, I think there's definitely a role for it. I think about it in terms of both formal education and informal one. I think if you had a semester long course I don't think that would be all that helpful but I think if you had these periodic humanities courses to teach empathy or different approaches, hands on role-playing where you get a difficult patient or you get a different circumstance, where you have to try to figure out how to show your humanity or be compassionate in your difficult circumstances, I think that could be a very valuable thing on a formal basis; and then again I think it's really incumbent upon the medical schools to recruit appropriate faculty. I'm sure you're the same. Many of my mentors, in terms of the success that you want to have, you tried to emulate: like for instance with my surgical training I can still hear the voices of my mentors telling me what to do, that you have to do it this way; so I think because medical training is at such an impressionable period of one's life and you have the opportunity to train with some really special people, I think making sure that they're more than just a great surgeon or great doctor, but to be able to show compassion toward their patients is needed.

RG: Role modeling and example are important indeed such as the amount of pressure to put on the eyelid during the examination…

JH: Yeah, and I think that small gesture for me forced me to really think about how I can make the eye exam as least as unpleasant as possible, and it's particularly important when you have someone who's scared or if you have a kid or a young person to gain their trust and to make it less unpleasant, that I think is critical.

RG: Thank you so much Jim if I may ask you a final question: who are you? how you would describe yourself with that background and what you're doing and the wonderful work you're doing overseas and at Hopkins, how would you present yourself?

JH: Let me say I guess in many ways I feel like I'm the luckiest guy in the world. I don't really feel particularly unique or special. I feel like I've been afforded plenty of opportunity and I've really kind of tried to take full advantage of all the opportunities I've had, and you know, I've kind of told other people that I feel I didn't really set my professional goals high enough, because I reached a lot of those probably a decade ago, and it actually forced me to think: well am I done with medicine? do I want to do something different than what I ultimately decided to do and it was to try doing some leadership and mentoring, so I focused more on that and that's wonderful. It has been very rewarding for me, so I guess that's how I sort of describe myself.

RG: Wonderful, a lot of gratitude, a lot of empathy and interest in the next generation.

JH: Because I have an active research lab, because I see patients and I operate and I teach and I mentor, I think when I look at some of my colleagues who are in private practices or do the same thing day in day out, and they made a ton more money than me, but they're all looking to retire, and each day is different for me. I think the variety of what I do helps me keep things exciting; and then of course being at Hopkins where you have really smart medical students and residents and fellows, they keep me on my toes: I think that the fear of being embarrassed by the people you're teaching keeps you on your toes.

RG: Well, no matter how great they are, Jim they've got plenty to learn from you. I do hope they realize it, they might not immediately, but they will one day learn what to do and certainly what not to do. Thank you so much, is there any parting words that I haven't asked you about that you think would be important to mention?

JH: No, I think this is a wonderful and needed idea that you're doing, so I really praise what you're doing.

RG: Well, thank you, thank you so much Jim.

Chapter 15
Shared Decision-Making

João M. Silva

15.1 Introduction

«Shared decision-making in Surgery: deconstructing myths» is intended to be a report on several issues regarding how patients and doctors behave nowadays and how they interact with each other. Medicine and Surgery have changed a lot over recent decades. Patients don't see doctors anymore as guardians of the secrecies of the body, and doctors have lost some leverage over the patients and see them more suspiciously.

There are many myths to be deconstructed.

This chapter will address the following ones:

1. Myths regarding "the Doctor";
2. Myths regarding "the Patient";
3. Myth of "Surgery";
4. Myth of "the System backing the Surgery";

The "patient–physician relationship," once seen as the cornerstone of Medicine, is challenged today by several factors. To mention three that are of paramount importance: generalization of the access to medical knowledge, development and widespread access to new technologies (CT, MRI, and other lab tests), and decreased quality of the humanistic education in society in general.

All this together is contributing to a profound change in the relationship between doctors and patients. Certainly, fewer mistakes are made regarding the diagnosis and the generalization of the access to medical care is something positive. However, what we should think of is the "quality of the diagnosis" and "quality of Medicine" overall.

J. M. Silva (✉)
Consultant Neurosurgeon at Unidade Local de Saúde de Santo António, Porto, Portugal

J. McFarland et al. (eds.), *Humanism in Surgery*, New Paradigms in Healthcare,
https://doi.org/10.1007/978-3-031-86018-8_15

Better and quicker diagnosis does not mean better Medicine. They mean more Medicine but not better! More Medicine means more appointments, more surgeries, more procedures overall. That is certainly good for the business of the medical world, but certainly not better for patients. How to distinguish and define the border between these two concepts? The section "Myths regarding Surgery" aims to find some answers to these questions.

How can doctors behave in a world where patients ask for solutions and employers for production? How to behave in such a circumstance where conflicting values are fighting each other? These questions are fundamental in the everyday practice of Medicine and Surgery.

There are four founding principles of medical ethics:

1. Beneficence
2. Non-maleficence
3. Autonomy
4. Justice.

To these principles, others have been added, namely Integrity, Vulnerability, Responsibility, Respect, Dignity, among others, as stated in the Universal Declaration of Bioethics and Human Rights [1].

When there are conflicting values at stake, it is up to the doctor to deliberate with the healthcare team and decide on the most prudent way to act. This means that the personal code of conduct as well as the inner values and beliefs of a doctor often plays a role when balancing the values mentioned above. The value of utility should be highlighted in this context, meaning the need to balance benefits and risks for the patient as an individual and for society as the community where the patient lives. When considering something (an appointment, Medicine, or Surgery) for a patient we must consider if any additional value for the patient and society is enacted by such an action.

Shared decision-making in Surgery has a small history when considering the History of Medicine. The paternalistic view of Medicine that was a dominant view until the twentieth century did not consider the patient's will regarding a decision to be made on his or her body. That was up to the doctor to decide, because that decision was embodied with the power of knowledge and the sense that something good is expected from that decision. Medicine was also profoundly different. Patients sought medical care when the disease was established and very often advanced. Also, the diseases were profoundly different since life expectancy was considerably shorter. The diseases that we see today, most of them related with an ageing population, were not a problem.

Infectious diseases were dominant until the late nineteenth century—cholera, typhus, smallpox, tuberculosis, syphilis, etc. There were no effective treatments for them until the mid-twentieth century. However, in the western world these are now treatable and curable diseases. By contrast, cardio- and cerebrovascular diseases were seldom a problem, as well as cancer or degenerative diseases. Nowadays those are the leading causes of death and disability in modern societies. Why did that epidemiological shift pose a problem to Medicine and to patient–physician relationship? The section myths regarding "the doctor" and "the patient" will address this problem.

We will then address the issue of "Surgery nowadays"? Why such a topic? Was Surgery in the past different from today? The answer is undoubtedly "YES." However, the details behind the answer are often hidden from public eye. Of course, we changed from a paradigm of surviving the Surgery to the paradigm of returning quickly to normal life after the Surgery. Surgery once viewed as a sentence of death is now widely seen as a sentence of cure. This has a profound impact on how the patients see the surgeons.

Finally, shared decision-making in Surgery: from the paternalism to informed consent. The profound shift in the role played by the patients and the resistance of many surgeons to accept that, especially when the desires of the patients do not match the opinions of the surgeon. We'll try to unveil the surgeon's behavior when this happens and why this is so important for the patient–physician relationship.

15.2 Patient–Physician Relationship

Patient–physician relationship is being challenged like never before. The super-powered doctor is not a reality anymore, and the super-obedient patient no longer follows the recommendations all the time. Patients question more: question their diseases, question the diagnosis, and question the treatments. They ask for second opinions, assuming that Medicine is an exact science, and they don't often understand when prescriptions and treatments vary from different doctors. What patients don't know is that Medicine tries to be scientifically based but actually is highly art-oriented. Doctors fear to be questioned, do not like to assume gaps of knowledge, they are not used to discuss and argue, frequently sticking to their dogmas, and they don't really consider that patients have the right to question their own problems. This is especially true in the surgical field.

All those problems pose a tremendous pressure on the patients who face different opinions and are told that in modern Medicine "they must decide!" How can someone rationally decide on something without a proper knowledge of the disease? We, doctors, don't have a good answer to this. We simply say, "this is my recommendation, now you decide."

'Myths regarding the doctor' are based on this. Patients think simultaneously that doctors know everything, but do not plenty trust them. When consulting a doctor, patients ask for answers for a very important issue: their own health. However, they have in advance an idea of their disease, they "googled it." From the myth of "super-powered" doctor to the reality of super-confusing doctors' opinions, the path is very narrow. Patients usually come to our offices with an idea of their disease; however, they don't know the rationale behind our thinking nor our thought process. And that rationale is not the same for every doctor/surgeon. That single fact generates confusion and makes that myth of super-powered doctor obsolete. Actually, doctors become super-confusing. How can we solve this problem?

The answer is in the "myths regarding the patient." Doctors/surgeons usually think their patients are ignorant and they don't know nothing about Medicine. Patients usually know nothing about Medicine, but they are surely not ignorant. That is the myth to be deconstructed about patients. Doctors need to understand that people care about their health; they want to be healthy, productive, and alive for as much time as possible. The "myth of ignorance" needs to be deconstructed by doctors because we are the ones that know this in advance. Patients are not ignorant; they just have a fair expectation, given by our society, that they can live longer and healthier.

We know that patients try to be informed about their diseases, we know that their information is biased, without a proper context, devoid of a rationale and very often wrong. But we also know that patients are asking for our opinion even though they think they already know what their condition is about. So, it is up to us to carry the conversation to a point where they can understand fully the 'reasons that fundament our opinion.

Additionally, there are three issues greatly challenge the patient–physician relationship in modern times:

1. Generalization of the access to medical knowledge.
2. Development and widespread access to new technologies (CT, MRI, and other lab tests).
3. Decreased quality of the humanistic education in society in general.

Generalization of the access to medical knowledge is a tremendous achievement of modern societies. If we go back only 50 years in time, in Europe for instance, the access to medical care was very scarce, especially in rural areas. It must be acknowledged that the economic transition from an agricultural-based society to an industry-based society and, recently, to a services-based society has facilitated the widespread to medical access. Despite all the problems, the societal and economical gaps constantly decreased over the last 150 years, and this paved the way for more people to have resources to pay their medical care. Moreover, the healthcare public-based system has greatly contributed to this increased access.

These achievements surpassed any difficulty that they raised. However, the more people are educated, the more people are coming to our offices. This factor has raised pressure on us, doctors, "accelerating our time." This had a tremendous impact on patient–physician relationship. The once standard of detailed clinical history and examination was abbreviated: "no one has time for that." Patients, then, feel abandoned, feel that what they say is not important, doctors do not examine them, don't listen to them, and don't even look at them.

And how have doctors filled the "gap of examination"? With more and more detailed tests! Even without talking or examining a patient, we can now know what his or her condition is and offer some kind of treatment. Replacing clinical history and examination with more and more tests has greatly damaged the patient–physician relationship. Nowadays, we could say we are living in the era of physician–tests relationship. Patients come to our office with a bunch of tests, and as time goes by they rely more on the test's results than on any other source of information, including the doctors. What happened then? We, doctors, don't have the time to talk with patients. The now standard 15-min appointment, sometimes less, has destroyed the trust the patients had in doctors. How can we trust someone that doesn't even speak to us?

This brings us to the last issue of this topic—the lack of humanistic education in society in general. With increasing access to technology, to a subspecialized Medicine, we have forgotten that we are still doctors, not technicians or mechanics of the body. Being a doctor is something much bigger than that. Being a doctor is being a confident of people secrecies (of the body), and the secrecies of the body often mirror the secrecies of the souls. But to be that gatekeeper demands time, education, learning how to conduct an interview, how to assess problems other than "body problems." Being a DOCTOR requires time, communication skills, empathy, the will to treat the person, not the disease. And this is about humanism, not technique or scientific knowledge. We need to go back to the old psychological and philosophical books and instead of focusing our attention only on the most recent scientific papers. Summing up, we need to see the persons who have the disease, instead of seeing only the disease. Hopefully, the future of medical schools will be one where evidence-based Medicine will walk side by side with Humanistic Medicine. A very strong scientific-based Medicine can only be possible if there is a profound sense of humanism in the Art of Medicine. Over the last 50 years, the curriculum in the med schools has been adapted to the new paradigm of Medicine, integrating all the scientific knowledge and all the new specialties that have appeared. Humanism has been neglected. Scientific knowledge allows us to treat patients but only humanism transforms someone who treats patients into a real doctor.

15.3 What Does Humanism Mean for Us?

Humanism mean the ability to feel the problems, to understand the patients, to speak the same language they speak. With current very specialized Medicine, doctors feel they are super-specialists, and they with lack of communication skills. Medical Humanities allow us to build therapeutic relationships with the patients; if we only use our scientific knowledge to understand the disease, we will lack the opportunity to understand the patient, the human being in front of us. This is especially important for young doctors—understanding that the current subspecialization has the purpose of serving the patients, not our egos. Knowledge without humanism is not useful when dealing with the patient.

Arriving here, it is of utmost importance to discuss the concept of utility in medical ethics.

We have so many expensive resources at our disposal that we must always consider the purpose and how they provide clinical meaningful benefit for the patient. So, beneficence and respecting the patient, addressing what really matters to them and can positively impact the natural history of his or her disease is a measure of our success and must be assessed for every procedure or Surgery that we do. If any Surgery does not respect this principle, it shouldn't be done. We, in the surgical field, are concerned with discharging the patient as quickly as possible and advise them to resume work as quickly as possible but on the long run do we assess if our surgeries have changed the natural history of the disease and have been translated to clinical meaningful benefits for the patients?

Together with beneficence and respect, we should consider the principle of utility, that is not used here as the simple integration of beneficence with justice. Utility means that, when considering a treatment or a Surgery, some benefits must be expected for the individual person and for society as a whole. When using medical resources, especially when they are public, and when speaking of non-malignant diseases, especially degenerative ones, we must assess our ability to modify the natural history of the disease when planning a treatment. The principles behind the treatment of different diseases must be valued accordingly. No one questions the personal benefit of treating a cancerous lesion in a 50-year-old woman. However, treating an 85-year-old citizen with a cancerous lesion is of dubious personal and societal interest. Utility must be used here. This is particularly important today. Because we spend a huge number of resources treating persons and diseases where a very small clinical benefit is expected; and those resources are lacking to treat other people or implement other policies that may have a greater impact on the society.

People are not ignorant; they understand what the reasons behind our decisions are. The policies must be clear, and a proper assessment of resources must be done. Then, with medical support and advice, it is up to policy makers to decide how far we should go in the treatment of certain diseases in different groups of patients.

So, what remains of the patient–physician relationship nowadays?

The remains of it are a bit destroyed by time and by the evolution of our society. New answers must be found, and old concepts sometimes help us to unravel those answers. We know that patient–physician relationship is not well but many of us fear to find the answers to fix it because we very deeply know the answers will lead to a profound change in our daily clinical practice.

15.4 Surgery Nowadays

As we stated in the introduction, in 50 years we have changed from a paradigm of surviving the Surgery to the paradigm of returning quickly to normal life after the Surgery. Once viewed as a sentence of death, Surgery is now widely seen as a sentence of cure. The paradigm of a 2- or 3-month hospitalization for any surgical condition is now surpassed by methodologies like ERAS "enhanced recovery after Surgery." It is not uncommon, for example, in neurosurgical meetings to listen colleagues saying that patients resume working the next day after a lumbar disk operation and some are discharged in the evening after a craniotomy for a small tumor.

So, conditions that once required prolonged hospitalizations or posed a significant risk of death are now seen as "little problems."

This has led to a false sense of safety in Surgery and people believe that Surgery is so beneficial that being operated in not anymore a problem, which is not true.

15.5 What is the Problem Then?

The problem is the "myth of Surgery," believing that Surgery is the "best treatment," the "most definitive" of all treatments at our disposal. Patients for several reasons and surgeons for others have fed this myth. Patients because they need something to stick with when other options are more inconvenient: resume a more healthy lifestyle, lose weight, do more exercise, solve family or work-related problems, among others. Doctors, because we want to keep working and to do so, we need patients willing to be operated. This has created the perfect match in our society. An unhealthy aged population with behaviors that enhance the problem of degenerative diseases and a group of people (surgeons) pressured by their employers to keep working at a high pace in order to increase the profits for themselves and their institutions.

Surgery is of course a wonderful tool that allows several conditions to be treated and some of them cured. However, it must be used parsimoniously and very carefully not to seed the idea that it is the best and definitive treatment, because it seldom is.

Surgical conditions and technical capabilities in the past were much more different than today. The widespread access to medical care allowed the detection of disease at an early stage, making their treatment easier and safer. That is the reasonable part of the explanation.

The dark side of this story, however, is related to the pathology. With limited resources in the past, those resources were oriented to real and significant pathologies. The patient selection of the past was determined by the diseases, not by the surgeon. A huge part of the pathologies that we treat today, especially degenerative disease can be managed conservatively. The healthcare resources are still mainly hospital-oriented and used to selectively treat a small number of patients. What we must think about is why this works in this way, who this benefits, and why those that become under threat do not complaint about that?

The very simple example is degenerative spine diseases. The large majority of those problems must be treated conservatively but resources are needed in the community: more access to physiotherapy and nutritionists, incentives to do exercise, and have a healthier lifestyle. This is not done at all and, in the opposite side, we see an increasing number of patients being operated in our hospitals to these problems. Numbers are unknown but we never spent so much money in these diseases as we spend today.

This has an obvious explanation: In many countries the healthcare became a business. And like in any business, the more you do, the bigger are the revenues. So, to the healthcare business world less patients means less money. Unfortunately this is done at the expense of people that are regarded as consumers, not even patients!

So, who are the ones capable of stopping the problem? The doctors!

Then, why isn't the problem being solved? Because doctors do not have the courage to stop it. Because the institutions and the industry demand more surgeries and we are committed to follow their wishes. Instead of being conservative, we try to be more and more aggressive—we "follow the literature, the tendencies." We are always trying something new because we became tired of doing the same again and again. And that something new is very often more expensive, sometimes more riskier… But we, surgeons, feel that we are doing something great to the patients. We did the first case of this or that, that's our goal. Our egocentrism is our biggest enemy because it often endangers our commitment with our patients well-being.

In areas like degenerative disease, the natural history of the disease is often benign and the life-expectancy of the patient is big. So, doctors feel sometimes obliged to treat that condition, even though we know those are conditions where no cure can be offered, only alleviation of suffering/pain.

However, in the natural history of degenerative diseases the patients are not suffering all the time. However, since we only have 5 or 15 min to listen to them, we only listen the part where they complaint of pain. The causes underneath that pain we don't listen because we don't have the time! Then, we often miss the social, working, and family problems that very often greatly potentiate the pain. So, we easily start the endeavor of treating pains that can't be treated surgically and this often is the starting point of a never-ending story.

Majority of surgeons act in good faith. They think they can help, clinical evidence supports their practice but what they often miss is that patients are not exams nor exams mirrors patients. Treating a CT or an MRI often has no meaningful clinical benefit for the patient other than the try to explore the placebo effect to alleviate patient suffering. And patient selection for Surgery takes time, sometimes more than one or two appointments and that is seen today as a waste of time and resources!

On the other side, patients demand solutions, and Surgery is seen as safer and a curative option. What patients don't know is that in majority of cases, and virtually in all degenerative disease patients, Surgery is not curative, only a bridge to resume a more healthy lifestyle. Patients don't know that any surgeon in the world can fix in a 2–3 h Surgery something that took decades to develop but, anyway, they hope, and sometimes demand, that this can happen. Then, we're back to the problem of time! With more than one or longer appointments this could be properly explained to the patients so they can understand the real magnitude of the problem. Instead we do not talk with the patients, we focus on main clinical symptoms (that everyone has), rely on CTs or MRIs and clearly overtreat patients because they want.

Afterwards, when the treatments don't have the expected result we say "we did everything we could, it's not anymore my problem" and the patient has nothing to do except to accept because he or she wanted that Surgery and now has to deal with another failure. A meaningful dialogue would spare hundreds of thousands of surgeries across the world every year.

This is what Surgery largely became nowadays—a way to institutions/companies make money, to surgeons keep working at a very high pace and patients feels that they are treated when they actually are flesh to keep the machine working!

15.6 Shared Decision-Making in Surgery

Now we must deter ourselves in the problem of shared decision-making, meaning, informed consent. What is informed consent nowadays? And what it should be in the future?

To those familiar with informed consent, in this new world of non-paternalistic Medicine, informed consent became a tool to pretend the treatment decision is of the patients and all the surgical or procedure-related risks are accepted by the patient while, in the reality and in the majority of cases, patients don't have a clear idea of the risks they are taking nor the decision is truthfully of the patient because a thoroughly discussion of the different treatment options did not take place. And it is not usually possible to do this—time doesn't allow!

Does this mean that informed consent is a lie? Yes and no.

Yes, because we do not respect the premises of it.
No, because patients do not complaint of the fundamental errors underlining it.

Shared decision-making takes time—to understand the patient, to understand the disease, and to shape the treatment to specificities of the patient. Without time there is no informed consent, there is no shared decision-making. Without the proper time what surgeons do is to give a paper the patient to sign with a brief explanation of the risks the patient is taking and that he or she is fully consenting something that he or she doesn't understand at all. This is done every day in the large majority of surgical departments.

So, how to change this?

Empowering the patient, release the doctors of the convenient paternalistic thoughts, giving them time to talk with the patients and taking them out of the center of the storm in what institutions and companies transform the surgical business. This brings to us to a very hot topic which is the discussion on healthcare systems. Public or private base, which one is the better?

Here we come to the myth of the "system backing the Surgery." We will focus on public-based systems. Private-based systems are more expensive and lack the sense of community since they rely on individual person ability to pay for their healthcare. When people can pay the system works perfectly because all resources can be used. The problem is when people cannot pay—then the burden of the disease fall down over the person but the society is equally harmed since it is deprived of a good resource to keep it working. Public-based healthcare systems live in a myth—the myth they will last forever. They won't if we don't make choices. It is not possible to give everything to everyone. Policy makers, advised by doctors, must do choices. And explain those choices. Very expensive treatments that give a couple of weeks/months more of live (sometimes in poor condition) must not be offered. And they don't because those resources are needed in other areas. Politicians should not be afraid to taking these decisions and doctors must understand that we can't treat all the people we see. There are people to whom a viable treatment option is not available. Doctors/surgeons are programmed to cure; the problem arises when the resources we spend with some treatments impair our ability to reach and implement other measures that can have a more profound impact on public health. There are areas, namely Oncology, where this problem is of paramount importance.

With surgeons freed from the constraints enumerated above a public base system have enormous advantages. Resources would be better canalized for prevention and lifestyle changes, surgeries would diminish, and patients would be happier and healthy.

Coming back to shared decision-making! All the facts enumerated above have a huge impact on it. The pressure over the surgeons, the disputable clinical evidence, the power of the companies that have an almost free access to the institutions create enormous bias in the decision process and also in the patient–physician relationship.

To have a better decision-making, in order to it be truly shared we, doctors, surgeons, must rebuild our Medicine, and we must rebuild the patient–physician relationship—with more time to talk with a patient, freed from external forces that shape our thinking and with more humanism, meaning, putting the patients at the real center of the decision process. Without that, Medicine will vanish as other pseudo-sciences vanished over time. Medicine is about humanity! We live in an era that whether with stick to that or we will definitely loose the Art of Medicine that our predecessors built to us.

15.7 Conclusion

This chapter intended to be a short reflexion on the main questions involving the Medicine and Surgery nowadays. The problems of today's Medicine are also the problems of our time—intense training, subspecialization, and acceleration of processes. Those problems were intended to address the question of preparing people to be able to deal with complex problems and diseases. However, we are creating a generation of mechanics of Medicine, half-robots half-doctors that are no longer able to do the basics of Medicine—collect a clinical history and do a rigorous clinical examination.

The topics discussed above pretend to be an alert to these problems in order to build solutions to fix them and carry our Science and Art to a path of compromise between humanism and science with the patients at the very center of this stage.

Reference

1. https://www.unesco.org/en/ethics-science-technology/bioethics-and-human-rights.

Chapter 16
Conversation with Surgeon 8—Judith Goh

René Génadry

Conversation with Pr. Judith Goh.
Recorded online on February 22, 2024, by René Génadry.

Abbreviations that follow

JG: Judith Goh
RG: René Génadry
VVF: Vesico-Vaginal Fistula

RG: Thank you again for taking the time Judith. I hope you're not too exhausted from the whole day's work. As I told you, I would like to have your perspective on humanism in Medicine in general, and surgery in particular. It is remarkable that there is less and less patient care and more and more technological caring for patients. The question is what is the best way to try to re include a curriculum into medical school in order to bring back the humanities into medical care. Is it possible? What would it take? and so on. I'm going to record this conversation if it's OK with you.

JG: Sure.

RG: We are following the definition of humanism in surgery as the application of the scientific knowledge and the technical skills to the acknowledgement of the social, emotional, physical needs of the patient. Essentially caring for the patient in her entirety. You've been very involved in humanitarian work for a long time. How did you get there?

JG: I think it started off when I was a medical student, when I had the opportunity to travel to India to do my medical training. A lot of my friends were going to Europe and to other places, and I had the opportunity via a lady at church who used to be a missionary in India, and I think that being exposed

R. Génadry (✉)
Carver College of Medicine, University of Iowa, Iowa City, IA, USA

J. McFarland et al. (eds.), *Humanism in Surgery*, New Paradigms in Healthcare,
https://doi.org/10.1007/978-3-031-86018-8_16

to quite a different setting in terms of medical care; and poverty because I was in quite rural India so it wasn't like India now but it was very rural, very poor and I suppose that brought home to me that I should be very privileged with what I have: I shouldn't I suppose take things for granted.

RG: It must have been a bit of a culture shock coming back home.

JG: Coming home was a lot worse because I spent three months in rural India. Coming home then I suppose with all the excess and the wealth, and I came home around Christmas time: I still remember this too, I came, this was many years ago now, I came home around Christmas, and I couldn't believe the waste and the wealth that we had. Yeah, I think that's why it's important for doctors to have that certain exposure. I mean the setting from my point of view and my experience is to do it at a younger age, because once we become doctors we are very much into training. You know we just want to get into the training, we want to complete our training, then after training you have to think about family, you have to think about the family, then you got to think about "am I going to set up my private practice," "where am I going to work." You can work many hours without understanding what is beyond your border, so to have that opportunity at a younger age when you haven't got all that pressure of specializing, getting through the programs, finding a job and setting up practice etcetera, I think that's probably a good time to introduce the humanities to the young doctors and medical students.

RG: So, you think exposure is critical at the youngest age possible.

JG: I think so. I think just having that concept that Medicine can be so much more… I think that's important that the young realize it. I'm sure a lot of students who go abroad might not continue with it, continue to think about it that way, but I think to have those who want to, to give them the opportunity. I think that's important.

RG: So that exposure to the lady in church was critically important for you, but it must have taken some predisposition or inclination on your part.

JG: Yeah, I think I've always believed that if the opportunity for me anywhere in life comes up, I should take it. I suppose as a migrant kid that's what I think the opportunity is there, you should just take it and run with it and see what happens.

RG: So, is there any specific background that medical students should have that would predispose them to be accepting of such a vocation, if you will?

JG: I think it varies quite a bit on the person; quite a few medical students go over to the so-called elective in Africa, and even in parts of Asia, and they come from varying backgrounds. Just recently in the last 3–4 months, one student came from a working family, she was working herself to get through university, but she wanted to experience and to look at perhaps volunteering doctor; and on the other hand, I had a couple of students, one her father is a cardiologist and the other's mother is a gynecologist. So, it varies quite a bit I think depending on their perspective. I think the parents are important to encourage the students to think about these things.

RG: Now how did you pursue after that Indian exposure and what happened to your journey?

JG: So, I went to India, and I did a fair bit of obstetrics and Gyn and I enjoyed it, and I did enjoy OBGYN as a student anyway, and then I thought OK, so I think I really want to do this, so I started my training. In Australia as you probably know the specialization pathway is quite different, and we become the intern, and then a medical officer for a few years before we actually specialize. But the other critical point for me is that towards the end of my OBG specialty, I also had the opportunity to travel back to Africa. So, I knew an Australian surgeon working in Ethiopia and the opportunity came up for me to spend 6 months in Ethiopia.

RG: Great, when was that?

JG: That was in 95 so it was a while ago. So again, I took that opportunity and spent five months in rural Ethiopia which was some hard work as you can imagine. I had to deal with situations that I did not have to deal with in Australia; but that also gave me the opportunity to visit the fistula hospital. I spent a month at the fistula hospital and back then no one wanted to do fistulas, so it was quite easy for me to visit. I spent a month doing training in Ethiopia then the other opportunity came when the year after, so there was 95–96 towards the end of 96 Catherine Hamlin wrote to me and said that one of her two Ethiopian gynecologists was on maternity leave, with sciatica and she couldn't sit down so Dr. Hamlin asked me to go over to help and back then no one wanted to do it (fistula surgery). So, I took the opportunity and spent six months at the fistula hospital as the staff surgeon there. From there I was in contact with other doctors who came over for training. So, I suppose when I am looking back when I started medical school, probably as a first-year medical student, I would not have thought that I would be a fistula surgeon, that I'd spend so much time in limited resource areas but having had the opportunities and taking the opportunities led me down that path.

RG: Certainly, it must have been quite challenging to make room, to be able to leave whatever you were doing, and go on to relieve somebody in Ethiopia.

JG: Yeah, it was quite challenging because I just took up a position as a specialist at one of the hospitals, but I was quite keen to go. So, I found a locum for me, and thankfully the director there was quite supportive. I think it's just worked out well for me so I'm quite thankful for that.

RG: So, you must be proactive, you're going to get resistance but if you're determined, you can make it happen.

JG: Yeah I mean it's been a little bit of work, but it's the same like right now: I've got private practice to run as well, but I try to organize my year 12 months ahead and so therefore it doesn't cause too much disruption in my practice; my staff know that this is what I do because I've always been doing this, and patients are quite accepting of it as well. Once they know that I'm not just going on a holiday somewhere, that I am going to help, I think a lot of the patients are very supportive; if they have to wait a bit longer to see me there, they're quite happy because they know that I'm trying to help other women around the world.

RG: It seems like you have done it primarily individually; would you think that getting connected to an organization, to a charity or to a foundation would make life easier? Or will financial issues fall in place once people realize that's what you need to do?

JG: Sure, I went to some places that I go to, like in West Africa, I went on the Mercy ship so that makes the organizing, the visas, etcetera a lot easier because they help you, but it just depends on what you'd like to do. I suppose that if you are quite happy with your organization then sure, but I find sometimes that I can be quite limited in doing things; like if you go with MSF for example, they might not do what I think I'd like to do. So, it's a bit more organizing and a bit more time-consuming to do it on your own, but it can be done.

RG: A lot of people are limited by family, financial situations and so on, would you have any suggestion as to how to manage that?

JG: I think financially it just depends on your outlook in life as well. I mean as doctors we do earn enough money, so I'm not sure how much money people want to make; I certainly live very comfortably. I've got a nice place, so I don't think I'm missing out by spending money volunteering. So, I don't think that's a problem. In terms of family wise, I think it potentially could be a bit more difficult for women, but I think more and more even in training we have our women specialists or subspecialists whose husbands are happy to stay at home; and I've got to know a doctor from the Netherlands who is very keen to volunteer: her husband is supporting her and even with a couple of young children she would come over to do camps.

RG: So, when there is a will there is a way. Judith let me ask you this, what have you learned from all your travels of the needs of the surgical patient? if you could just give me an idea of how you conceptualize your approach to a surgical patient in a different environment, different culture and so on?

JG: So obviously I do my fistula work when I go overseas, and again as a migrant kid, I think "that girl or that woman could be me!" if I haven't had the opportunities that I had, That's how I see it, and that's how I've always thought: it's more than fixing the hole if you know what I mean right?

RG: Yes, absolutely. Judy, it sounds like the pivotal activity for you had been that trip to India initially. Is there anything in your childhood that you can think of that might have contributed?

JG: Yeah. I grew up for the first 12 years in Malaysia, multicultural, so it was quite normal to have people of different color, different face, different languages etcetera… so in terms of travelling and going overseas, it wasn't as daunting for me, because I might not be able to speak the language, but even when I was a child, I couldn't speak some of the languages that people around me could speak. So that wasn't too much of a problem that you think you can get by. I'm not sure to be honest, I mean I know some of my siblings would not volunteer; they will support me, they'll support what I do, but they themselves would not be doing the volunteer work.

RG: Now, has there been any mentoring that has played a significant role in your journey?

JG: Yeah certainly. I suppose that in the church that I went to, people would go east. When I went over to India, certainly there was an OBGyn there who was very kind, was very good and she taught me quite a few things. And so, I thought that's quite a good thing to do, yeah.

RG: As you were going through medical school, did you get any encouragement or any support from any of the faculty there?

JG: Not really, no. Because a lot of friends were, like I say, going to Europe or somewhere to do the elective surgery, so if I hadn't been at church I think I wouldn't have had that opportunity but I think having something for the students would be excellent: like an interest group or something, and then having someone who's been overseas like yourself or someone like that to be a contact person or to be a mentor for the students who want to go, that would be good.

RG: Great idea, so that would be a kind of channeling before mentoring if you will. But from the people you have been exposed to, do you think that there is any way to identify people that could be made more humanistic or humanitarian in their approach to patients or is it something that's innate?

JG: I think it's a little bit innate. I mean some people, once you finish your training, they fall into the trap of needing to run the practice and then the cost of running the practice that all becomes a bit of a problem; and then you know like it or not, being doctors and surgeons we're quite egotistical, others like to be looked to be busier than the other person etcetera so, you know, there can be a bit of that happening as well. I think it is important for students who are interested, to be given the opportunity before that happens. I call it the distraction of going to the specialty, and setting up practice, whereas I think if students who have that interest, if they've had a taste of what they can do during this training, there'll be the opportunity for them to volunteer as well. I suppose you must set it up as part of the routine almost.

RG: In your environment there must be people that come and ask you "how can I do what you're doing" how do you nurture the interest or is there any way to pass it on?

JG: Yeah, so I certainly talk about what I do if someone asks me, and I do have some young residents who are coming over with me to try to do some work, some of them have not continued to volunteer, but I've got a couple who are quite keen to continue to do the work; and I've got a second year doctor who was an intern last year and he's been to Uganda once and he came over to Cambodia with me in December and he went over again this year: So you know if they want to come over, I try to make it happen for them, or put them in contact with one of the places that I know, and they can if the times that I'm going doesn't suit the term or the holiday break or whatever then they've got the opportunity to go there by me trying to make contact for them.

RG: Are they usually self-supported or is there any way to help provide for them?

JG: Usually they are self-supported, but the OBGYN College here do have travelling fellowships which I think will help; the pharmaceutical companies also do provide travelling fellowships as well. I think that would help for those who would like to come here.

RG: From an educational perspective, is there any way to instruct/entice people in volunteering or is it just exposing and letting the chips fall where they may?

JG: I give lectures to the medical students. The universities close by here do have an interest group, and every now and then, they'll ask me to speak about volunteering which I think is good. So, I inform the people working here and if any of them contact me then I'll try to help to support the travels.

RG: Judith, would you recall a patient that has impressed you significantly during your humanitarian travel, someone that stands out, that have taught you something?

JG: I suppose the patient that I was actually thrilled about was a lady that, when I first saw her on the Mercy ship in Sierra Leone with a fistula, wouldn't speak to anybody, she wouldn't make eye contact, and I knew because I spent a bit of time with her that she was obviously highly embarrassed about the situation. We operated on her VVF and the first few days she still would not speak to me whatsoever but at about day 10, I remember she started to open up because I think she believed then that she could be dry; and she could see the other women also having dry beds. And then I remember that we couldn't shut her up. That provided me with a lot of satisfaction with what I was doing, and I think that just makes everything worthwhile for me anyway. Some patients that, I suppose in the last 30 years of doing fistulas, I've tried to look at a few things for the patients, to look at their mental health. I'm still looking at the problem of urinary incontinence after fistula surgery, and that was because I remember a patient quite early on in my fistula career where she essentially had anorexia. She was very depressed, and she eventually died because of anorexia, and I just felt that they wouldn't believe me when I said look, she's depressed and the comeback I had was "but we all care for her." You know the concept that you could come from a loving environment but still be depressed that was quite a new concept for some of the local people there. So that prompted me to look at some mental health studies et cetera which I then published. Just so when caring for fistula patient don't just look at the hole but the patient as well.

RG: That certainly illustrates the point that needs to be made that you need to take care of the patient as a whole not in part.

JG: Also, the ongoing incontinence. I remember early on again in my fistula career that the dye test was negative, but the women would not believe that it was negative because they were still very wet; and so that prompted me to again try to look at ways to help these women. Back then, some of the doctors would say you know but the whole is closed. That's it, she should be thankful. I said but she's still wet so that again prompted me to try to bring attention anyway to these women that continue to have issues with incontinence.

RG: Can you tell me a bit about your most challenging case? I suspect the one with anorexia is one of them.

JG: She was extremely challenging. I suppose the patient wasn't under my care, but I had to do the ward rounds from time to time, and just seeing her over a number of months melting away to nothing just about, and I suppose feeling very frustrated that no one was paying attention to her mental health; that was extremely challenging yeah, and yeah extremely frustrating yeah, and extremely sad.

RG: So how do you deal with that: lack of resources, different culture etc.

JG: Yeah, different culture, lack of acknowledgement. The doctor's looking at her felt that I was criticizing them, saying that are you trying to say we don't care for her. I was trying to say no, well anyone can get depressed. I mean she's had a dead baby; she's been leaking urine: I would be depressed too. So, they just took it personally, rather than looking at the patient, they sort of looked at that. They took it personally, and again with the incontinence as well they said but the fistula is fixed you know. So, I think that it has been extremely challenging certainly in the fistula world to have fistula surgeons look beyond the fistula.

RG: The whole as opposed to the hole (right yeah alright yeah)you bring back all that experience with you when you come back, how do you pass on all that to the younger physicians? What would be the best way to pass on that kind of information to the students and to the residents and to the making of the of the humanitarian surgeon.

JG: I'm hopeful that more and more of the students through the medical school are exposed to the psychosocial aspects of the patient, and I'm also thankful that more and more we do have the multidisciplinary team approach, and so we do get a lot of input from social worker, from the psychologist etcetera. I remember even just the last couple of weeks when, because here in Australia this is now summer, and so we have our new residents and our new fellows and one of the first year fellows said ohh Gee it's really good to have the team approach, because she understands that we need to think about the patients family, the travel, the finance and all the other aspects of her care. So, I think it is important for students and for young doctors to be involved and to understand. It is not just looking at the medical aspect but looking at the whole patient. That highlights the need to look at the whole patient, and having the experience for this young fellow to hear the concerns the psychologist has, the concepts the social worker has, etcetera and then to understand perhaps yeah that's why the patient might have missed the appointment rather than ohh she just didn't want to come, but to understand perhaps there's another reason why she might not want or be able to come, apart from that she might have forgotten. So, I think that's important. And also for me try to teach the young doctors to think about what's happening at home for the patient and whether she has a home, she might not have a home, and to see the psychosocial aspect: that's part of the history taking and when they present to me, I ask them what's happening with her whether she got a job, what's going on at home, et cetera so that it becomes a bit of a routine for them to think about.

RG: Yeah, but it's a critical routine. Because again I agree with you but as such it could be a double-edged sword: Would people who see a multi team approach just give up their part to focus on their technical skills? Then I see your position as the most critical, the most pivotal one in trying to direct the approach to the patient: a young doctor seeing the psychologist and the social worker might just forget about that aspect of the patient and only rely on their expertise. I really do appreciate your being there for that because it is critical to put the whole process into the proper perspective. That is wonderful. So, what is the biggest lesson that you've learned Judith from your lifelong humanitarian activities?

JG: I suppose I can do a lot more than I think I could have. But I try! If I look beyond the medical condition, there's so much more that we can help patients with. And for me in terms of volunteering, it was to be available and take the opportunities. It might be a bit challenging, but I believe that if it doesn't work out, it doesn't work out; then that's fine then I move on, but you know if it works out you know then that's great.

RG: So, you must be open and available, and develop the proper attitude. Do you think again as a rule that humanities have a role? Besides proposing and exposing, do you think educating is possible, and do you think you can educate someone to be more humanistic in their approach to patient care?

JG: Yeah, I think a lot of students come in just thinking about, ohh I want to be a doctor, I'm going to be operating, I'm going to just be doing this and doing that, but I think to help open their mind, and just to increase their thoughts about the humanity is critical. And one thing I do worry about a little bit even in surgery: now we can sit on the robot and not even touch the patient. I wonder whether we are decreasing our contact with the patient now, so if you're operating, at least you are touching the patient and the tissues. I don't know I just feel sometimes that we're just moving further and further away from the patient, even at the time of surgery we're not even in contact with the patient.

RG: That is exactly what is happening and is going to continue to happen unless we do something about placing Medicine where it should be as regards to the patient. I'm fascinated by your journey Judith, and I'm sure now volunteering runs after you, but for a while I'm sure you had to run after these opportunities. Any suggestions as to where to look for volunteering opportunities for medical students or even premedical students, people that are still in college trying to figure out where they want to go and so on.

JG: Yeah, certainly I think websites are available for students depending on what they want to do and what they want to volunteer, which is fantastic because you know obviously you know when I was going through medical school there's no Internet. So, I think it's a lot easier, and certainly you know the organizations now like MSF etcetera they've got websites that you can look at. Even the charity hospitals and different hospitals in Asia and Africa have got websites that you can contact. So, I think even to direct the students to just have a look on the Internet. I think that's a good start.

RG: Thank you. Now Judy let me sum up with a personal question: who are you?

JG: I'm Judith, I'm a fistula surgeon, an Urogynecologist and I spend a lot of time helping women overseas and trying to train the next generation of people who are interested in helping these women.

RG: During all this, have you found any fascinating person outside your area that has inspired you, that you have worked with, that has really been a "role model" that shaped you a little bit?

JG: Still in the area that I work with, I suppose it would have been Catherine Hamlin, but she's in the same area she's because I spent a fair bit of time in Addis with her, and just the way she looks at life that was a big role model. And just the way she cared for the patients taught me a lot about caring. And even in my time in India this particular OBGYN doctor that I spent a bit of time with just the way she cared for her patients as well, yeah so that was good, and I learned a lot from them.

RG: Do you think we're on the right path to try to push for an improvement in the humanistic approach to the surgical patient?

JG: Yes. Like I said I worry more and more that the doctors and the residents, we call them registrars here, are looking more and more about getting numbers! I don't know what's happening in the US, but they're very interested in getting the numbers, and like I said thinking about robotics essentially moving away from the patient, and I think it is important to bring things back into proper perspective. It's more about just the patient: there's so much more to Medicine than just seeing the medical condition I mean, or seeing the surgical opportunity, or can I do the operation?

RG: To be humanistic do you think one has to be religious?

JG: No. I mean I'm a Christian, but I know a lot of people who volunteer who are not religious. So, I don't think you have to be.

RG: So, what are the characteristics of someone who wants to volunteer.

JG: It depends on the perspective in life. One was in Medical School and became a young doctor, and she said to me I am not sure this is what I want to do. She believes that there's a bit more to Medicine than just what she was doing, and she said that she heard a lecture or a talk that I was giving about volunteering, and she said, yes this is what I want to do. She then contacted me, and said you know can I come over. So, I think it depends on the person, but for the individual it is important that they have that opportunity if they want to do it.

RG: Right, are there any criteria by which one can identify those people that are going to be inclined to become volunteers?

JG: Some people ask me about volunteering, but I have my doubts in the sense that if they can't adapt to being flexible at work, then I doubt very much that they can adapt to being even more flexible in a limited resource area; so if I see that they want for example when they walk into theatre they want every single thing opened up, because they might want to use it, I don't think this is going to work out great; if they jump up and down because they haven't got a specific instrument that they often use, I also think that's not going to work out, because often you have to make do with what you've got. So, if they can adapt and think outside the box in terms of problem solving, I think there would be a good chance for volunteering. Look also at caring for the patient, because when they go overseas, they need to think about the patient as a whole, because the support systems aren't as good, there's no social worker to help the patient, there's no psychologist to help the patient so you know they need to be more caring for the patient.

RG: Yeah, so from what I understand empathy, flexibility, adaptability, cultural adjustment and all that requires a big dose of humility. Is that correct?

JG: Yeah, Yeah

RG: Anything that I have not addressed, that you would like to share or state?

JG: No, I think you covered a fair amount. I hope it's been useful.

RG: It's wonderful, it really is great to talk to you and it's so good to see you again. Thank you!

Chapter 17
Do Surgeons Dream of Robotic Sheep?

Paolo Casella

This short story is dedicated to medical undergraduates dreaming of becoming surgical trainees, expecting to have a smooth transition from student to an expert surgeon.

It beguines misquoting Philip K. Dick's dystopia as a surgeon's life sometimes seems to be, and is intended to share with all of you my somehow peculiar insight on the history behind becoming "a surgeon," which is almost mythical and so many times misunderstood as a human who cares of wounded and other patients by the use of his hands, brain, and feelings.

As George Smiley said: "(…) now that I have the leisure to remember, that's what I mean to do for you, so that you can share my voyage and ask yourself the same questions."

17.1 Surgeon's Hands

The word surgeon is derived from Chirourgos, a composition of the Greek noun Chiros, meaning "hands," and Ourgos, from the verb "έρδω," which means "make or act." So the surgeon seems to be, by default, he who heals through the action of his hands, without any suggestion that neither knowledge nor feelings are required for the job…

There is evidence that "surgical healing" has been practiced in the Paleolithic, as shown by the discovery of a fossilized healed femoral fracture in an adult Homo sapiens, suggesting that at least one individual of that species, in some way, splinted and took care of another wounded member of the same clan that otherwise could not

P. Casella (✉)
Paediatric Surgeon Senior Consultant at Hospital Lusíadas, Lisbon, Portugal

J. McFarland et al. (eds.), *Humanism in Surgery*, New Paradigms in Healthcare, https://doi.org/10.1007/978-3-031-86018-8_17

survive. To some anthropologists, this seems to be the earliest proof of the beginning of human civilization.

Besides brain growth, civilization seems to be linked with the evolution of the Hominidae hand which has a primordial differentiating function, by the presence of a well-developed opposing thumb, allowing the "fifth ape" proficiently perform very skilled tasks. Through acquired experience, humans developed specialized tools as an extension of their hands, enhancing the discovery of new skills and actions.

From the surgical history point of view, specialized tools with the intent of healing or practicing other surgical procedures are very well documented since the Bronze Age through ancient Egyptian and Roman civilizations.

Surgical instruments, such as human hand extensions, have evolved over the centuries as surgical practice increased, with a progressive sophistication achieving an almost technological perfection in the last years that is epitomized in the success of robotic surgical procedures that may evolve, or maybe not, toward a Brave New World in which some procedures will be performed without a surgeon being required.

Unequivocally manual skills are essential for surgical practice.

17.2 What Do Surgeons Think?

Surgical evolution has always been a consequence of the practical thinking of generations of surgeons because, in my opinion, they are essentially empirical scientists. Probably most of the surgical progress came from repeated observations and tryouts with an incremental change in the traditional practice according to the better outcomes obtained.

In a very commonsensical statement in 450 B.C., Hippocrates explained that surgery depends on the patient, the surgeon, his assistant, the instruments, and the light, and also how many things and how we're to be mended, at what time and place, and in what way. All these concerns are so actual but seldom explained in medical schools, in an era where checklists are mandatory for a correct surgical practice they may suggest that we should return to the classics and the basics.

Throughout the centuries, many members of human society discovered how to care for the wounded and perform procedures that corrected some anomalies, establishing a traditional way of performing those operations that evolved in many different places of the world, like stone extraction, cataract surgery, or nasal reconstruction.

Until the eighteenth-century, empiric trained barber-surgeons were excluded from traditional university education, where trivia and quadrivia formed the basis of classical knowledge for physicians. But it was the "cutter" that performed practical interventions such as bleeding, cutting the stone, amputations, and bone or joint reductions, under strict supervision and prescription by the physician. Like other skilled workers, barber-surgeons belonged to guilds with formal rules of tutorial training and examination, keeping secrets of their skills and trying in some way to regulate their practice.

It was the untold silent work of eminently practical barber-surgeons that contributed to the development of fundamental knowledge in fields like anatomy and physiology challenging classical knowledge like Galenic anatomy, which allowed an evolution of medical practice establishing the basis of scientific surgery.

Later, those scientific-thinking surgeons also fought against the major limitations of surgical practice: pain and infection. Until then, only skills and speed could differentiate a surgeon from another, but with the introduction of anesthesia and antisepsis, and further on asepsis, the surgical practice became much safer.

So, humanity reached the nineteenth century, to be known as the "surgeons' century," and through the spreading of the Halsted principles of modern surgery, it has been possible for most future generations to benefit from the present-day practice, like open heart surgery or organ transplantation. So, it seems that surgeons do think a lot.

17.3 Do Surgeons Write?

According to oral tradition spread by many, vox populi says that surgeons do not like to write at all, but many of the early historical documents, from Ebers Papyrus to Galen writings, all of them concern mainly surgical case reports, their evolution, outcomes, and surgical techniques employed. Many of those old documents were lost in the Dark Ages, but the classical texts have been preserved by the Arabic and Jewish cultures. In the tenth century, in the cosmopolitan city of Salerno, many of those documents, both ancient Greek and Roman, were translated from Arabic and Hebraic to Latin, renewing the lost knowledge that rapidly spread across Europe.

From thereon surgical books evolved through the centuries mainly describing patient records, procedures, evolution, and outcomes, but also discussing theories on the causes of the anomalies found. In the eighteenth century, the more enlightened way of looking at Nature shifted the surgical literature toward previously misunderstood subjects such as embryology, pathology, inflammation, infection in a pre-microbe era, wound healing, and pain control.

New typographic techniques recently developed allowed the introduction of almost perfect images, some in vivid colors, describing pathological specimens and surgical procedures, many of them only attempted but certainly very similar to the modern ones.

The Industrial Revolution brought a shortening of distances and faster ways of spreading knowledge outside universities and so the medical press flourished.

The Lancet, one of the most prestigious and widespread medical publications, was created by a surgeon in 1894 and started the plethora of medical journals available in this century that, exponentially, explore every obscure aspect of surgical knowledge. As a consequence of this actual meta-universe of data, only reachable employing complex algorithms on giant databases, we have seen a transition from a sound and holistic knowledge of surgical practice toward an almost mandatory surgical super-specialization.

We must agree that surgeons do write a lot, mainly trying to keep accurate and time-consuming records of what they do and what they explain to the patients, trying to prevent litigation with them or their lawyers, but also with the ubiquitous health management organizations. Unfortunately, this enormous amount of clinical data is no more intended for the sharing of practical knowledge as it used to be, but for those of us practicing in very competitive academic hospitals, the actual mantra is to publish or perish, writing every day more on everything less.

17.4 Do Surgeons Talk?

Surgeons talk essentially with patients and their families and about those same patients with other surgeons. After achieving a somehow correct diagnosis, surgeons explain why and how they intend or not, to treat the patient in a more invasive and intrusive or less intrusive way, even, soundly speaking, convincing some patients that doing nothing could be the best option.

They spend most of their time discussing the risks involved and the hopes of a cure that the surgical treatment can offer, always keeping in mind that a no risk procedure do not exist even in simple cases.

But surgeons also talk with other surgeons, discussing those same patients, sharing tips and tricks of how they solve difficult cases, or even sharing funny events of their daily practice, mostly remembering facts of their training years and the ways of doing of their masters and often complaining about their professional career or personal lives.

Some of us also spend some time discussing wages and status cars, even gossiping about everybody or everything. To those gossip oriented, I always remember Baruch Spinoza's quote: what Paul says about Peter tells us more about Paul than about Peter.

Yes, surgeons talk a lot, and by listening to what surgeons say, we can deduce that there are essentially three different styles of surgeons: the scientist, the clinician, and the entrepreneur. Each of these styles influences directly the decisions that each of them takes, either the more aggressive versus the more conservative approach to the surgical treatment or obviously the way they communicate the risks and the choices available to the patients.

17.5 Do Surgeons Dream?

Surgeons are inveterate dreamers, dreaming of perfect operations performed in a perfect and always available operating room, with a complacent anesthetist, skillful scrub nurse, and compliant assistant, with unlimited access to top-notch technology on demand, in an almost healthy patient that will have an uneventful recovery with a perfect outcome.

We all know this is a never-ending utopian dream indeed.

Surgeons keep dreaming of new ways of doing surgery, changing practice toward better procedures and techniques, decreasing complexity and suffering for patients, and trying to emulate Leonardo's quote "simplicity is the ultimate sophistication" according to the well-known surgical aphorism: KISS, keep it simple surgeon!

Even if they dream a lot, practice will confront all of them with a much somber reality of unexpected events and outcomes, with unsatisfied patients and a lack of support from those who should share the burden of modern surgical teamwork. So, some start dreaming of the desired change in their lives or practice.

17.6 Do Surgeons Suffer?

When everything goes awfully wrong, we do suffer a lot. This usually occurs at the worst moment, when the patient and family are worried and start losing their trust in you as a surgeon, and when whatever you do seems to be completely hopeless in what we call a failure to rescue, which is the worst KPI for a surgeon. We suffer in silence, becoming a secondary victim of our failures, developing feelings of guilt, sadness, and anxiety, in need of strong support not only from friends and family but also from our institutions.

Surgeons are over-self-confident by default; otherwise, how could they cut through perfectly healthy tissues to correct congenital anomalies or treat diseased organs? Coping with failure or unexpected outcomes is often omitted and should be an important issue in surgical training.

Failure is part of our job description as the great French vascular surgeon René Leriche said: surgical failures are like tombstones in a small cemetery that all surgeons carry inside themselves. Even if we enjoy being a surgeon, we must be trained for suffering.

17.7 Surgeons Are Human

For all the reasons mentioned above, we must agree with Henry Marsh that in his fascinating book "*Do no harm,*" he unequivocally states that surgeons are human, just like the rest of us.

This pearl of wisdom encloses all that a surgeon in training and in his professional life must always have in mind because we are programmed for error, and errors will occur unexpectedly.

Much of what happens in hospitals is a matter of luck, both good and bad, and success and failure are often out of the surgeon's control, even in a perfect environment, because serendipity is part of human life.

Serendipity has been a permanent companion of my practice as a paediatric surgeon, always dealing with the unexpected in a life spent correcting congenital anomalies. This undisclosed driver of a surgical life confronts each one of us every day with an enormous number of choices to be made. The correct choices to be made are always based on our knowledge and experience, skills, and state of mind, depending on social and personal life.

As humans, we do have pleasure in what we do every day in and out of operating rooms, attending an emergency department or outpatient clinics, discussing with others the options, and every day learning new ways of doing a better surgery. And yes, we have fun in doing things this way, so much fun that so many times we overlook our personal life, neglecting our health and relations.

Finding a perfect balance between a highly competitive professional life and personal life is an acquired skill just learned by personal experience and never taught in medical schools. We must always be remembered that there is another kind of life outside hospitals, even if not as demanding and rewarding, there is a lot of fun in arts, sports, and family life.

Being able to look beyond the everyday concerns of our practice, enjoying family and friends' company, engaging in social causes, sports, or music, or simply reading a good book is the only way to prevent emotional exhaustion and professional burnout so frequent these days.

Otherwise, surgeons get exhausted just like the rest of us, and when exhausted, they may dream of robotic sheep.

17.8 Moscow Rules for Residents

To all who dream of becoming a surgeon, I share some rules that I developed through my long years as a Paediatric Surgery instructor, training many residents now excellent surgeons, and this is a kind of wisdom that avoided them many troubles.

These acroamatic rules are ultra-cautious tactics for operating in the most dangerous circumstances, and residents as spies alike are supposed to work in very hostile environments and should be advised to use Smiley's People "Moscow rules" to survive along their training years as spies survived in the cold war.

Moscow rules teach us that we must always watch our back, but when we became consultants or even chief residents, "London rules" described in Mick Herron's satirical Slough House series are perhaps more straightforward. In short: cover your arse.

- Assume nothing. Take nothing for granted, neither patients' or family's goodwill nor some colleagues' advice, and certainly not surgical outcomes.
- Murphy is right. If something can go wrong, it will go wrong at the worst moment, when the patient is sicker, and the family is really worried.
- Never go against your gut; it is your operational antenna. Follow your instinct and experience, if you are afraid of an unsafe anastomosis, use instead an ostomy.

- Don't look back; you are never completely alone. Ask for help whenever you need it, and if you make a mistake don't try to cover it, because everybody will know soon.
- Everyone is potentially under opposition control. Your most faithful supporters will whistle blow in certain circumstances.
- Go with the flow, and blend in. Follow the new surgical trends and fashions but listen always to the old guy's opinions.
- Vary your pattern and stay within your cover. Follow the rules but use common sense when you intend to bend them.
- Any operation can be aborted. If it feels wrong, it is wrong. There is always a palliative surgical option that can save the patient's life or body function and your reputation.
- Maintain a natural pace. Lull them into a sense of complacency. Never despair or act meaninglessly, and keep calm and act professionally even in distress.
- Build in opportunity but use it sparingly. Use your luck but don't abuse it; it seldom occurs twice in an operation.
- Float like a butterfly, sting like a bee. Surgery must be not only elegant and detailed but also effective, and to the point, do not linger in unnecessary "surgical arabesque."
- Don't harass the opposition. Don't be unnecessarily brave, or otherwise, in due surgical circumstances, you can produce serious bleeding or irreversible damage.
- There is no limit to a human being's ability to rationalize the truth. There are infinite ways of feeling guilty and suffering the blame for it.
- Pick the time and place for action. Keep your options open. Don't believe in dogmas and absolute certainties; use your imagination and creativity, spiced with a lot of common sense.
- Once is an accident. Twice is a coincidence. Three times is enemy action. In surgery, there is a place for bad and good luck and many coincidences, but if you fail, look obsessively for the causes of the failure.
- Carpe diem.

Chapter 18
Conversation with Surgeon 9—Michael Breen

René Génadry

Conversation with Dr. Michael Breen
Recorded online on February 17,2024, by René Génadry

Abbreviations that follow

MB: Michael Breen
RG: René Génadry

RG: Hello Michael, I just wanted to have a conversation about the issue the humanism in surgery. You are in a good position with all your commitments and international work to look at it and see where medicine is and where it's heading and try to find out how one can look at ways to improve the way things are proceeding. To define it so that we are on the same page, it has been defined as the application of scientific knowledge and the technical skills to the acknowledgement and respect for the emotional social cultural needs of the patients and their families; so, it's basically addressing the person in its totality, physical, emotional, social along with its distress and weaknesses. With the technical aspect and the scientific advancement and all the Artificial Intelligence and so on, I think you get the impression that medical care has become a bit dehumanized. So, I just wanted to see your take on that.

MB: Sure, but you have to extract everything from me, like you're a dentist basically.

RG: So, what do you think determines the humanistic approach? What from your perspective contributes to making a humanistic physician and surgeon?

R. Génadry (✉)
Carver College of Medicine, University of Iowa, Iowa City, IA, USA

J. McFarland et al. (eds.), *Humanism in Surgery*, New Paradigms in Healthcare,
https://doi.org/10.1007/978-3-031-86018-8_18

MB: Yeah, working overseas, you're working abroad…

RG: Tell me about your path; how did you get to be where you are, how did you get involved with working overseas?

MB: Yeah, somewhere along my time in medical school, I can't pinpoint it, but I had the idea that I needed to go abroad and work in a place where I was needed. I mean whether from parents or talking to other people, there's usually a kind of a Christian element in your desire to basically be helpful. If you look at the Hamlins, there used to be a statement at their hospital in Addis Ababa that says "whatever you do to the least of these, you do to me"; that used to be a big sign for Reg Hamlin and that was his favorite quotation. You also see that most people who stay a long time in Africa, tend to have a kind of a Christian you could say Calling to stay abroad, as opposed to doing it short term. I remember Jerry Putnam who's also another fistula surgeon, he said that anybody who stays overseas long term, there's usually a Christian element in their work.

RG: Did that start in childhood? Did it go back to that or is it something else that moved you?

MB: No, it didn't. It wasn't the reason I became a doctor shall we say. I just didn't have always had this knowledge. I've always gone to church regularly and that type of thing, but like somewhere along the way in medical school was firmly implanted in me that I was going to go and work somewhere in Africa; but it wasn't that pinpointed, but that would have been it. And then literally, when I remember finishing my job in Dublin, not finishing but when I was planning to go abroad, a nurse came up to me and when I was working in one of the maternity hospitals, she said to me, would you be interested in going to work in Kenya? and I said yeah! I would be, and it was as simple as that; and she put me in contact with the doctor there. That was my first approach in 1984. So, I did two years in Kenya, did everything there. Somebody had told me even before I went to Kenya that anybody who goes to Africa always do Obstetrics and Gyn when they come back. I didn't pay much attention to that but then, I haven't been two years in Kenya, my plan was to specialize and go back and work in Africa. Initially, I went to South Africa for a while because somebody also put me in contact, and said it was a good place if you wanted to learn how to do things like ruptured uteruses and actually have somebody teach you how to do as opposed to being on your own. And then from there I went to Zambia where I stayed most of the time and then eventually to here, Madagascar, six years ago.

RG: So, what are you doing now in Madagascar are you part of a hospital or institution or a clinic mission.

MB: No, it's purely fistula work; it's run by an organization called "Freedom from Fistula" which is basically run by a fairly rich Scottish lady who uses her money to run it here in Madagascar, and the unit in Malawi, and there's also a unit in Sierra Leone. We were based in the hospital here in the main port city of Madagascar, but we're kind of independent of the hospital. She doesn't like wasting her money on building things, so she always tries to adapt; you know you can spend an awful lot of money building, and then there's nothing left for running things… but from many points of view you could say she's a fairly shrewd businesswoman, but she also has a medical background: she used to be a nurse. So, she knows what you're meant to do and she's one of the few organizations that actually employ surgeons.

RG: How did you get involved with that particular group, did that come naturally?

MB: Well, since 2011 I've been involved because sometimes, they call me and ask me to go to Malawi initially, actually before Jeff came there, and so I used to do sessions in Malawi and sessions in Sierra Leone before Madagascar you know that was a short term 2-week sessions.

RG: Michael in your medical education was there anybody that was particularly influential in your decision, besides the nurse that opened the door for you?

MB: No, no I think it came from within really. I mean when I was in Kenya I met John Kelly, you know John, and so when I was looking to go back more full time before I got to Zambia, it was actually John who put me in contact with the hospital there, and it was John really who taught me how to do fistulas properly. He used to come once or twice a year, so if there was anybody influential, it would have been John.

RG: Anybody else that influenced you in that sense, outside of the medical system or the medical community, family wise or friends or students or any circumstance?

MB: Not really. Nothing comes to mind. It was very much as I say from within, rather. John was the only one who would have helped me along the way…

RG: So, from what I get from you it really was innate: I mean it's the environment obviously, the family values, your Christian upbringing, your commitment, and circumstances that really you look for because of your convictions.

MB: Yes, that's right. When it comes specifically to fistula work, you encounter the patients wherever, like first in Kenya and then as you say there is no great outside influence.

RG: Well, it certainly does take a lot of humility to accept all that you have to go through to do the work that you're doing.

MB: Yeah, I had a fairly easy ride I would say in the sense that you know doing medicine was easy, I didn't have to make any great sacrifices: college wasn't that expensive, and we didn't end up with any great financial stash or anything like that when I finished medical school, so I was pretty much a free agent you could say. (You probably would enjoy this: there's a missionary chap I know in the northwest of Zambia, and he always says **half-seriously** a missionary **married** is a missionary **marred.**) I have seen many doctors who basically want to work full time in Africa, but once the wife and the kids come along, that's the end of their dream.

RG: So, you made a conscious decision not to get married.

MB: No, no, no, as I say I was just lucky.

RG: Even luck must be prompted. Michael let me ask you another question about medical students or pre meds and so on: is there any way do you think there is any particular character besides background, or upbringing that could help identify people that you might think would be likely to become a more humane surgeon? is there any way to inculcate that kind of a culture in someone, or do you think it's all innate?

MB: Well, people look for role models all the time; I think when you're invited to speak to certain groups, but the reality is that modern society, even the links for people like me or other people working in Africa even those links are fractured. I've never been invited to any places or to anywhere in Ireland to talk or anything like that, which I would do, I know I won't terribly enjoy it, but I would make the effort, because people need those role models; but I think they are so preoccupied with shall we say the modern world and just all the things that they're worried about, litigation and all these things, I mean that's about it. When you talk to other people, you realize how important it is: I remember one time talking to a girl that I know who has been out and was planning to come out again, and she said she heard Andrew Browning giving a talk at the Royal College and she said it changed her life…So that's the type of opportunity you need, but you can't invite yourself to these things…

RG: We talked about role model; can you think of anybody else besides John Kelly that has been a good role model for you?

MB: Well obviously the Hamlins were a very definite role model. Nobody else springs to mind. Yeah, they were clearly a great role model to a lot of people. It used to be a great Center for people to go and learn.

RG: Michael, can you think of any event or patient that has influenced you and/or has made a difference in your life in your years practicing there?

MB: Nobody springs to mind. It's not one particular patient, it's just all the patients. That's everyone because fistula patients are particularly grateful to what is done for them and they've also had very little help over time, that's how they end up in the situation. Getting back to John Kelly he was one of these people who would kind of plant seeds in many places: he would just persist, and he never did things on a big scale in the long term. I remember in Angola now it took him about two years even just to get a visa to get into the country, but he never gave up: he was persistent. He went to the place down where he was, and you know things were tough there and what surprised them was that he came back the following year because everything was so terrible the first year, they thought he'd never come back. That was what he was like. Now Paolo is doing fistulas there now. That's just an example you might say it didn't make a huge effort in John Kelly's part, but the end result was very productive you know so planting that seed so that somebody else could take it up.

RG: Michael, you talk about planting seeds but how do you pass on the information to the next generation?

MB: The best way is preferably hands on training. That's the idea, but writing is definitely a big help. it's one of the nice things that happened to me when

I was just in Addis, one of the doctors there came up to me and she said: I want a photo of the man who wrote my favorite obstetric fistula book. You can write but you don't get much feedback you know. You just don't know who is even reading it. So obviously writing and videos are obviously another great way to doing this.

RG: It's a very comprehensive and a wonderful book, how long did it take you to put it all together?

MB: Well you see I can't go to time on it, because I always start writing from the time I started learning, because I actually remember when I was at Addis for training and you know I wrote up my notes, and I actually gave them to Catherine Hamlin to read and she was able to correct things and tell me I must show you this and I must show you that; so it's a process overtime, I just kept adding to it. It just takes time and obviously getting other people to read it, both people way above you and people way below you. Yeah, so that's how I did it.

RG: So, it spans at least twenty years or so.

MB: Or so yeah exactly yeah that would be very correct yeah, you're spot on there.

RG: Do you think one could evaluate the degree of humanity in physicians?

MB: Well, I suppose as it says in the Bible, by their fruits you shall know them, that's the only way I suppose. I think that's the best way to do it. I mean because if you think of Kees, like a lot of people don't like him and his approach whatever but you know at the end of the day this is what he's produced. You might not like his style but the fruit he produced is good. That's the only way you can evaluate it, and then humanity is something you discover; it's not something you can inculcate you cannot train someone in getting that humanistic attitude towards a patient; it's part of your personality and your abilities and I cannot think of any way to identify that personality. Usually, it's the interest of the person in the person that will show you their humanistic bend, because like people who are interested in working overseas generally speaking, they have that human element. I am sure you know the old expression that an African doctor told me years ago when Europeans spend a long time in Africa, they are either a missionary or a mercenary…

RG: Is there any way to differentiate beforehand?

MB: Well, the mercenaries are very much more focused on what their salary is or what they are getting out of it, that's their reward while the more missionary type are more focused on the human aspect: the reward is in the work rather than the salary.

RG: Do you think humanities have a role in the making of the surgeon or the surgeon is just a technical person, and you let other people deal with that aspect of the patient?

MB: You must have a human element to manage the patient properly, you have to take in the whole patient you're dealing with. I'd rather much more be treated by a doctor with a human element, but obviously the technical skills are important: you need both. But you know there is a tendency which I've noticed over the years that with some missionaries their primary interest is the religious side rather than the medical side. I have seen guys who are very much into the religion side with to the detriment of the medical side, in that they obviously spend so much time and then they make excuses like we can only put things together, but God has to do the healing: that was the excuse whenever your repair fails. I think there's a kind of a danger there. You must decide you're either a doctor or a missionary. There is an overlap with being a religious person, but I think you should primarily be one or the other.

RG: So, what would be the characteristics of a humanitarian surgeon? what would you expect as a character or attitude that would help you identify that person as really being humanistic in its approach?

MB: Well, you know as I said it's not looking for rewards, I think the main thing is that they give you a bit more. I think that's probably the only thing. I can't put it any better.

RG: Michael, you've been in situations that are very challenging, resource wise, patient wise and so on, is there anything that is particularly useful in advising on how to approach those situations?

MB: That is probably not terribly different from the situations you'd have anywhere else obviously, yes better resources, but from that side, you plan to manage that, you work within that framework. So, it's the usual things like dealing with different personalities and sometimes people can mistake your behavior because you are an outsider, and you're susceptible to be seen sometimes as racist in your behavior, and that type of things. So, you just have to kind of work around them: They're probably easier to deal with than what you'd have to deal with at home.

RG: Michael since you have been in Africa have you got a chance to go back home regularly?

MB: Yes, I go regularly at least every two years sometimes earlier

RG: Any change in the reception that you get there? have you had any experience with somebody coming approaching you saying you know Michael I'd love to do what you're doing?

MB: Surprisingly not. I suppose the only contact I would have had over the years, apart from a few friends who come out and they are not the ones I would influence in the sense that like some of them have worked abroad anyway, the only other group would be medical students, but I've not seen any of them come back, or at least I am not aware of any of them.

RG: If you were approached by your medical school to talk and try to express your thoughts and ideas that to medical students, how would you approach it?

MB: Well, I have never been asked. I'm not aware of other Irish doctors working overseas. There may be guys who do short term things in one or two specific places. I don't think anybody knows about me and that's OK. I've never asked either. When you went back say 30 years ago there would have been another missionary nun who was linked up with home more, and you would hear about them. I think that would be a good way of influencing medical students in university or hospitals where I've worked in the past.

RG: In hospitals sometimes, some nurses or social workers are willing to support you, to provide you with material equipment and so on for your missions. Is that the group that could influence medical students, or do you think that it's just an individual decision?

MB: I didn't hear of anybody working overseas and over here you hear them talking about things, but they won't be inspired because as I said I would go back to that girl who heard Andrew talking in the Royal College and giving a talk about his work. So yeah, I'm not sure how we do that. That obviously is a way to influence people but as I say it's harder in life for any place to invite you and you can't invite yourself to anything.

RG: Michael from your lifelong practice in that environment what lessons have you learned about the patient requiring surgery?

MB: You know the first thing is whether you should be doing the operation; and another thing is that, generally speaking, most of the surgeries we do are elective: so, don't be afraid to wait for your outreach for help, to ask somebody else to come and help you to do what needs to be done. I remember John Kelly saying: just save up those patients for somebody you know that way you'll benefit, and the patient will benefit. Don't be afraid to wait and get help there are a lot of people who are willing to come and help on a short-term basis. Another big thing you could say in this humanitarian work is being a facilitator for other people to come because like when I was in Zambia, I used to have a pediatric surgeon come with the urology team once a year and a colorectal surgeon. You need somebody to facilitate, who can lead to the areas with them and organize things. You must have the humility to accept the fact that you can't do everything, it's very much a win-win because the patient benefits and you benefit because you learn from these guys. and they benefit because they enjoy their trips, they enjoy helping you. I remember reading a report of one of the urologists who did this camp recently in Zambia, he said "this is a trip that is good for the soul and reaffirms why I became a physician." You sometimes lose track of that.

RG: Can you remember the most challenging interaction you have had with an individual patient?

MB: The difficult thing is maternal death and here that's a different situation. Litigation is not part of the scene here which makes it a bit easier you could say. Once the problem is over, we don't think about it too much.

RG: From your perspective I don't get the impression that one can educate someone in becoming more humanistic, just take the person and expose it and see what happens.

MB: I think that's true, yeah. You need to lead people in the right direction you know because everybody needs their own models along the way.

RG: Is there a good role model outside of medicine, anybody in your experience that has influenced you in becoming who you are.

MB: I suppose you could say along the way you get spiritual advice, but I can't think of anybody else

RG: As a way of concluding I just want to ask you who are you, who is Michael?

MB: I don't think about these things, I'm just a simple guy, just trying to do some good. I always thought this word humble means you have been humiliated along way.

RG: This is true, but it takes one to appreciate it: to learn out of a humiliating situation you must be humble enough to accept it and grow from it.

MB: Yeah, I think it's much easier for somebody else looking from the outside to decide who I am or what I am. You can do that alright.

RG: Is there anything else that you think I did not address that we should be talking about regarding humanism in medicine?

MB: On a more general level, coming back to the fistula work, you can see all these organizations which are doing "humanistic" work, but their primary concern is always "numbers", great quantity. And that's the thing which separates our boss from all the other big organizations: she has no interest in quantity, but if you only treated one patient in the year, she wouldn't mind that, you know. It's the bigger organizations, their focus is very much on numbers, numbers, numbers, which lead to problems: it's just like what's happening to a lot of NGO's, a lot of these decisions are made by non-medical people who tend to be "very humanistic" and whatever, and all concerned about the patient, but in reality their primary concern is always the numbers which should be less of a priority. It really makes you angry: when you're on the ground and seeing the damage that is being done, and the millions of dollars wasted that's just to no benefit to patients.

RG: How can one change that was or is it possible?

MB: Yeah, I think you need bigger medical input into a lot of these organizations, you know. The big decisions should not be made by people who are somewhere in the USA or Europe or wherever. That shouldn't be the way, they are often not medical, they don't know, they claim to understand this, but they don't.

RG: You need more humanistic physicians in on boards.

MB: Definitely, definitely! because they're making their careers on the back of these patients, they kind of hitching a ride, kind of hijack the work that is being done and that's wrong. That's what I would say is the biggest wrong I'm observing from the system side.

RG: Michael what we're trying to do is try to see what it would take to include in medical school curriculum some form of humanistic training. Do you think that possible and how could that be done?

MB: Well medical students do come for their elective; I think that's been a good thing in the long term. Although most have never come back, they at least gain some exposure to humanistic work.

RG: So obviously as medicine is getting more scientific and more technical, the patient and her personality are lost in the process, and the question is how we can put the patient as a person back in the equation.

MB: It's just basically focusing on the patient not just her problems.

Thank you!

Chapter 19
The Aesthetics of Surgery

Pia M. Sorto, Hrvoje Baric, Magnus Tisell, and Antti Huotarinen

Beauty is said to be the gateway between the nature and the spirit [1], and beauty's mystery has inspired philosophical inquiry throughout millennia. The study of aesthetic experiences—those created by the senses and the imagination—has led to questions about the ontological nature of beauty and about the qualities of the subject experiencing beauty. Originally, the ancient philosophers saw beauty as a road to the divine and to the Absolute Good, equating it with moral virtues. Later, this objective nature of beauty was questioned by the eighteenth-century aesthete, who separated beauty from religion. Questioning the concept of taste arose; who had the best taste? who were able to perceive beauty in its purest form? In the twenty-first century, aesthetics continues to cause debate, linking aesthetics to other areas of human activity such as politics, as well as bringing into question the established interconnectedness of beauty

P. M. Sorto (✉)
Helsinki University Faculty of Medicine, Helsinki, Finland

Oulu University Hospital, Oulu, Finland

H. Baric
Department of Neurosurgery, Clinical Hospital Center Zagreb, Zagreb, Croatia

M. Tisell
Department of Neurosurgery, Sahlgrenska University Hospital, Gothenburg, Sweden

Institute of Neuroscience and Physiology, Department of Clinical Neuroscience, University of Gothenburg, Sahlgrenska Academy, Gothenburg, Sweden

A. Huotarinen
Institute of Clinical Medicine, University of Eastern Finland, Kuopio, Finland

Department of Neurosurgery, Kuopio University Hospital, Kuopio, Finland

J. McFarland et al. (eds.), *Humanism in Surgery*, New Paradigms in Healthcare,
https://doi.org/10.1007/978-3-031-86018-8_19

and art, and giving the latter an independent role as a means of communication. Whereas the conceptual framework of aesthetics has witnessed a shift, such as from the religious and the righteous towards secularity, some phenomena related to beauty such as the implicit pleasure in the subjective experience of beauty remain an unquestionable property of beauty.

We can approach the beauty encountered on all the planes of existence through the lens of aesthetics with medicine being a surprising source of beauty since beauty appears at the meeting of the human spirit and the strong spine of natural sciences. The vast tradition of the philosophy of medicine still has room for the specific aesthetic phenomena only encountered in the field of surgery. The idea of this text was born within a small group of Finnish surgeons wanting to contribute to the academic discussion on the philosophy of surgery, and our thinking inquiry was further contributed by colleagues from Sweden and Croatia. And it appears that surgery more than perhaps any other medical field can be discussed through aesthetics. Even though it is an unnatural act and considered by some to be an act of violence, different types of aesthetic phenomena are intrinsic to surgery and are experienced by surgeons, rendering aesthetic experiences as an important window into surgery, at a comparable and complementary level to emotional, cognitive and analytical viewpoints to surgery. Often while operating, both beauty and pleasure appear in some form or another. The surgeon, classically described as a cold-blooded machine-like calculating creature who is able to cut into his fellow man with a knife, might be intuitively guided by a multifaceted sense of aesthetics. The objective and the subjective realms are connected in a very concrete way within the surgeon, giving birth to a beautiful and successful surgical operation.

This text describes three different dimensions of surgery—the sensory, the intellectual and the moral, discussing their aesthetics in the light of classical and contemporary philosophical traditions. The hierarchy of this text loosely follows Plato's and later Plotinos' description of the development of aesthetic understanding. First, one sees the beauty of the physical and perishable, but later, we learn to see the beauty in the rational, immaterial level containing ideas of great beauty, and eventually, we learn to appreciate what was considered to be the highest form of beauty—the Good. This journey parallels the development of the appreciation of the aesthetic in the growth of a surgeon through the different phases in his surgical career, starting from the mere excitement of being able to open and directly modify the human body, proceeding through to understanding how to operate and how to perform surgeries and treat diseases, and culminating in the ability of a master surgeon to adopt a holistic viewpoint that considers the patients' needs in order to reach the best possible treatment outcomes. The gift of having a mentor able to mediate and mentor the aesthetics of surgery to the developing, less experienced surgeon is discussed at the end (Fig. 19.1).

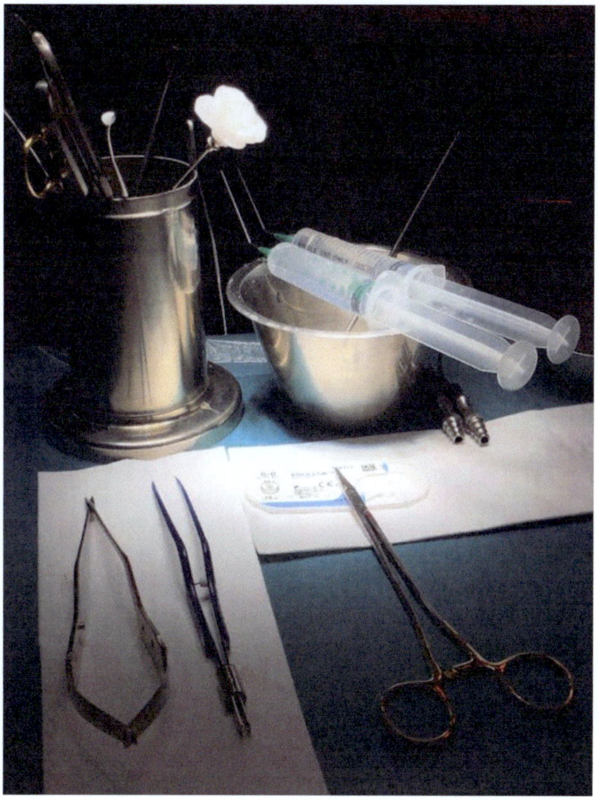

Fig. 19.1 Surgery contains multilevel beauty

19.1 The Beauty of the Physical Dimension and Love of Nature

The simplest form of beauty is the beauty encountered on the physical level and can be experienced via the sensory system. Along these lines, the first skill a surgeon develops is the ability to truly see. The career of the surgeon starts in the role of an assistant, who is often only allowed to observe the master's work. The assistant's hands are burning to use the instruments, but it is made clear from the beginning that this is not yet allowed. The novice surgeon will then have time to enjoy the beauty of the human body, riding safely through the operation with the master surgeon, whose focus is fully on the operation; the sightseeing being in the background of the master's cognitive landscape, who already has developed a great sense of the visual field and is capable of pointing out all that is abnormal or suspicious.

In ancient times, the beauty of an object was seen as a reflection of the highest form of beauty, the Absolute Good and the divine. The eighteenth-century philosophers started drawing a distinction between beauty, virtues and moral, and established a new vision by which the immediate sense of beauty can be caused by the

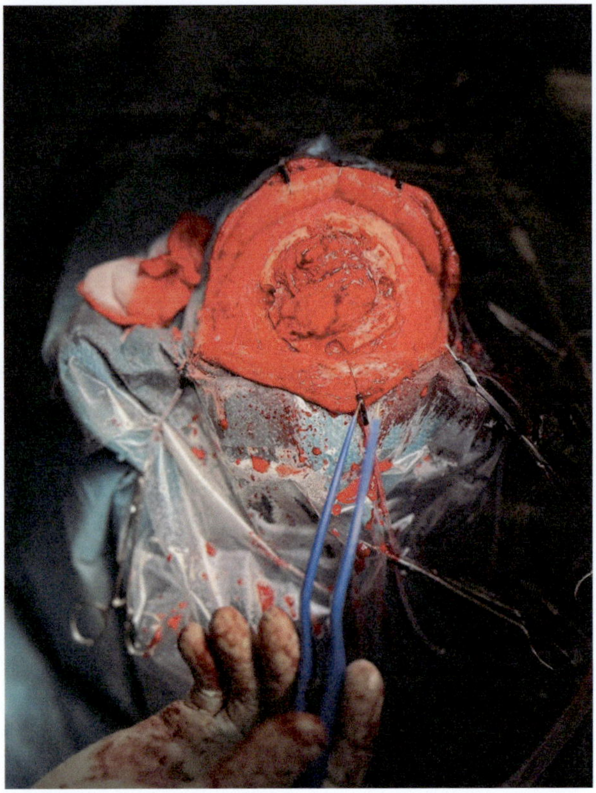

Fig. 19.2 Beauty of the bright colours is pleasant to the eye

objects themselves [1, 2]. The beauty of bright colours and regular shapes internalized via the sensory system is available without any intermediacy even to those individuals who had not yet developed higher cognitive capabilities or appreciation for higher values [3, 2]. Most beauty was said to belong to the area of vision, where the colours [4] and 'decorative pictures projected to the matter' [4] awaken pleasurable sensations [1, 5]. In surgery, this visible beauty can already be appreciated during the first moments of a surgical procedure. The skin with the underlying bright-yellow subcutaneous fat spindled together with the spiderweb-like connective tissue, the oily surfaces of the fascias or the intense red of the oxygenated arterial blood can arguably have aesthetic value in and of themselves. Harmony, a classical quality of beauty, is linked with the concept of health [6]; thus, the untouched, healthy anatomical vistas on the way to the pathology, such as to an inguinal hernia, to the intracranial space or to a hip joint, can be appreciated from the point of view of aesthetics (Fig. 19.2).

Anatomical views can feed the imagination, the place where aesthetic experiences are born according to the views of the eighteenth-century philosophers. A thoracoscopic view of the infected hemithorax might be compared to a trip to the planet Mars, and brain ventriculoscopy to a voyage to an underwater labyrinth. The movements of the vocal cords seen during a laryngoscopy, or the mysterious inner

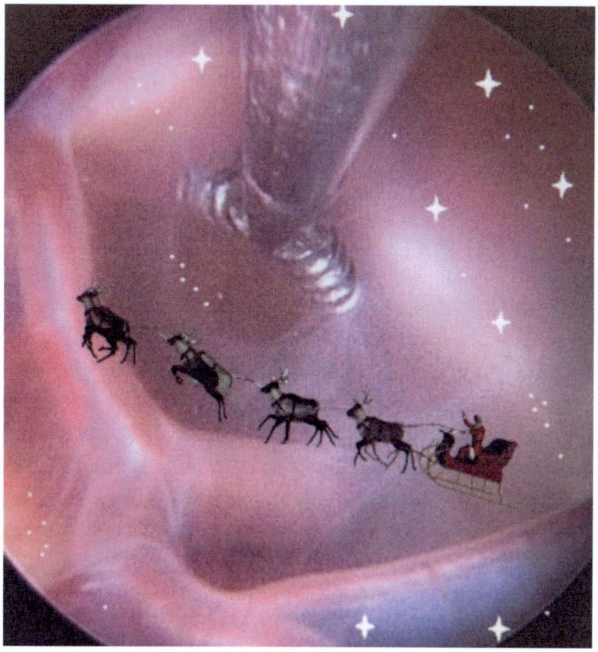

Fig. 19.3 Surgical views can feed the imagination. (Image credits: Neurosurgical Christmas card of the Helsinki University Hospital's Department of Neurosurgery, Finland, based on a brain ventriculoscopy by Dr Päivi Koroknay-Pál & Dr. Nuutti Vartiainen)

atmosphere of the eye is only a few examples of the complex yet harmonious unity of the body, and a person with a background in anatomy can appreciate this beauty at an even deeper level [2]. Anatomical knowledge is important for a successful orientation in the surgical field, and finding the wanted object such as the dura during spinal surgery is like meeting an old friend; on the other hand, for those with more experience, finding an anatomical variation or exploring a more obscure environment may cause excitement and wonderment. Both qualities of beauty [1] are available for those with much expertise. Knowledge has even been considered a prerequisite for love [7], and anatomical knowledge is fundamental for all surgeons (Fig. 19.3).

Beauty invites further exploration [8] and serves memory and learning because emotional experiences are always remembered better. The quest for curing the surgically treatable disease is an invitation to enter and learn. A child has a need, or tendency, to break things to find out how they work, and it might be argued that a surgeon feels a similar sensation when exploring the intricate biological system in which functional parts are segregated into meaningful anatomical compartments and organized into a coherent whole. In the times of Aristotle, harmony and unity were considered standards of beauty [9]. The principles of the divine order were considered to be evident in beautiful objects and the idea of perfect proportions [4]; and the idea of perfect proportions was carried on into Renaissance [1]. Each part of the machine has its specific purpose; there is nothing too much or too little in the healthy human body. The more complex the anatomy, such as in the neck or in the brain, the greater the pleasure of observing the harmonious whole composed of muscles, nerves, blood vessels and other structures. The perception of a functional whole invokes a sense of beauty at a higher level, and at the same time, anatomical and functional wholeness are necessary prerequisites of health. Mini-invasive surgery does not always promote the understanding of the whole, and to gain a larger understanding, one needs re-exposure through repeated surgical operations of hundreds of cases.

The pleasant feelings caused by beauty indicate a positive judgement of the object [2], and seeing something beautiful often gives an idea that it is also Good. Besides shining in the biological complexity of a functional system, the living body contains yet another type of beauty. This positive value, being seen as either divine or not, is life itself. The eye has an intuitive understanding of freshness, the body is fully alive, and it functions continuously. The two-phasic venous pulsation on the neck of the supine human is a small but certain sign of life. The snakelike movements of the clean mucous bowel surface during laparotomy might evoke the same type of pleasure as seeing fish moving in a lake. Muscle fibres move in an elegant fashion when reacting to stimulation by bipolar cautery. During surgery, the entire operating field pulsates in the rhythm of the beating heart and breathing lungs, which leaves an impression of just how profoundly the human body is imbued with life. With larger magnifications such as with a microscope, this effect becomes even more intense. The beauty of the life calls for our love and adoration [1], and it would be narrow-minded to consider this call only as an external one and not as the internal one experienced by the surgeon. Answering this call can lead to an appreciation of the healthy tissues needed to build the next steps of surgical aesthetics.

19.2 The Intellectual Beauty of Aesthetic Acts and Reasonable Surgical Decision-Making

There are higher levels of beauty beyond the beauty of the physical level; the classical views of Plato or Plotinos [4] or the eighteenth-century philosophers such as Reid [2] both described the hierarchy of beauty in relation to the subject experiencing it. While only the sensory pleasure was enjoyable by those who are on the primitive level, to learn to see the beauty in acts and deeds is a way to learn to see beauty beyond this level [2, 4]. There is beauty in movement, in power and in presenting skills [2]. Leriche described a good surgeon as '…a person equipped with pleasure of movement, attracted to risks, carrying a different type of soul' and continued to say that: '…their works are perfect from the beginning to the end, giving the impression of an art'. The ability to operate on the body aesthetically is then a higher skill than the ability to only observe the beauty of the body. Despite only being one part of the surgical treatment, the procedure itself is at the heart of the surgical process. This is craftsmanship and has nothing to do with science; performing masterful surgery can cause physical aesthetic feelings. The naturally high concentration needed during surgery, the immediate response of the setting and the high cognitive value of the process are all prerequisites for this pleasurable state of flow, which

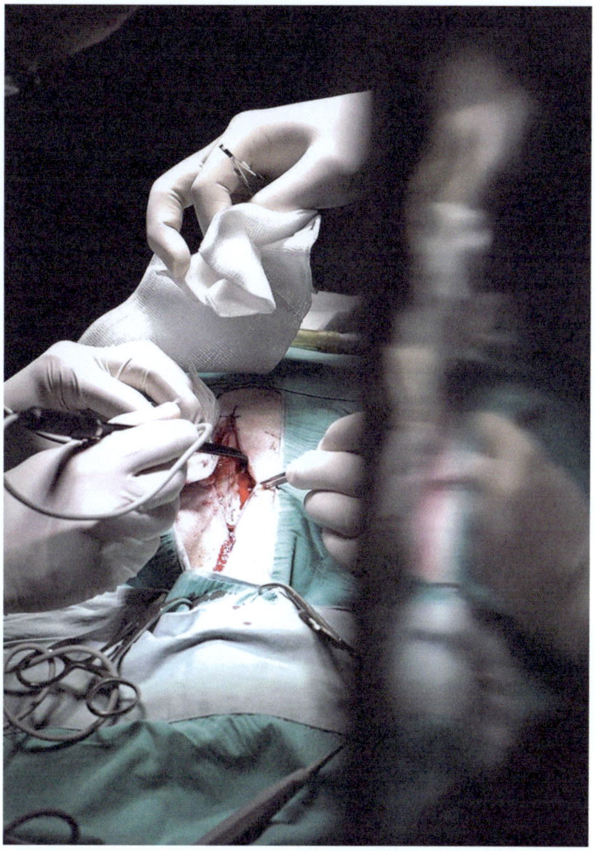

Fig. 19.4 Four hands working in concert—poetry in motion

causes the transcendental pleasure of forgetting oneself for a moment. If something is performed especially well [1], it could be called art. Art is not synonymous with absolute control of everything, as some of the best surgeries might appear to be aggressive messes, and the controlling style is only one way of operating [10]. Perhaps this is best highlighted in severe hyper-acute cases where safe control can be only achieved through speed when approaching the crucial anatomy to avoid excessive bleeding or the manipulation of tissue (Fig. 19.4).

The surgeon's work then is to make everything in the field more beautiful, to remove unpleasant pathology and reconstruct the natural aesthetics, to clean up the abdomen after an intestinal perforation, to empty an abscess, to remove a tumour, the antithesis of beauty, to reduce a fractured back to the 'hairline' and to return everything as close to normal as possible. Yet, balancing this hairline is sometimes not obvious as the skill of determining the pathological from the normal healthy anatomy usually requires repeated exposure to the pathological and not only normal healthy anatomy. Dissecting the gallbladder off the liver without bleeding or resecting a glioma without extra white matter suctioned is the result of hard practice, which can lead to heightened sensitivity of the visual and haptic clues available in

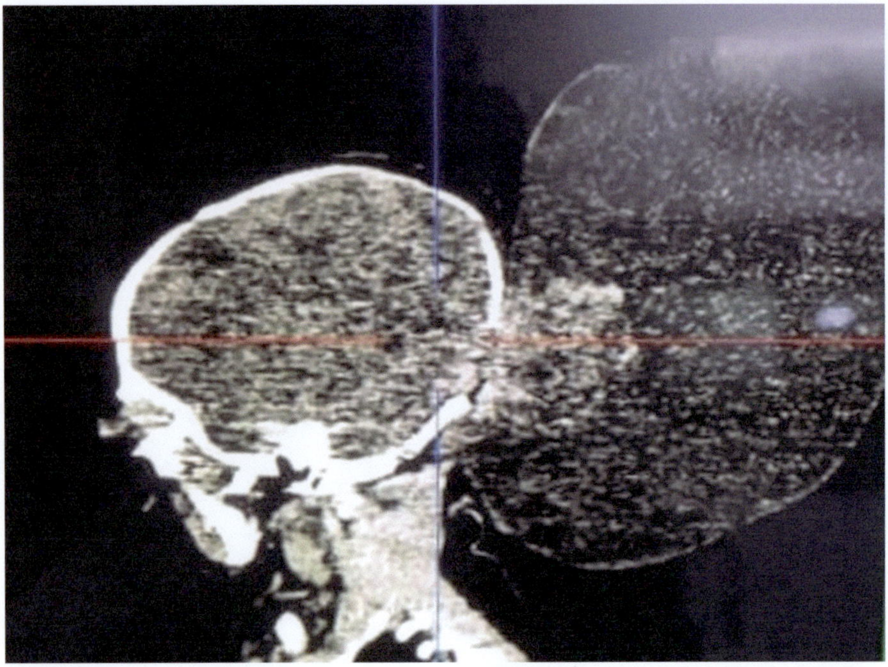

Fig. 19.5 Undoubtedly, pathological processes such as this giant encephalocoele can be considered ugly. (Image credits: Dr. Lamilton Lchikafa, The Queen Elizabeth Central Hospital, Blantyre, Malawi)

the surgical field and tender purposeful moves with proper angle and proper force, securing maximum achievable function with minimum collateral damage. At moments, this control also contains the skill to determine the pathological from normal healthy anatomy. Thus, the act of conducting beautiful surgery also includes the notion that, in beautiful surgery, dissection entails haptic sensing of tissue properties to define proper anatomical planes and, sometimes, extent and nature of the pathology itself. This is seen in the capability to find and naturally define the presented corridor limits of the pathology. It is the internal harmony of the different senses of the surgeon and the anatomical knowledge and external harmony of the surgeon and the surgical field (Fig. 19.5).

A surgeon's soul can experience the even higher level of aesthetic pleasure, the intellectual pleasure of well-planned surgery—'beauty born of reason' according to Plotinos [4]. Surgery starts with the indication, and this requires rational, scientific thinking. The developing surgeon collects not only the technical but also theoretical skills to be able to produce well-planned and thus beautiful surgeries, with nothing to add or to remove. Besides beauty being contained in reasonable acts, Aquinas [1] and Hume [5] linked beauty with good composition, with integrity, due proportions and clarity, which could all be the properties of a good surgery. As minimum entropy is one of the definitions of beauty as suggested by the modern theoretical physicist

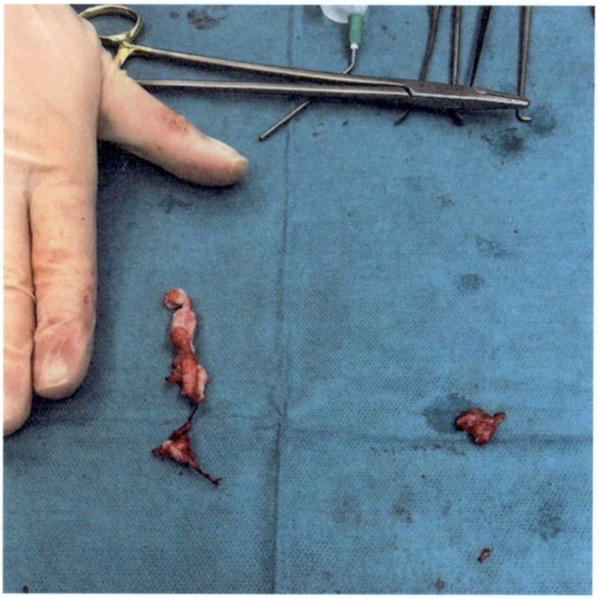

Fig. 19.6 Satisfactory catch from lumbar microdiscectomy—beautiful!

David Deutch [11], the most elegant of surgeries might be those with no extra movements; as simple and straightforward as possible. This may imply more beauty in fast and minimally invasive surgeries but could also contrarily be understood as perfect proportions of safety margins in required exposure and confidence in the identification of anatomical landmarks. Many times, well-planned surgery is very safe but fluent. Contradicting this sometimes-well-planned surgery might look repulsive, as after a damage-control surgery with the Bogota bag, but the beauty then lies in the reasonable plan, something that is not visible to the bare eye alone. Intellectual pleasure accordingly entails a higher level of judgement in proportion to the goals of surgery for a particular patient and what are the realities when treating the pathologies at hand (Fig. 19.6).

19.3 The Beauty of the Virtues and of the Absolute Good in Surgery

The craftsman can feel the satisfaction after the wound is beautifully closed. However, in surgery, the success is measured only by the outcome and no operation is finished until the postoperative control visit. Sometimes devastating complications appear, and the surgical indications weigh heavily especially in these situations. Performing the right surgery at the right time for the right patient is the difficult part in the art of surgery [10]. In decision-making, one should be as scientific and rational as possible, but sensitive to the patient needs, striving for the best solution for each individual as possible, as our duty is to rise to the Good, as stated by Plotinos [4]. In aesthetics, higher and more general considerations rise above listing the level of scientific evidence for a certain case. Usefulness [1] is one of the qualities linked to beauty especially in the eighteenth century, and the greater the value of both science and artistic activities has been considered, the more peace and well-being are increased [12], as seen by the Epicureans. With regard to Plotinos [4], the things that we eventually become are the Good which is the highest in the hierarchy of the beautiful things, the Absolute. What feature included in the most beautiful surgeries is the Good (the highest moral truth)? How is the surgeon, whose virtuosity shines without colour? Longinus in De Sublimitate describes the truly beautiful and sublime as that which always pleases all people, and in human history, it is the wish for the 'other' to be well and help the 'other' in distress. A surgeon who has high moral values and is motivated to develop himself as much as possible for the best of the patient has this quality. These are most beautiful surgeries—aesthetic experiences with a living shape of a moral truth [13]. With this in mind, even the heaviest and ugliest decisions such as amputations or the decision not to perform any more operations in the face of a terrible prognosis become beautiful. If art is the ability to communicate feelings [14], what else is surgery if it is not born out of true and good intentions towards an 'other' fellow human. Therefore, beauty in virtues in surgery includes both the art of operating skilfully and knowing when not to operate.

The moral skills are the last to develop in the human [2], and they might be the last step in the development of the surgeon; the one who blends the useful with the sweet has gained every point [15]. To develop the good moral sense is eventually to develop good taste [16].

19.4 The Master as the Standard of the Good Taste in Surgery

Some tastes are better than others, as stated by both Hume and Kant [5, 12], and the experienced one is sensitized with the most developed taste to be the best critique of certain skills [5]. To encounter a good teacher is a blessing for the young surgeon; an experienced and wise mentor, with noble simplicity and silent greatness, can transfer and initiate an understanding of what is the beautiful and the Good in surgery and teach the standard of the good taste in surgery. As stated by Blaise Pascal, to have a good taste means the ability to make good choices, and the master can thus teach the learnable skill of rational assessment of beauty, as formulated by Reid. Beauty can be shown to those who cannot observe it by themselves, and they will also be able to understand and enjoy it. The surgical stories of the mentor can live up to the Aristotelian standards of well-written dramas, containing all the pain and the fears of the profession to teach the unreal feelings when the irreversible has happened, to encourage integrity in the face of unfair treatment and to teach the clarity of avoiding complications.

The experience of beauty has an important social dimension, as it wants to be shared, and sharing beautiful experiences is an intensive form of communication [1]. The relationship between the teacher and the apprentice can become highly emotional, especially if the connection is built through aesthetics. It is possible that the whole surgical community is more connected through the aesthetics and the pleasure than they themselves can understand. Besides the values that health care provides, the most important being health and well-being, surgery contains an inner value in itself. It could be that the mysterious connection between surgeons might be partially mediated by the artistic dimension of the profession.

19.5 Surgery Is a Perfect Field for Inquiry into Beauty

Aesthetics may be considered as an epistemic approach to the analogical reality of rational thinking and scientific knowledge [17], and these can support each other. In surgery, where sensory experiences connect with motion through knowledge, the beauty coincides with wisdom. As stated by Plotinos [4], the nature of the Good has dressed itself into Beauty. To develop an understanding of the beauty is a way to become more rational [18], as only through the rise from understanding can sensory beauty to rational beauty and eventually the beauty of the universe of ideas, and of abstractions and virtues be grasped. Surgery with all its dimensions is an excellent starting point towards the mysterious, abstract essence of Beauty, and the career of the surgeon can easily parallel the inner road towards the highest Good.

Beauty causes inner happiness [2], as the soul is said to remember itself again when it encounters beauty [4]. The same light is said to brighten the mind, the nature and the matter [19]. This could considerably help many surgeons in bearing their strong and strict responsibilities and naturally occurring hardships. Those who see the beauty and feel it the deepest are called lovers [4], and the love of surgery could be taught and communicated through the beauty of the phenomena encountered in surgery, especially for those who are naturally prone to approaching the world through aesthetics but also importantly for those who are not. Their paths might be enriched. (The authors of this chapter are Finnish (P.S., A.H.), Croatian (H.B) and Swedish (M.T.) neurosurgeons.)

References

1. Beauty - The Stanford Encyclopedia of Philosophy, 2022.
2. Thomas Reid, Essays on the Intellectual Powers of Man, 1785.
3. Alexander Baumgarten, Meditationes philosophicae de nonnullis ad poeama pertinentibus, 1735.
4. Plotinos, Enneads 1., 6, on Beauty (Peri Tou Kalou).
5. Hume, of the standard of taste, 1757.
6. Pythagoras according to Diogenes Laertios, The life and teaching of significant philosophers.

7. Erich Fromm: The Art of Loving.
8. Alexaner Nehamas, Only a Promise of Happiness, 2009.
9. Aristotle, De partibus animalium.
10. Akça A. René Leriche and 'Philosophy of Surgery' in the light of contemporary medical ethics. Ulus Cerrahi Derg. 2013;29(3):131–8.
11. Deutch: Q&A. David Deutch. Nature. 2015;526:S16.
12. Reiners S. Vuorinen: The classiques of estheticas from Platon to Tolstoy. Helsinki: Gaudeamus; 2009.
13. Johann Sulzer. Stanford Encyclopedia of Philosophy: 18th century German Aesthetics. Plato. stanford.edu/entries/aesthetics-18th-german/.
14. Leo Tolstoy, What is art, 1898.
15. Horatio: Ars Poetica.
16. The Third Earl of Shaftesbury. Internet Encyclopedia of Philosophy. iep.utm.edu/shaftes.
17. Alexander Baumgarten, Aesthetica, 1750–1758.
18. Denis Diderot, Beau, 1753.
19. Marisilio Ficino, De Amore, 1469.

Chapter 20
Conversation with Surgeon 10—Steve Arrowsmith

René Génadry

Recorded online on February 6, 2024, by René Génadry
Abbreviations that Follow:

SA: Steve Arrowsmith
RG: René Génadry

RG: Hello Steve. I would like to have a conversation about Humanism in surgery. With your experience and your active involvement in international work, I would appreciate how you view the humanistic part of medicine, where do you see it heading and how do you think it should be managed.

SA: So let me go into psychiatry mode here and talk about humanism: tell me how you would define it, so I know exactly how to respond.

RG: It has been defined as the application of scientific knowledge and the technical skill with the acknowledgement of and respect for the emotional social and cultural needs of the patient and their families [1]; so basically, addressing the person in its totality both physical, emotional, social along with its distress and weaknesses. I think the best place we see that is in the patients that have not been exposed as much to the latest technology and science of medicine.

SA: Yeah, I can already think of a bunch of thoughts on this, but I think my perspective is unique because, among all the expat fistula surgeons, there are not too many of us who actually lived in Africa for any significant period. And I did that and as such, I got to be something other than just a visitor; and I just found that what really floated my boat day after day after day was getting to know the patients as incredible human beings and not just as challenging pelvic reconstructive cases. And one of the

R. Génadry (✉)
Carver College of Medicine, University of Iowa, Iowa City, IA, USA

J. McFarland et al. (eds.), *Humanism in Surgery*, New Paradigms in Healthcare,
https://doi.org/10.1007/978-3-031-86018-8_20

things I love about you is I know you feel the same way but at times I felt like we were in relational Siberia and some of our international colleagues, you know, fix the hole and that's it. 'Don't talk to me about success'. The same in training, it is all about relationship and modeling and mentorship and not about having somebody stand 10 feet back from the operating table in a group of 60 'trainees'. It's interacting with that person trying to pass along this thing about how important it is to connect personally with our patients and that's what's the key to enjoying yourself in this frustrating world of fistula care; but then on top of that, whether I liked it or not, for the past 6 years I've had my goodness stuffed up to the gills with being a patient myself and seeing how both individual providers and the system interacted with me and then reflect on that as well. That's why I say my perspective is a unique position.

RG: Tell me about your training and your experience in Africa.

SA: So you know in retrospect I just think I could not have had any better training whatsoever as a surgeon than what I received in my program and our chairman who was a phenomenal surgeon: he had his residency interrupted by two or 3 years at Danang hospital in Vietnam at the height of the war, so he was like you could throw off a hand grenade inside the patient in the middle of the case and he was just like: 'well, look at that…' and he knew exactly what to do and he knew how to do it elegantly and everything, but the guy was a fanatic about the relationship between the surgeon and the patient: as soon as you touch that patient with any kind of instrument it becomes a covenant, you know, that whatever happens to that person as a result of what you've done to them that's on you, and you take responsibility for that, and as much as you're able to, you continue to interact with that person as time goes on to make sure that everything is OK. You don't think of it as who can I dump this person on now that she is having a problem; and so he even made us do the whole transplant program: we had to go retrieve the kidneys, we had to do our own chemo for cancer patients; and one time a patient had a GI bleed and he even made one of our residents go do the endoscopy, the idea being that you have this unbreakable bond with this patient when you engage with them to have an operation. And that's what I came out away with, as being the norm because that's what I was expected to live by through my whole five-year urology program at the Medical College of Ohio. (I trained between 1982 to 87.)

RG: So, the chairman was a very important influence on your development.

SA: Right, but I mean I guess also because it resonated with what I thought that doctors were supposed to be when I signed up to go to medical school you know, that it's not just like being a plumber or a carpenter or something it has to have a terrific amount of close personal investment in it because we are dealing with whole human beings and not with uteruses or gallbladders or you know fill in the blank…

RG: So that interest usually precedes basically the exposure to the medical sciences…

SA: Yes, that is correct, but don't get me wrong, my residency was brutal because he made us do broad training: I had to do 6 months of internal medicine and Pediatrics because I had to be able to do it. You didn't get a consult unless something bad was going on, otherwise you managed it yourself, and your post op patients, and then we had to have a terrifically broad surgical background and I had to do vascular and chest and plastic surgery and all this stuff. Then I ended up in Jos, Nigeria, and my first 2 years I was the only surgeon on staff and most of that time the city and the federal government hospitals were on strike. I was the only surgeon available in the city of 800,000 so I was having every night to do chest stuff, head stuff, pediatric surgery but my training set me up for that, even though I wasn't even a general surgeon.

RG: So how did you end up in Jos, Nigeria?

SA: When I was in residency my first wife, she had gone to medical school in order to be a single woman medical missionary in Africa and so, she was willing to erase the word single but none of the rest of it. So, when I got to my last year of residency, we started shopping for jobs overseas, and the only mission that really got back to us when we made inquiries as husband-and-wife physicians, I couldn't believe it was this one called SIM (Society for International Ministries); and their medical director said 'you know you're never going to know whether this is for you or not until you go over and give it a try. So why don't you try to set that up'. So, my *** kicking boss of whom I was totally in awe and afraid of at the same time said: 'oh yeah sure, let's see what can be done;' and he let me go for a month during my residency! That was in January of 1987, and we went to Liberia, to Monrovia. I don't know if you've been there, but in my first night there at 3:00 in the morning, the general surgeon came and tapped on the window to wake me up, because there were no phones, and said 'excuse me, my name is Bill and I am glad to see you and have you, but I got a case for you. Let's go'. He had a lady with typhoid with an acute abdomen and he said, 'well, let's operate on her and if she doesn't have a typhoid perforation we can go ahead and fix the other problem', without telling me what the other problem was! I was so jet lagged I couldn't argue. So, we opened her up and there was no perforation, but she had a big old vesico-vaginal fistula. I had never heard of the obstetric fistula thing… I kind of knew that it was possible to happen as a surgical complication; and just the week before I left, I was looking at my, like urology for dummies, textbook with pictures and saw a description of an O'Connor abdominal repair of a fistula, so I started in doing that, and the general surgeon who kept saying ohh do you always dissect this far laterally, but I was like ohh it's one of the most important things you got to do that every time you know, just totally pretending like I knew what I was doing which I did not and it was like a big fistula too. But it went great, and she did fine. and then you know she was so happy I thought this is pretty cool because I had been concerned about whether I had anything to offer in urology in resource poor settings where they just need a surgeon and so anyway, she did great. Then we went home…and I started planning on going back to work at that hospital until they buried me when I was 85 you know. I had a military scholarship to pay for Med school which retrospectively left me debt free, otherwise I never could have gone over. And then 6 weeks before we were scheduled to move to Monrovia, the civil war finally reached the city and the hospital kind of got partially blown up and there were 20,000 refugees on the hospital compound, and so that didn't work out. Our mission said WellOK why don't you go to Nigeria, and we got a hospital there that needs a surgeon and this thing in Liberia that's going to blow over. I mean you know how these African countries are, so naturally it lasted I think 17 years total and then I ended up in Jos and so that was how I ended up there.

And then one day, a few women with fistula showed up. (they've been this British lady named Una Lister, I don't know if you've ever run across her, but she was already in Zaria which was not too far away) so one day, I had a whole van load of women with fistula failures from Zaria show up looking for help; I was a brand new fistula surgeon and here was a bolus of 15 impossible cases, but I muddled through and then the incredible thing was I didn't have any kind of a program or anything and all these ladies couldn't pay; and in our place we didn't have any government support. It was a Mission Hospital so people had to pay something, and so I just wrote home and said this is really cool, is there any way you could help support the surgery which only costs X amount? I wrote to all our financial supporters, and I know this sounds cliche, but I never had enough money in the account to do more than one or two more cases, but I never turned a single woman away because there was always enough to do one or two more. So, I ended up doing 100 the first year and then it was 200 and then that program has done over 20,000 repairs there now.

RG: Was your wife with you at that time?

SA: Yes, OK and so (she's in family medicine) she went to a family medicine meeting, and they had books on obstetrics because that was when family docs were trying to do deliveries and there was this book on obstetric fistula, that Zacharin book, that she bought for me and said that I know you're into this. And so, I kept seeing this Hamlin and Hamlin, so I wrote to Catherine Hamlin fistula hospital Addis Ababa, mailed it and she invited me to come for a couple weeks; when I got there, she was 3 hours late picking me up because Reg Hamlin was having the malignant sarcoma on his femur removed that day. And so, it was obvious he was never going to work again, and I really liked it there. I really, really was drawn to the idea of only doing fistulas after having to do something every night that I didn't know how to do.

RG: So what year was that again?

SA: This would have been around 92. It turned out my mission had a strong presence in Addis, and so they agreed to second me to the fistula hospital, of course as long as Catherine provided me with housing. She forgot to do so.

RG: Where did you end up?

SA: Well so she regretfully said, ‘I didn’t do that!’ but she knew everybody in town, and she knew this guy whose dad had been the first British ambassador to Ethiopia, and he was a diamond merchant in South Africa and had lived in Addis with his dad and so he built this gorgeous house; he was never there because he lived in Johannesburg. Catherine wrote to him and said can I stick this family in your house until we figure out where to put them? So we moved in and word got out in the neighborhood, there’s this wealthy new American family here; so within 3 weeks, we had eight unemployed paratroopers come break into the house, and they murdered the next door neighbor and hung him in the tree in my front yard to let us know that they were serious, and my kids had seen AK47 pointed at them and the guys had hand grenades and machetes and just spent the whole night with me separated from them, so I never knew if they were alive or dead or being raped or whatever, and they finally stayed like 6 hours, and then left when it started getting light: well it was ‘welcome to Ethiopia!’ and then we stayed 3 years but you know gradually our kids were having some school issues and even physical problems that clearly were PTSD. and so, we decided to go back, and we ended up in New Mexico because it was as close to third world as we could come in the US, but anyway that’s how I ended up in Nigeria and then in Ethiopia. We were doing 1200 fistulas a year when I was there, and I think that was the absolute peak time for the Hamlin hospital. (and I think it’s just totally gone to crap since because of adorning international attention which is interesting.)

RG: So, you ended up in an Indian Reservation in New Mexico?

SA: I was at a private hospital and then my wife worked partially in the private hospital and partially for the Indian Health Service hospital. It was a Navajo Hospital, and I could literally throw a baseball out my office window and hit that building, so and they had no urology help so they sent me all their urology cases, and then I went and did remote clinics at all their facilities and everything, so I think the biblical term is, I was in the IHS but not of the IHS. Anyway, so that’s kind of where or my geographic journey was.

So, this thing about relating to the ladies, when I went back, I negotiated a part time job so that I would have, not part time between noon and five, but a 0.75 FTE, and I spent the 0.25 FTE in Africa. I would always be out sitting around wherever the ladies sat around, and letting them try to braid my hair and stuff, and just trying to learn from them and I always came back saying that I gained a lot more than I ever gave them just from learning about how to be a person in hard circumstances; and little did I know that not too long after all that, they were my best trainers in how to cope with the idea of having incurable metastatic cancer in all that was going to mean as far as being able to keep smiling, realizing that you know the presence of God in all of it, and trying to sort through all that, they walked and talked because they're still like destroyed their lives, but they weren't dead… So where else could I get a set of tutors better than that. So, I owe them a lot and I just don't hear a lot of fistula people acknowledging how much of a give and take it is to work with them. You know they love to talk about what they're bringing and everything. I had a guy write to me one time. He said you know, 'I'm about to retire and I can go over there and help them black ladies with my fine surgical skills.' And I said 'really?' I wrote back and I said tell me more about your training. He said 'Well, you know I've been doing surgery for about 32 years now, and he said mostly small animal but some large animal too:' he was a veterinarian and he considered himself to be fully qualified to do fistula surgery. So, talk about the opposite of humanism in medicine there you go. And there's such a temptation in the kind of work that you and I have done you know to get turn into that, because you feel so unbelievably important going over there to do what they don't have access to. You can lose sight of the fact that they are imbued with the same human rights as our patients in Baltimore you know and like lot of times, they're a lot easier to deal with than in Baltimore. But you know as I said that my transition into cancer life, I had a 12-hour debulking surgery and I almost died from a cytokine storm afterwards because of all the ablation of 35 liver metastases, a temperature of 107.1 from my storm, and prolonged ICU stay and sleep deprivation. I had to have pleural effusions tapped and just one after another after another.

My surgeon was great I have a great relationship with him, and I can call him anytime and he's back on the phone with me within 10 minutes but every other place that I've been to Mount Sinai, Sloan Kettering. I just saw my sixth oncologist the other day, and last thing he told me was 'great to meet you, by the way I'm retiring in September'. None of those people feel a sense of ownership, but for me as a patient because they're a part of an interdisciplinary team I get that, I understand that, but the dangerous side of that is that no individual feels like they're the captain of your ship.

RG: Can that sense of ownership Steve be taught or is it innate, either you have it, or you don't? what determines someone to be taught to be more humanistic or is it possible?

SA: Yeah well, I get what you're asking, and I would go back to my boss: everybody in my program had to behave that way whether they had internalized that or not, and I think behaving that way through your whole training program has to rub off on you. Maybe you don't fully embrace it, but so seeing it modeled is huge! and then being expected to live up to the most of what's being expected of us usually and so if we live in an environment that expects us to produce a certain financial rate per year, to see this many patients per day, to not spend more than this many minutes per interaction, to limit liability by never talking to people about complications or whatever, that's exactly the opposite kind of input and I think that inevitably wears off on people too; where they don't feel the same kind of connection and so when I show up as the patient they don't realize that I'm expecting a covenant relationship with them that so it's like unrequited love. I had a well-known oncologist at Yale, and she sent me this e-mail: by the way, you got a met in your spine too… and I wrote back: tell me more… and she never called me back. I called, I emailed and everything like 19 times never once did she call me back, so I said goodbye. At Mount Sinai, I had a great oncologist there, he is kind of the father of neuroendocrine carcinoma care in the US and I really loved him, for we were both old school and everything but the system at Sinai was so hard…that's about four and half hours from here so I would get my scans done at Dartmouth which is an hour from here and everybody was fine with that. And so, I was due for a pet scan, and I got a call from Sinai saying when do you want to do your pet scan. I said no no, I get that done elsewhere because I live far away. I got 11 calls saying when are you going to do your pet scan with us, and finally I talked to my oncologist coordinator, and I said why do you have to call me 11 times about this very simple issue? She said you should feel 'honored' that we call you at all. She said that right out loud. During the pandemic I had a whole string of virtual visits and the same person said we're not going to renew your cancer medication anymore, and I said why not, and she said well you've refused to follow up we haven't seen you here for 14 months and I said I did that because your doctor told me to do the visits virtually; and they said no you haven't shown up, we're firing you!

RG: Was that a physician or was that a 'health care provider?'

SA: It was a nurse. I've had experiences like that just over and over and over again. I just marvel at the fact that as a physician, I have a terrible time figuring out how to get basic things scheduled and paid for. I wonder if it was somebody with no education and no savvy about the system how do they negotiate that? There's a certain amount of obscenity to it all too: my treatment is one injection per month IM of a somatostatin analog that tricks my body as it binds up receptors and puts my system at rest. I still have a liver full of mets: one of my recent MRI's called my Mets 'innumerable' but none of them have grown in 6 years at all because of this injection. The medication is fairly small target audience so it's a little bit costly. Dartmouth got up to cost charging me $36,000 a dose, so I told everybody my motivation to survive my cancer was that I heard that Jennifer Lopez, the pop star, had insured her butt for $1,000,000 and that I wanted to live long enough to have a **** full of medicine that was worth more than her $1,000,000 policy. So, I went over that mark two years ago by the way, so I have a million-and-a-half-dollar butt now. In Geneva, the insurance paid for everything, but they said this is so expensive you got to find a cheaper place to get it. You know that makes sense except in American medicine you can't. So I went down to our tiny little Community Hospital down the road and I said would you mind ordering this and giving me my shot in the **** once a month? and they said let us look it up, we love what you have done with your garden cause I drive by your house every day but I've got to check with the chief pharmacist, but I'm married to him so that's no problem. So, she called me back and she said I found out that we can do that, but you know we must mark up our medications and we generally do 50% but we'll do yours 40 cause it's cancer care, and I said Well how much is it going to be then, she said you're not going to like this, $11,000. Dartmouth was doing a 600% markup on my cancer treatment they were clearing $25,000 a month on my care, and then I wrote and complained and they said well we have all these other expenses to give you that medication; like what, I walk in and I pull my pants down and bend over, somebody goes and then I turn around walk out, and Erin (my wife) had to do it for me all through the pandemic, so how can you say that's $25,000. That's the degree to which the business side has taken over which I would say is the main force against a humanistic bent to medical care of any kind. It is just that it happened on our watch you know. When I started if somebody really needed something you know everybody figured out a way to get it for them somehow.

RG: Steve, it sounds like on a certain level you've given up on changing the attitude of physicians in this society.

SA: So, what I've done is I've trained probably 60-70 to a hundred of fistula surgeons, and I can think of about four who have understood what it was that I am talking about. I'm extremely proud of them they're out there doing this better than I could, and I think I must be satisfied with the fact that I got four out of 100.

RG: It's good that we got the four, but the question is: would education help enlist more than four, and could we reach 10%? and what would it take to do that?

SA: What would it take? Let me go back also to the expectation side you know that it's a non-binary thing. You don't educate or what's the word for having accountability, you must do both at the same time I would say. For instance, I have gone twice to Bangladesh to survey every institution doing fistula care in the country to help them write their national policy. I found one day there was a group of ladies sitting around and I got talking to them and the first two that I talked to, one had some dyspareunia, went to the doctor who said without any exam you need a hysterectomy and got booked: she showed up the day of her procedure and they said sorry we're running way behind, but we'll get to you. Eventually, they turned her off, did her abdominal hysterectomy and she got an iatrogenic fistula. It turned out the surgeon was too busy, so he sent the clinic manager in to do her hysterectomy. Then the next lady that I talked to, same thing some very vague GYN complaint got scheduled for a hysterectomy without an exam, got a call saying we're running way behind today, just hang out at home. Later they knocked on the door, a surgeon showed up to do her hysterectomy on her own kitchen table. And she ended up with an iatrogenic fistula. So, I would contend that being willing to let your administrator do surgery or to do someone's elective surgery on their kitchen table is not a training issue. That's something where an execution or two done in public on TV would be really effective in reducing the incidence of that kind of behavior, but short of that I don't know what you can't say ohh they didn't know that was OK.

RG: Doesn't happen in this country…

SA: Well in this country what we have is lawyers, and you know whether we like them or not and I don't think any of us think of them as morally upright right, but they impose that kind of system financially on us that we have to pay attention to outcomes and things like that, that doesn't address how people are treated you know subjectively, are they treated respectfully and all of that kind of stuff. But there is the level of accountability that you know you don't do blatantly awful things to them. I think that's one of the things that is a western concept more than it's African or even Asian concept that you have somebody looking over your shoulder all the time and you better watch out.

RG: Steve, do you think it's possible to identify someone who is going to be within that 4% that we've talked about?

SA: No. I think you got to give it your best shot on everyone and then hope for the best, and then as time goes on, and your interaction with them goes on, you start to think this person gets it, and he or she really not only is smart and capable but really cares about these ladies and then once I get to that point then I spend all my time with that person and I tell the other ones to go to lunch and come back 6 h later.

RG: How long did it take you to identify those that are recoverable?

SA: Just really like my number one right now is the secretary of ISOFS I don't know if you've met Itengrae. If you were going to be abusive to one of his patients, he would tie you up and put you in the trunk of his car and dump you in the bush somewhere because he will not tolerate it. Plus, he's a very very capable surgeon. And so, I first met him, and he was very shy and all of that but working with him like on two separate trips there, I thought this is the real deal.

RG: So, from what you're telling me that kind of attitude is innate!

SA: You know you cannot inspire someone to be like that. I think you can only discover it.

RG: So, there is no way to put criteria or to put some identifiers that would predictably allow you to decide that this is a person that is going to proceed with his care in a humane fashion?

SA: I think that's an accurate statement you know that it's completely subjective: you know you can say how fast can he do an abdominal hysterectomy and would stand there with a stop watch click but how likely is this person to really go to bat for his patients and all of that? and I have to say too sometimes it's not whether you like the person or not: have you ever been to Hope hospital in Bangladesh? so there, there's this guy Biswas there who's been their fistula surgeon forever and just immediately drives me over the wall being around the guy. OK he's just so aggravating somehow, and he doesn't know it. It's mostly just cultural. One time they picked me up from the airport after 40 hours straight of travel and said hurry, hurry and I said why hurry, we already put the spinal in your first patient… So then one day I was doing a case and the lady started bleeding like crazy and Biswas was with two important university gynecologists who had shown up and just shoved him out of the way. I didn't know the system there, and usually they didn't have a blood bank and I said we need to get this lady some blood, and we need it now. And they said ohh; and I said what do you mean ohh. How are we going to do this? ohh the doctor has to do this. Well, I said where is the doctor? and they said ohh! and I said you know we're going to stop until you tell me where Biswas is, and we had the lady all packed up. Like 20 min later he walked in with two units of blood and handed them to the anesthesiologist, and they were his blood... He disappeared and donated two units to take care of the lady, so he got it in his own cultural way. And he's doing the right thing. He still drives me crazy: I run the other way when I see him and everything. So that would be the thing: if I like somebody then I know they're going to turn out well, but that's not a criteria there, but to see how they are, are they willing to make choices that are costly to themselves in order for their patients to do well, that's the number one criterion: how you generate, I have no idea, you can only observe it when it happens.

RG: What I am getting from you is that although education does have a role, the end result of such an education is never predictable, you just must try and hope for the best.

SA: Right. There are many docs out there who are doing way better in their capital city UroGyn private practice which is not the same as them being out here, soldiers in the army against fistula. And then, I just have to depend on Itengrae to find his four and each one of those four to find their four. This is why change is so slow when we want it to be rapid. I don't know of another answer.

RG: Have you had any experience with any patient that have made a difference in your outlook?

SA: You mean has my philosophy been shaped by patients. Yes, there's this lady Hadiza in Nigeria. I operated on her like seven times she had shown up with like three previous surgery but each time we each actually did make some headway: there was a clearly definable thing that we were shooting for, and so I felt OK about trying in, then I heard that she was cured: she was dry and I was like hot dog and I went to go see her but she'd been discharged by the time I got there. I thought well crap and I knew that she lived like 15-hour drive away and she was a Muslim and she had become a Christian just because we treated her like we cared about her, we did not try to proselytize or anything and she had begged for a Bible in Hausa when she said where I'm going there aren't no other Christians or whatever. So, then a week later I walk into the clinic, and there's Hadiza sitting there, and I thought well crap she's broken down, or she's wet again after all of this: and she walked in, and I asked her what was going on and she said ohh no no no no I'm fine, still dry. And I said Well what are you doing here? And she pulled out the Bible and handed it to me and she said my family had found this, and they were going to burn it, but I knew somebody else needed it, so I brought it back. She made a 15-hour drive to give me the Bible. So, you can argue about the horrors of missions and all of that, but as far as her being willing to sacrifice her own discomfort, time and expense and everything because she was generally concerned about people right, that was humongous! for me to do that and that kind of thing was alive and well with the population of fistula ladies.

RG: How did you pass on the lesson from this lady to those you've trained?

SA: So, to me you know you can say well you've got to use 3-0 Vicryl not 2-0 because you know 2-0 is too big causes too much tissue reaction etc.... that's one way to try to train them, and they forget all that, and they go right back to doing whatever they did before. But I keep an encyclopedia of personal stories in my head and whenever any situation comes up, I start spewing those because to me one of them illustrates the point that's far more on the spiritual psychological side of patient care than the technical. And believe me, I'm all over about the technical side while we're operating and all of that, but I feel like if I can get those fine little prompts in our day-to-day life to tell them stories about people, those things they remember, and they're changed by and then they can apply all the technical things in the future.

RG: I see you are a strong believer in storytelling in educating in that people remember the point you want to make.

SA: Yes, I think that's well recognized by speakers and by anthropologists: people remember stories whereas they might not remember the reasons why the CT2 needle is the only needle to use.

RG: It has been stated that background is important: do you think someone's background have much to do with the making of a proper physician?

SA: Um, do you want me to go out on a limb here and say I think that people who've been comfortable their whole lives are less likely to be able to relate to uncomfortable people, through your own experiences with suffering and I don't mean unless you had a fistula you can't be a good fistula person but I mean the idea of feeling vulnerable, feeling like you're dependent on those around you for things that you ought to be able to take care of yourself, feeling like you're not appreciated even though you do your best to be appreciated, and those kind of things if you can connect with that personally, then you have the capacity I think to carry that on to your patient care; whereas if you come from a line of eight generations of successful surgeons, and you know learn to swim at the Country Club,- and I went on a trip once with a lady who learned how to drive in her father's Bentley and when we were telling stories about airline misadventures, she was ohh we were in the Learjet and landed in Aruba one time. And there was this really bad storm... she just had a hard time getting it, about what we were talking about, because she hadn't had that experience… that is not being judgmental of her, - but I think that the hard things that we go through in life prepare us to go through hard things with other people. I'm getting more and more qualified all the time with this hard crap.

RG: I just need to review what the points you've made that are all very important and see what I can find in trying to get a sense of who Steve is, and what are the main points that would allow one to learn from his experiences in trying to shape some sort of a curriculum that through stories would give physicians the ability to develop into a more humanistic person, using their scientific knowledge and their technical abilities to deal with the patient in a holistic manner. I think from what I get from you, it is background as much as environment in addition to being exposed and expected to follow modeling of proper care that determines success in such endeavor.

SA: I think humble people make the best caregivers, but if you want to teach that it takes humility on your part and that's sometimes in short supply in our world.

RG: You've just hit it on the head. I mean you just really need the humility to recognize first that there is a lack of it, and two that it should be the driving force behind being a physician, that if you don't approach it with humility, you're not going to be able to be successful no matter what you do, you can pretend but patients will recognize that it's fake.

SA: Right. And then, how to counsel people today where all the inputs they're getting within our system here in the states are to push you away from doing these humanistic practices; you can do it so long as you do it in the five min follow up appointment. and then I think people are demoralized but because maybe they have a desire to practice this way and they are actively persecuted if they try to do it.

RG: Let me summarize a bit: if you were to describe yourself (and I know that you have told me a lot about you), who are you?

SA: Who am I? I have a hard time doing this without doing a spiritual talk. I don't believe in spiritual being, I think there's plenty of that around, but I feel all the time as if my life has been an embarrassment of grace, that you know grace is unmerited favor, it's stuff that is given to you whether you desire it or not. It has nothing to do with that and I just feel like my whole life I've been a very imperfect human being, but yet I've been put in perfect place at the perfect time with the perfect background to interact with these unbelievable women, to be able to not have to vaguely conceptualize what a loving God can do in the world but actually see it, and actually feel like a little part of it, and that is riches beyond measure. And so like I always say the way I've spent my life has been financially suicidal, and that's true but even there I mean on the great side I'm sitting talking to you right now in an 1810 farmhouse in Vermont on 115 acres of rolling forest, in one of the most beautiful valleys, and one of the most beautiful States: and this place just fell in our laps and it was just a total grace thing, there's no way I could have expected to have. This is always like my dream place to live and then boom, so I never expected that or whatever, but I would say the same thing professionally once you get a taste of the system as it exists today I think all you can expect is to go away frustrated and hope that maybe 2% of what you've done is meant something in your practice in the US; whereas I had a urologist from Augusta GA come work with me in Nigeria, and he had a tremendously lucrative private practice and after day one he said 'I thought today, if I never had another day of working, today made it worthwhile' and then I thought, well crap I get this every day and so that I thought that was great too, because it was a reminder to keep recognizing that every day was a gift. Some of the gifts were really hard, but still. So, I am a person who has had an unfair dunking in the grace tank, and I don't know why that is I can't describe; if I were God, I wouldn't pick me to do that, I would pick somebody far better than me, but that's just not how it works. So here I am.

RG: Steve, you know in a way we all feel the same way, but I think you are a wonderful human being, and you have a wonderful way of expressing it.

SA: Thank you for saying that.

RG: As a final question do you think humanistic training has a role in the making of a surgeon?

SA: Right. I think it should be mandatory! to make sure that people are practicing that way with an eye towards how we deal with people, with human beings, and like I said I'm on my sixth oncologist right now and I have a highly specialized condition; I need very specific help by some of the best people in the world, but I would go with a local dude who I could really relate to and feel cared for than somebody with terrific data team qualifications.

RG: Should that be part of outcome measures?

SA: Yes absolutely! but try to come up with a way to introduce that into the curriculum and you'll be… because this is what I said to you in this whole talk, what we all want is a 7-step process to come out with a well-trained, technically astute, humanistic surgeon: I don't know how to do this. But at least we can try things out and see what works and what doesn't and provide opportunities. Maybe all surgeons should get sent overseas to work with Itengrae or whatever, not as helping them but learning from them. To have the people in other settings be their mentors. That's the difference that I had a lot of time when I was the only surgeon in whatever place when I was really depending on the local guys to bail me out, so that I didn't kill people.

RG: Well to do that, it takes a lot of humility doesn't it?

SA: Yes, but humility is easily driven out of you. I think it's easy to make somebody humble by putting them in a really nasty circumstance. Maybe we should have a 'nasty circumstances' rotation.

RG: It does take humility to accept being put in that position, doesn't it?

SA: Yes, to accept that you can't do everything for everybody. But I really feel another great thing was having a boss who had that covenant concept. I've never heard anybody else say that. I think he was not a spiritual person at all, but I think he even used that word the minute the scalpel touches the skin, that's a covenant between you and that person.

This is something that I wanted to say too about the way that you do training. I think on the technical side it has echoes in this, that the thing that I think most fistula gurus do the worst it's the idea of the last step of handing over and getting out of the way of the person so that they can put things to use and then that brings about humility for them when they find 'ohh I've got to do this all on my own'. So like for instance in all my work with Mercy Ships, the docs didn't realize it, but there was a TV camera in the ceiling, so after I got the idea that they kind of knew what they were doing, we'd have a case and we'd be scrubbing, I would say: 'I'm very interested to see how you do this case' and I let them go in and then I'd say: 'I got to call out here' and I would leave and never come back but I would be sitting in the office watching on the monitor and if they started to do something I would come running because I also check the patient. So, like what doctor Kropp did to me was the ultimate paradigm for training. It wasn't with me but there were two of us each year in my training program. So, my colleague was doing a horrendous fourth reoperation for primary retroperitoneal fibrosis where everything back there gets encased in scar, and they were trying to dig through and figure out where the anatomy was, and my colleague now reached in with an Allis clamp and came out with a piece about yay big of the wall of the inferior vena cava. So immediately the whole abdominal cavity was filled with this dark red drainage, you know as we call it, and so even though this is close to the end of our training, he looked up at doctor Kropp and Dr. Kropp looked at him and he went and he took off his gloves and he said I really need a cigarette and he walked out… and so Peter had to get his thoughts together, he had to get organized, he had to think how am I going to deal with this? what do I do first? while he's holding his whole hand over the hole in the Cava. and he did it. But imagine the balls that took doctor Kropp to accept the risk, but what he was saying is, I trust you Peter in a way that you could say that in words, but it would never have been communicated so effectively. So that's the kind of communication I think that leads to this deeper level stuff.

RG: That's modeling and teaching by example.

SA: Yes, not like some of our Dutch colleagues: last time I heard him talk about it, he had banned asking questions while he was training because he found it annoying, so he would have all these guys standing back against the wall not asking questions and then he'd say I trained 6 surgeons today. So, then I think of doctor Kropp, I need a cigarette! Polar opposites so that's the way to demonstrate on an emotional level our own commitment to our trainees too, to get out of their way and to allow them to succeed on their own. Now that's what I've done with Itengrae very quickly. I got to know that he's probably the best urethral surgeon in the fistula world for sure. If there was a case like that, I would leave him and say, 'I'm going to go and do some emails' and I would walk through but it's one thing to say that you admire your trainees but it's another thing to walk the walk and prove that you trust them.

RG: Steve how have you dealt with difficult situation where in a different culture with lack of equipment, material, lack of ability and to do that in a positive and efficient way?

SA: I have a different attitude about all of this. I'm so thankful that I started out with six years in Africa before I got into the traveling expert mode: we would buy fishing line at Kmart and bring it back from the States and wrap it around a piece of wood and throw it in the autoclave and we will close the abdomen with fishing line you know, and we would rewash catheters and use them until they fell apart. We used the urethral catheters 100 times each. We had a backup lighting system which was two pieces of pipe with a Peugeot headlight hanging down and a car battery on the floor, and we made it work somehow: it was not ideal, and I would never choose to work like that… When I go around, I think there's a lot of entitlement that has come with the fistula surgery movement. People assume they're going to get a whole bunch of money to remodel their theaters and everything, and I say you don't need that, and they have to listen to me because they know that I had to live that way surgically in an environment probably worse than what theirs was. So that's where that credibility comes from being committed enough to live in the situation that they live in, so that you can speak to that. I still would advocate hard at home for bladder scanners, and stuff for our ladies and try to get that, but to say well we can't do this because we don't have the materials…

RG: So, ingenuity, humility, acceptance and adaptation… you must be easily adaptable to whatever circumstance.

SA: But to buy the platform to preach that sermon, I had to live in the nasty situation first so otherwise why would you listen to me? and that's the principle filling the blank whether it's resources or cross-cultural care or whatever, you have to walk the walk, you have to do it yourself otherwise I wouldn't listen to somebody else telling me that unless I knew. I've always said if I wouldn't go to a new church lest the pastor had been in prison.

RG: So, what else did I not ask you Steve that you would like to say before I close it?

SA: I guess what I would like to say is if you think of six other things, I'll do this four times if you want to. This doesn't have to be a one-time interaction. Please anytime.

RG: Thank you!

Reference

1. Swendiman RA, Marcaccio CL, Han J, et al. Attitudes and habits of highly humanistic surgeons: a single-institution, mixed-methods study. Acad Med. 2019;94:1027–32.

Chapter 21
Open and Closed Heart Surgery: Reality and Fantasy

Mark Mekelburg

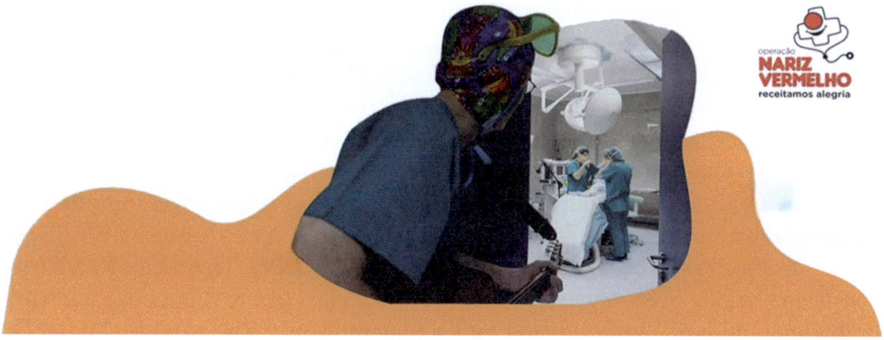

Reality and fantasy. What do these terms have to do with each other? They are opposite and disconnected from each other. When separations like this exist and things appear distant and incomprehensible, it is necessary to call in an expert, a specialist.

That's where a doctor clown comes in. In the practice of medicine, a specialist is a professional who continually increases his knowledge and experience in an area of practice that is constantly diminishing in size but increasing in focus. Eventually, as his reputation expands and his knowledge expands, his area of expertise becomes so specialized that he can confidently declare, as the doctor clowns do:

> "I know everything there is to know about nothing."

I know that one should not use personal pronouns in professional papers, but I am breaking that rule because that is what clowns do and, in this case, what doctor clowns do. It's not that we throw the rules out the window. We just look at the rules

M. Mekelburg (✉)
Operação Nariz Vermelho, Lisbon, Portugal

J. McFarland et al. (eds.), *Humanism in Surgery*, New Paradigms in Healthcare,
https://doi.org/10.1007/978-3-031-86018-8_21

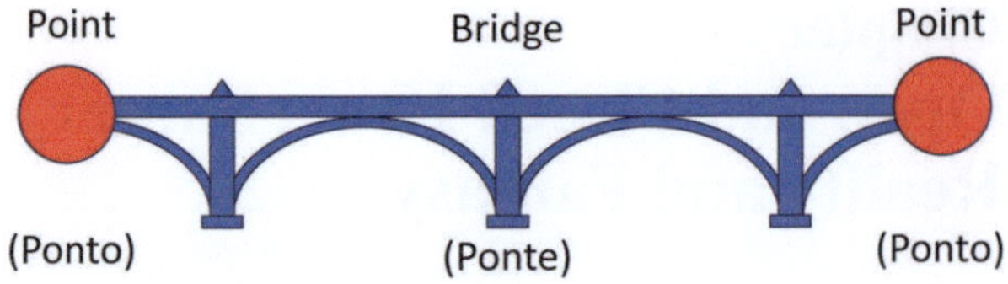

Fig. 21.1 Bridge illustration with play on words in Portuguese

through a different window. We hate boxes so we just use them for play. We "think outside the box."

Human beings are specialists in creating boxes. Unfortunately, many times, the boxes end up limiting growth, learning, progress, and the development of innovative ideas. Routines (often boxes in disguise) frequently become the determining factor for creating feelings of comfort and security. This can be good up to a point. But when routines begin to close the door for courage to risk trying something new or different, the sad result is often gradual stagnation in the work. Stagnation is not synonymous with life. Learning, growth, development, and enthusiasm begin to slowly deteriorate. Joy or excitement fade away. There is nothing "fun-tastic" about it. The most amazing thing about this is that it is accepted as normal.

Well, I invite you to step "out of the box" of normal and take a walk into the surgery ward with this doctor clown and maybe discover that this specialist knows more than he lets on. He knows something that just might make you want to leave normal behind.

The doctor clowns of Operação Nariz Vermelho (ONV) (Operation Red Nose) have been working in Portuguese hospitals since 2002. I like to summarize our work as "building bridges." In Portuguese, it's a play on words. The word for "point" is "ponto." A bridge is built between two points or "pontos." The word for bridge is "ponte."

You begin with two "points" (pontos) and then seek to build a "bridge" (ponte) (Fig. 21.1).

In my lectures and workshops, I always begin by playfully seeking to build a bridge of empathy with the audience. I "feel their pain" as they have been sitting in chairs for such a long stretch and I decide to relieve them of their suffering! I clap my hands and immediately command them to stand up, get rid of everything in their hands, and turn to the left. Surprisingly (not really!), everybody immediately jumps to their feet and turns to their left. I promptly set them "right" stating that it should be to my left and not theirs! Everyone lets out a hilarious groan of laughter as they turn to "my left."

I ask the people on my left side of the audience to put their "car" in reverse and ask the people on my right side to put their "car" in first gear. Then I ask the people on my left to begin moving backward and ask the people on my right to move forward, everybody putting a squeeze on the people in the same rows in the middle. I join the fun going to the end of the line of people in the front row. Now, we are ready for the fun to begin. I ask everyone to place their hands on the shoulders of the person in front of them and start massaging. This is what I like to call "the massage before the message"!

If you want people to listen to you, it helps to "get in touch" with them. Starting from this moment, everything we do is to the person in front of us. Sometimes we use "force" so we pat the sides of the person's upper arms. At other times it is necessary to be more "sensitive" so we gently squeeze the neck. Still, at other times, we need to "rationalize" with people and "activate their neurons," so I insist that everyone "knead" the head in front of them. Be careful with the bald ones! To conclude, I admit that what we really desire from other people is to "gain their ear." Joyfully I request everyone to gently pull the ear lobes of the person in front of them and make them look like "Dumbo" the elephant! Of course, there are always a few super enthusiastic people in the audience so I ask everyone to turn around and pay back the favor as we repeat the whole series of massages!

This is "serious play." It's a very playful moment but there is a serious purpose in it all: It breaks the ice and brings us all together on common ground in a fun and pleasurable way. Everyone is more relaxed which helps to open the door for better communication. It's not a new idea in communication. But it may be new in the operating block.

> "Medicine, after everything else, is summed up in communication." [1]

I don't believe that the immediate response of most physicians would be the same. Medicine is a serious science and hospitals are serious places in which to work. At least in Portugal, that has been my understanding after presenting lectures and workshops to thousands of healthcare professionals and medical students about this subject. Their academic course load and professional experience do not demonstrate this statement to be true. If you ask most of the health professionals, family members, and hospitalized children who are familiar with our work as doctor clowns, it is very doubtful that they would respond that "Doctor Clowning, after everything else, is summed up in communication." On the surface, it would appear not to have much to do with communication. But at the underlying hidden root, it is the very basis of our work.

Being an American living and working in Portugal for over 34 years, I have learned a lot about my mother tongue, English, through learning Portuguese. Communication comes from the word communicate. Communicate comes from the Latin root where we get the word "common." In Portuguese, this is the word, "comum" from which you get two other words: "com" and "um." "Com" means "with" and "um" means "one." Therefore, "comum," (common), essentially means to be "with one." The basis of all communication somehow has to do with this idea of "being with one," being, having, finding, or building something "in common."

I began to learn this as a clown before I began working as a doctor clown. The normal position for my shows illustrated this concept. I am standing up while the audience is sitting down. We are looking in opposite directions. The clown's objective is to use his art to build a bridge, a relationship, with his audience. Building a bridge is a process that may take a long time. Sometimes it can be almost immediate.

As doctor clowns, we always respect the space of the children, family members, and health professionals with whom we work. We must learn to be continually conscious of where we are (ponto) and where the other is (ponto). Then we have a much better chance of building the bridge (ponte). We begin by seeking to discover or create something in common with the children. In a hospital environment, bridge building can require much empathy and compassion as you try to "walk in someone else's shoes." "Empathy" has a smaller word in the middle, "path," which illustrates this principle perfectly. To empathize with someone, be aware of and share another person's feelings, experiences, and emotions, you need to know, understand and "walk their path," even if that is only mentally. Then you will be better equipped to build a bridge, a "path," from where you are to where they are.

Compassion touches on the same idea but especially in the sense of "suffering with." The connection of suffering with another person brings compassion beyond sympathy into the realm of empathy. In the case of surgery, these would appear to be fundamental.

So this brings me to the seeming irony of the title of this chapter:

> "Open and Closed Heart Surgery: Reality and Fantasy"

Instead of referring to "heart" in the physical sense, I am referring to one's character, feelings, inclinations, the center, the most intimate part of a person's being. In this sense, you can have an "open heart" or a "closed heart." The status of your heart will influence your communication, empathy, and compassion. It will either inhibit or facilitate your capacity to build a bridge from one heart to another, to be with, to walk with on a path, and to be mentally and emotionally sensitive to another person. One's heart condition affects one's capacity and intention to share hope, confidence, security and tranquility, life, from their heart to another person's heart.

So, is this "reality" or "fantasy"? What's the difference between the two?

Now you might think that it is necessary to choose one or the other. But you need both! My favorite characteristic about the clown is that the clown puts one foot in reality and the other foot in fantasy. If the clown puts both feet in fantasy, he will kill himself. He will think and try to do something impossible like trying to fly like a bird. He will go up to a high place and jump off as he flaps his "wings." As I was reflecting on this many years ago, I came to another conclusion: If a clown puts both feet in reality, he will also kill himself. It will simply be a slow, painless death as he stops right where he is. He will stop learning, stop dreaming, stop trying. He will be safe, satisfied, and comfortable right where he is.

Reality is where "real things take place."
Fantasy is where "fun-tastic things take place."

You need to put one foot in reality and the other foot in fantasy.

As doctor clowns in hospitals, these artists must adapt their art, image, and play so that they can function within the limitations, rules, and hygiene of the hospital without disturbing the work. The doctor clowns in the surgery ward have even stricter limitations and rules that they must follow. They must learn to keep one foot in reality and the other foot in fantasy. That is why we call our work, "serious play"!

Maybe a little history of how we came to work in the surgery ward may help. Building bridges does not refer only to people but also to organizations, businesses, schools, and other institutions. In this case, the same principles applied to building the bridge between ONV and the surgery ward of the hospital.

The doctor clowns had been working in Portuguese hospitals for over 10 years. The biggest compliment we could ever receive from the health professionals was when they would begin to treat us as members of the team. The bridge between ONV and Dona Estefânia, the main children's hospital in Lisbon, was well intact. In 2012 we were surprised to receive an invitation to do a six-month experiment in the surgery block. After defining the conditions, the regular visits began in May of 2013 with two doctor clowns, each one working alternately 1 day a week.

It was a major change and challenge for the two artists who would alternate weekly in this project to begin their work and adapt to the conditions of this completely unfamiliar environment. They received warm smiles and enthusiastic greetings from the nurses and other auxiliary help. As for winning over some of the doctors, surgeons, and anesthesiologists, the objective was for things to go as well as possible, considering that, in the beginning, some were very skeptical about our work.

The head nurses decided that the doctor clowns would use the same surgical gowns, caps, and clogs as provided by the operating block for the other professionals. The doctor clowns would not use any of their clown clothes, clown shoes, or their white doctor coats. They were limited to using their makeup, a red nose, and any props that could be disinfected and kept in their pockets. The doctor clowns decided that they would use a guitar, kazoo, and rhythm instruments like shakers or drumsticks. Finally, the artists would dress in the same space as the parents of the children who would be operated on.

ONV's artistic director, in collaboration with the head nurses, instructed the doctor clowns to intervene in three primary areas in the block. They were to receive the children at the entrance to the surgery ward, then accompany them halfway down the corridor leading to the operating rooms, and, finally, interact with the children in the postoperative recovery area.

It would be very pleasing to say that in the beginning the doctor clowns just fit right in and everything went very smoothly. However, one thing you learn about clowning is that many times you end up being a clown even when you are not trying to be one! Here are a few stories to allow you to experience the reality and the fantasy!

21.1 Dr. Pipoca's First Visits in the Operating Block

It was the first day on the block. Our artistic director explained everything about how visits should be carried out. She had called attention to one important detail: When starting to accompany the child to the surgery room, the doctor clown, upon reaching an "imaginary" red line halfway down the corridor, would stop at that point. It was simple and concrete. So, Dr. Pipoca was already dressed, got oriented with a nurse in the recovery room, and then went to the reception area at the entrance to the surgery ward where the first child entered. Dr. Pipoca immediately became very attentive, a little nervous since it was his first visit there, but confident. After all, he was a specialist! He watched from behind the nurses as they prepared the young girl to go to the operating room.

The opportunity arrived and Dr. Pipoca playfully but calmly approached her and playfully staggered at the sight of her colorful pajamas. She simply smiled back. That was a good start. So far so good! Soon she was transferred to another stretcher and the nurse began to push it down the hall. Dr. Pipoca started playing his guitar and accompanying them as the nurse began to shake her body to the rhythm of the music. Another encouraging sign! Even though she was on her way to the operating room, she was calm and just smiling at Dr. Pipoca. He thought, "So nice! How wonderful! This is so much easier than I imagined!"

The trio followed the corridor to the door of the surgery room and the nurse pushed the stretcher inside. Dr. Pipoca said goodbye to the little girl and the door closed. Dr. Pipoca stopped playing, took a big breath of relief, and thought, "Yes, Madam! And that's that!"

Then, just proud of himself and his head held high, he began to head back toward the entrance. Suddenly, he stopped in fright and screamed inside to himself! He thought, "Oh my God, I completely forgot the red line! What a clown!!!"

All nervous and disappointed, with his head down and worried, he went to confess his incredible mistake to the head nurse. She just rolled her head back and laughed out loud. Gently she told him not to worry about it. After all, she thought it would be better for the doctor clowns to accompany the children all the way to the surgery room door.

Well, that was a relief! Maybe she was right. But if that wasn't enough, on the third or fourth visit, as Dr. Pipoca arrived at the door of the operating room with a young boy, a nurse inside began signaling for him to enter the room. Dr. Pipoca just gazed at her with his mouth open and signaled, "Come in? Really? You want me to come inside?" And the nurse signaled back, "Yes, come in!" Then, full of doubts, but smiling, he entered the room and continued to play the guitar while the young boy was transferred to the operating table. Dr. Pipoca, completely out of his comfort zone, played his guitar and watched, for the first time, as the boy went through the process of being anesthetized.

What a first day! As the work began to develop, we soon discovered that we had a lot more freedom and opportunities to play in there than we anticipated. Entering the operating room became the norm during all our visits unless a nurse or anesthesiologist asked us not to go in due to some special circumstance.

21.2 No Way! Professionals Would Never Do That!

A baby, around 1 year old, entered on a stretcher accompanied by his parents. A huge, tall nurse decided not to take him to the operating room on the stretcher and picked him up. Dr. Pipoca got the cue and started playing a jazzy tune on the guitar and she began to take the baby down the corridor, just wiggling her booty all the way. Upon arrival, they entered immediately into the operating room only to discover that the anesthesiologist was late. Not sure what was going to happen, Dr. Pipoca just continued to play the guitar while the nurse continued to dance and rock the baby in her arms. It seemed like everything was ok when another nurse began to take notes from a paper on the wall as she began moving her body and feet to the music. Suddenly, Dr. Pipoca was surprised as a male nurse grabbed another female nurse and they started dancing! Dr. Pipoca, as he continued to play the song, looked at this whole scene and said to himself, "No one could believe that this was happening in an operating room!"

21.3 Now That Guy's Got Some Rhythm

A 4-year-old African boy entered the surgery block and demonstrated that he had already drunk "a cocktail" before entering the block! As soon as he saw Dr. Pipoca, he let out a loud laugh and started giggling and rolling over at the same time. Dr. Pipoca went into action and this little boy could not understand why there were red noses behind his ear, under his pillow, and even by his feet. His gentle laughter and amazement continued as Dr. Pipoca showed him a shaker and drumsticks and asked him if he wanted to be part of the band. With great enthusiasm, he nodded his head and chose the drumsticks. Immediately, he took to the stage revealing a natural talent accompanying Dr. Pipoca who played the guitar and kazoo.

They started down the corridor, nurses and doctors laughed and smiled as the two-man jazz band passed by with a dancing nurse pushing the gurney. When they entered the operating room, that's when the scene took off. As the nurses lifted him over to the surgery table, he just continued to play. They needed to take his T-shirt off, but he just kept playing. While they removed one arm, he played with the other hand. Then, he switched playing while they removed his other arm! The boy was so happy that no one believed he was going to have surgery.

They prepared to put a mask on him for the anesthesia and showed him a green anesthesia balloon. Dr. Pipoca stopped playing for a moment and asked him if he knew how to blow up a balloon. He enthusiastically nodded his head, yes. Dr. Pipoca then explained that if he blew in the mask, the balloon would inflate. The anesthetist took the cue, gently placed the mask on his face with one hand and showed him the balloon in the other. She signaled him with a nod of her head. He blew, the balloon inflated, and he wiggled with joy! Dr. Pipoca began playing his guitar again and this little four-year-old boy began blowing into the mask repeatedly while beating his drumsticks to Dr. Pipoca's rhythm. In a few extraordinary minutes, smiling and serene, the beating of the drumsticks became slower and softer as he peacefully fell asleep with everyone in the operating room astonished with unbelief as they watched this scene.

Every encounter is a story.

Every surgery is a story.

All stories have four basic components:

- Character.
- Situation.
- Problem.
- Solution.

Which of these four components is the most important?

For over 15 years I have had the privilege to lecture and do workshops with medical and nursing students in a variety of schools here in Portugal. For the most part, in every group of about 30–40 students, most of their responses either focused on the situation, problem, or solution. That simply revealed that their primary focus was not on the character, the patient, the person, or the human being they were caring for.

These results have been from medical and nursing students, people who were/are being trained to work in health care with people. This has been done without any intention on the part of the professionals who are teaching and training them and this does not state in any form or fashion that there is no sincere caring for the people in the hospitals. However, it has helped to understand some of the basic causes that helped to create a need for humanization in hospitals.

When we began our work, the humanization of the hospital was very much in the air. It didn't make any sense to me at first. If hospitals were created to care for human beings, why would there be any need to "humanize" them? However, as the work developed, our eyes began to open and understand the meaning of the term. The first thing we noticed was that they began painting the walls of the pediatric wards with color! Well, of course! We had been so used to seeing "white hospitals": white walls, white ceilings, white bed sheets, white uniforms, white doctor coats, and sometimes even white shoes! We began to wonder why everything was white. Then we noticed other changes as well: they began to paint figures and designs on the walls and ceilings. Nurses began to use colored coats with designs on them.

It began to make simple sense. Children live in a world filled with color from their surroundings, clothes, toys, pictures, cartoons, etc. What kind of effect does that have on them when, already feeling sick or in pain, they enter a completely white world? Without going into details, it surely doesn't help them feel comfortable and relaxed. Most probably, it contributed to causing tension, fear, and resistance in collaborating with the doctors and nurses who were caring for them. It was easy to begin to "do the math" and understand the need to make the hospital environment more natural, comfortable, and pleasurable.

The most important component of a story is the characters.

It is the characters that draw our attention and interest. We get to know them, who they are, what they are made of, and their qualities, strengths, and weaknesses, as they go through the situations, face the problems, and search for solutions for their problems.

The focus of the work of the doctor clowns is on the child, the other "character" in the story. Their focus is not on the problems of the child (although they learn characteristics of the basic pathologies of the children in the variety of situations in which the children are found). When they focus on the child, doctor clowns must train themselves to learn to use the "3 H's": their head, heart, and hands. This requires learning self-knowledge and humility. That doesn't mean that he puts himself down. It just means that he raises up the other. The clown gives away his power. This comes out in the hospital as they give power to the children. If a child does not want their visit, they accept that. The child is in control. That doesn't mean that the doctor clowns give up. It just means that they respect the space of the child. They seek to build a bridge. As was stated earlier in this chapter; to build a bridge, it is necessary to know where two points are: the point where the doctor clown is and the point where the child is. If both are not recognized, then any attempts to build a bridge will literally "miss the point." But if the starting points are identified, building the bridge can become a fun-tastic experience!

It can be immensely challenging but well worth it. Why? Because in reality, real things take place but, in fantasy, fun-tastic things take place. Both are necessary! The serious play of the doctor clowns in the surgery ward is realized, not only without disturbing the work, but it helps to improve the work attitudes, atmosphere, and actions. It requires one's head, heart, and hands. Seeking to humanize the hospital with this work requires all three.

Using one's head represents thinking through situations, defining problems, and searching for solutions. Using one's hands represents doing the physical part of the work. Many people use their head and their hands but leave their heart at home. It can be very easy for any professional to be extremely professional in their work by using their head as they use their hands to apply them and do the work. They can win significantly in their work but lose in their work relationships. They leave their heart at home.

The doctor clown's art needs a heart, an open heart. It is fun-da-mental that they develop the right attitude and read the atmosphere before going into action. This starts from the inside, opening their heart, becoming vulnerable and accessible to each other and to the child, family members, and health professionals. From their attitude inside, they begin to read the atmosphere on the outside. They pay attention to everything they see, hear, and feel around them in the present moment, in the here and now. This is where the doctor clowns live and become conscious of the first "point" of the bridge, who and where they are, and what they are feeling physically, mentally, and emotionally. From this point, they discover where the others are, the second "point." As these two points are recognized, they can respect the space of the others and go into action to start building a bridge. They start from the outside building to the outside, but they desire to get close enough to knock on the door of the other's heart. They hope that the other will open the door of his or her heart to complete the bridge.

This is the process of the doctor clowns, playing to bring fantasy and reality together to create a community where fun, pleasure, imagination, and collaboration flourish.

Open heart surgery refers not only to the relationships between the professionals and the patients. It also applies to the building of healthy work relationships among professionals. It can be very easy and almost automatic to make the same mistakes by giving priority to the situations, problems, and solutions and forgetting the people with whom you are working. All of them are characters in the "surgery stories" that are being written. Each one of them has a fundamental role in how they are going to develop their character, influence the other characters, and help write the story. Here is one example:

One day, between visits with the children, Dr. Pipoca noticed a nurse sitting in the hall with her head down. His reading indicated that there was some stormy weather going on inside her. On impulse, he walked up behind her as he softly played a song with the kazoo and started tapping the rhythm on her back with his sticks. She flinched in surprise as she let out a soft laugh. Then, she began to relax and enjoy the music and rhythm softly tapping on her back. The sound traveled to other parts of the surgery block. Upon hearing all this, the head nurse came out of her office to see what was going on. She looked at this scene and said, "Now, this is real work!"

Dr. Pipoca did not solve the problems that were occupying the nurse's attention (He did not even know what they were!). But his attention given to her as a "colleague" produced some relief and distraction for a few moments in which she was able to catch her breath, regroup, and then continue her work. It was simple head, hands, and heart.

Over the almost 34 years living and working here in Portugal, I acquired a lot of knowledge about my mother tongue, English, through learning Portuguese. Portuguese is much closer to the original Latin roots. The root of the Latin word for heart is "cor" from which comes the Portuguese word "coração." Interestingly, the word "coração" and the word "courage," both come from the same root word in Latin. This reveals an incredible insight between the two words. The literal meaning of the word "courage" is "big heart."

The doctor clowns have big hearts. They wear their hearts on their sleeves. I like to summarize a clown as "a human being, naked in his humanity, but exaggerated." This openness, vulnerability, sincerity, and simplicity of the clowns reveal their humanity. It is not so much a "head" consciousness but a "heartfelt" consciousness of their humanity that enables them to freely identify, empathize, and sympathize with others. The word "clown" comes from the word "clod" which is a clump of dirt. A clown was a man of rustic or coarse manners, a peasant, someone "down to earth."

Clown doctors use serious play in surgery wards to create a fun atmosphere which helps improve work attitudes, actions, and relationships. Every surgery is an encounter, a new story. Using one's head, heart, and hands, Open Heart Surgery builds a bridge between reality, where real things take place, and fantasy, where fun-tastic things can take place. Both are necessary!

Reference

1. Nunes, PMMH, Work of the doctor clowns in Portuguese hospitals. [Press conference with Operação Nariz Vermelho, 17 Feb] Lisbon, Portugal; 2005 (Unpublished).

Chapter 22
Conversation with Surgeon 11—Ana Pastor

Jonathan McFarland

Recorded online via ZOOM—28th April 2024

Participants

Jonathan McFarland (JM)
Dr. Ana Pastor (AP)

JM: Okay, fantastic. Well, today gives me enormous pleasure to interview Doctor Ana Pastor, who's Head of Neurosurgery at the Complexo Hospitalario Universitario de Ourense in Galicia. Hi, Anna. Thanks very much for coming.

AP: The pleasure is mine.

JM: Can you tell me a little bit about your background?

AP: Yes. Well, as you know, my name is Ana Pastor. My married name is Ana JMPenrose Stevens. I'm a neurosurgeon here in Ourense in Galicia, northwest of Spain. I did my medical studies in Santiago de Compostela, which is one of the oldest university in our country. But I spent most of my youth between Morocco and France. I was sent to France at the age of nine to a boarding school to further my studies. Then when I qualified in Santiago Compostela, I went to do my full training as a neurosurgeon in the UK.

JM: That is fascinating because, of the interweaving of different countries and different cultures. You were born in Galicia but studied in France and then went to train in England. Do you think this has made an impact on you?

J. McFarland (✉)
Faculty of Medicine, Pompeu Fabra University, Barcelona, Barcelona, Spain

Faculty of Medicine, Autonomous University of Madrid, Madrid, Spain

J. McFarland et al. (eds.), *Humanism in Surgery*, New Paradigms in Healthcare,
https://doi.org/10.1007/978-3-031-86018-8_22

AP: Of course it has. It has made an impact because I could learn and I've learned from different people. And I think it makes your insight richer. Your insight is much richer because you are living with different type of culture. I think we should all travel and live in different parts of the world to know the way life is around the world, especially regarding medicine. We live in a part of the world where we are quite lucky, and I think traveling around and working around is something everybody should do as a personal and professional experience.

JM: I completely agree with you. And I think it's very interesting that you bring in medicine into that vision or viewpoint. And so, did you always want to study medicine or was there some trigger that made you want to study medicine?

AP: I always wanted to study medicine. As far as I can remember as a young kid, I always wanted to be a doctor and a surgeon. You know, I shouldn't say that, but when I was younger, I used to open the bellies of pigeons or rabbits or chicken, and fish. I used to study all the digestive tract. I was impressed by the inside of the animals. I know that is not proper to say today. In that time, we could do that.

JM: That's absolutely fantastic. So, what age would you be when you were, let's say, kind of 'politically incorrectly' opening the bellies of pigeons?

AP: Well, I think I was, I was around 6 years old, 6, 7 years old. And I was quite young, you know. Yes. And that was to be a doctor. I wanted to become a surgeon watching the Vietnam War when I was young the Vietnam War. And I always remember, that always impacted me to see the Vietnamese American running towards a big helicopter they had in that time, carrying all the wounded soldiers to the helicopter. They were shot while they were running, and they were put in the helicopter, and were taken away. And then there was a magazine, a French magazine called Paris Match. And they used to, they used to tell us that the surgeons were saving lives, putting tourniquet or operating on those soldiers. So that impacted me when I realized that surgery could save lives, especially in an emergency, and also remember the poor Vietnamese on the floor bleeding, dying, bleeding. So that impacted me when I realized the surgery could, was a good tool to save lives. So, I decided to become a surgeon.

JM: It's fascinating. I remember, well, two images that come to me. I'm not sure whether they came to me at the time, but you never really know whether memories are real memories or memories that you've been told. But I remember the, the helicopter taking off from Saigon with people hanging onto it.

AP: Yes.

JM: And then the horrific image of the little girl escaping that I think was probably in Paris March as well. Those made an impact. So, you must have been young when this happened.

AP: Yeah. Yes, yes. I was born in 1959, you know, so, yes, I was 5 or 6 years old. And I remember that. I remember that, you know, I remember reading about the surgeon, you know, putting in chest drains and taking those soldiers to the hospital.

JM: I mean, that's fascinating, Anna. And so, from a very young age, you wanted to be a surgeon because you saw the way that surgeons could help. So, from a very, very young age, you wanted to help. And also, it's probably true that surgeries through the ages have grown or come out of wars, really.

AP: Yes. Oh, yes, definitely. Yes. The triage was with the wars of Napoleon Bonaparte. And then, well, the American, the war of Vietnam, taught me a lot about bleeding and dying and people dying from bleeding in the belly, in the chest, anywhere.

JM: And then I'm thinking of Sir Charles Bell in the Crimean war, who was, as well as being a surgeon, a painter who painted the soldiers, wounded soldiers, and he was probably more famous as a painter than a surgeon, although Bell's palsy comes from him. And then I'm also thinking of Doctor Josep Trueta, who was famous for the saving of limbs during the Spanish Civil War, am I correct?

AP: Yes. It was amputation of the limbs too. Yes.

JM: So, it's very interesting. Do you think this is some reason why a lot of the metaphors used in medicine, but particularly in surgery, are bellic metaphors?

AP: Yes, they are. Yes. Yeah. It's very sad. The war helped us a lot. You know, it's very strange. We learn, we are killing each other and then we have Red Cross and others. I don't know, amazing.

JM: It's amazing. But it's also fascinating how such a young girl at the age of six or seven, as you, was so determined to go into surgery, and you said you studied, you studied a lot in the UK. What was that experience like?

AP: Well, first of all, it was big. As a professional, it was a personal experience. Although I lived in Morocco and I lived in Spain, it was a big change in culture, I think. I first worked in Scotland for 3 months, and I went to England and there were big cultures changed. I think the English, they live differently. They see life differently. The communication between them and their friends, and family and work is very, very different than the Spanish way. So, there was a big culture difference. They were nice to me, but they had different way of seeing life and human beings, you know, to see human beings.

JM: And when you say seeing human beings, that obviously touches on the professional side as well.

AP: Yes, yes. The Spanish people are used to touching people, to crying with people. You know, we are quite a warm people. The British are very good doctors, but the relation is colder. It's more distant.

Yes. More distant. They explain to the patient what they have very well. The patient trusts the doctors very much. But I think the way they see life in the human aspect is quite different from us. And also, I think the English patient, the British patient, accepts illness or death better than the Spanish, although we are Catholic, and we believe that we will be better after death. But I think the British, especially the English, accept illness and death better than we do in Spain.

JM: This is fascinating. Why do you think this is? Do you have any theory about this?

AP: I thought it was religion, but no, it is not religion. I think. I don't really know I think I prefer the way they are. It is easier to explain about their illness to an English patient or British patient than Spanish because Spanish tend to cry. I think because the English are less emotional than we are, I think they are taught to control their emotion, not to cry. I think it's educational.

JM: It's maybe educational; at home as well. Maybe it's both at school and home. But what you said about the fact that the British people are, I wouldn't say less afraid of death, but they take death as some being something more normal, maybe even more natural. And is this something that can be universally taken into other cultures? Because I have a feeling that death is still a taboo here in Spain. What's your opinion about that?

AP: In Spain, it is a big taboo. I mean, we fear death. We don't speak about death, although there are laws that especially, you know, people can decide if they want to die because based on the law. But we fear death. We don't talk about death. We think we are never going to die. You know, a Hindu accepts death. They stay with dead people, you know, and Spanish, when somebody dies, they need to get them away very quickly, you know, recently my father-in-law died and his daughter stayed with him for a few hours. That would never happen in Spain. They would have taken him away straight away.

JM: This is curious. One thing which amazes me, although it could be something to do with the heat, but the funerals in England are maybe 2 weeks after the death. And the funerals here are like the day after the death. And I've never really understood that because it seems to me that to have a funeral 2 weeks later is more a sign of, I'm not sure whether respect is the right word, but you have more time to 'take it in'. You are able to organize a memorial of the life rather than just the death. And this is something which is very, very different between the two cultures. And because I think death is a normal thing and we need to assimilate that. We are humans. We are mortal.

AP: Yeah. I mean, sometimes I speak to a son or daughter. They come with their dad who is 90 years old, with a head injury, where you say I think he's quite young, you know. So we in Spain, although we are Catholic, you know, we should not be like that. But as you say, somebody died or they want to bury them. And I think we should stay with the dead longer, because it is the last time we are going to see them. So, we should stay the necessary time, because the it is the last time you are going to see them. You could even touch them.

JM: It's very strange. So, it's definitely not something religious. And in terms of England, did you become a neurosurgeon in England or in Spain?

AP: Well, I wanted to become a neurosurgeon in Spain, but I did my training in the UK. My fascination for neurosurgery is because the brain is totally unknown. The brain directs us, and we don't know anything about it. The way I am is because of my brain, because of my education. I don't know anything about the brain. So, I always wanted to see the brain, to touch the brain, to see the way the brain is inside. And that could explain why I'm like that.

JM: I completely understand you, even though, as you know, I'm not surgical. But the brain for me is miraculous. Well, the human body for me is miraculous. Not from a religious point of view, from a point of view of the complexity. And I always remember, I think it was Henry Marsh talking about the brain, this, what, two pounds, three pounds, small muscle. No, I think it's a muscle. You call it a muscle, really?

AP: Yes.

JM: And all of the thoughts, all of the paintings of the Renaissance, all of the great works of literature have come out of this two pound muscle.

AP: It's amazing. I mean, I love the body because, you know, you are born there, you come out of somebody and then you appear in the world and then you start moving, you start to breathe, your heart beats, and it's all magic, you know, it's wonderful when everything is working, but, you know, I know how a muscle works, but I don't know how to breathe. I don't know why I'm hungry, why I like, why I love, why I hate. I don't know that. And these elements of life are all directed by the brain and it cannot, I mean, no, no, it's all transmission between neurons. I don't know. It's not as simple as that. It's more we don't know about it. It's more that still escapes us.

JM: Yeah. They say that there are lots of advances in neuroscience and lots of advances in imaging techniques to see into the brain, but I still believe that we are nowhere close. We're very far away from understanding the brain.

AP: I say to patients, an MRI is like a photo of somebody. When you see somebody, you don't know if they are a nice person or a bad person. So an MRI is only a picture. It's not a function like a city scan. You know, you only know. You can only see a structural lesion, but you don't see, because sometimes you see, some people have brain, very atrophic brain, you know, and they are well, and this is people with a full brain and they're not well. So, you know, is. It's only a picture. Sorry.

JM: No, no, no, continue. It's fascinating.

AP: You can do functional MRI, but no, it shows you how. Where you move, when you move or when you feel, but it doesn't, or it cannot, show you about your emotions. No, no. It's amazing. The brain is amazing.

JM: The brain is amazing. And when you talk about functional MRI, everybody thinks this is a great breakthrough because you can see which part of the brain is active when you're quoting Shakespeare or whatever, but in reality, all I see is a part of the brain working, but they don't really know what's happening.

AP: That's it. That's it. You know, there's a big unknown. I Wanted to become a neurosurgeon, and I asked one of the consultants, I want to be neurosurgeon. He told me was. He told me, listen, Anna, women should be GPs because to be a neurosurgeon is very hard for a woman. Maybe I shouldn't say that.

JM: No, no, you should say that, definitely.

AP: And I said, well, you'll see. Only one consultant told me that.

JM: In the UK?

AP: Yes, it was in the UK. Yes.

Because, you know, in Spain, you have to do an exam, a national exam, so they don't know whether you are a woman. It doesn't matter. In the UK, your training is based on interviews.

JM: So it was terrible. This is terrible. Because I have the feeling that in terms of surgery, England, in terms of women, surgeons have been more advanced than other countries. No.

AP: When I was there, when I was in Europe, I was doing my neurosurgical training, neurosurgery. There were only a few women. There were four or five neurosurgeon who were female.

JM: Yeah. There was no money.

AP: No, no.

JM: I think it's incredible. I've heard women students saying that they were advised not to do surgery. And this is in 2022, so. 2024.

AP: So it's just me!!!!!

JM: I think it's incredible.

AP: I was advised not to do it in the UK. So that was another strong reason I wanted to do it, you know.

JM: Ah, so you have a rebellious streak in you, Anna, is that correct?

AP: I wanted. No, I want to be neurosurgeon. And then I started my training as a neurosurgeon. And then I did my exam or they told me that was that, you know, the doctor that comes very hard, was it, to be a GP for a woman? It's a much easier life to be with children, you know, because being a surgeon is quite a hard life, you know? But Sorry.

Sorry, I wanted to be a neurosurgeon before that man told me that anyway, so.

JM: So, but did you have anybody who was a mentor or anybody who you had this one consultant who said, you should know it's not. But did you have people in favor in helping you and supporting you or not?

AP: Some consultants did, yes. A female neurosurgeon. Ms. Bannister. Mister Laget also helped me. Mister Hockley. Yeah, I had a few consultants who helped me a lot. Yes. Yeah.

JM: Okay. Do you think the role of the mentor, I mean, I'm thinking now of education and medical education, which I think has come forward in some ways very strongly, in some ways is lacking a lot.
And I think that. I'm not sure. Do you agree that the role of the mentor is important?

AP: It is very important. It is very important to help you in medicine a lot. You know, that's why there is a lack of humanization because first of all, in medical school we don't learn about humanization. And then you are 18, you go to medical school, you study and you study and study and nobody looks after you. They only know about you, about your marks. They don't know you as a psychological person, and I think we should have mentors to help us to solve all the questions we have. Because when you're a student, you have many questions in your head, especially as a doctor, you have many questions. I think the mentor is very important. You have to pay them, they have to spend time with you. It's all money, all money.

JM: Money seems to come down to a lot of it. But I think the role of the mentor is having good examples and learning from watching. So this is my point and I think that maybe the medical education is too crammed full with facts.

AP: I think as we have in Ourense, we have 6 year - medical student and we look after them very well because I think in many places there are many of them and they go there and nobody looks after them or talks to them. Here, in Ourense, the students go with us to operating theater, they go to see patients. Well, we all make sure they feel well looked after and that we are teaching them.

JM: Experience about hospitals, you know, and they are, because very often the medical student, the person is kind of as soon as you become a medical student it's kind of the person is isolated, the personality, which is just as important as the education in medicine because everybody's a person and sometimes we forget that both the patient is a person and the surgeon or the doctor is a person as well.

AP: Definitely, yeah, we are all persons. We always do our problems. I think medical students have to from a young age. I don't know the ways in the UK, I think when I was a resident I used to look after medical students also in Spain for example, as we teach students but we don't get paid for it so we don't mind. But you know, if you want things to work you have to put money in. It is the way it works. You know, the world has changed a lot. You know, for us work was a question of dignity and we used to give our time to everybody but now people don't give time. If they don't receive something back or money or I don't know a diploma or something like that. So, I think if you want to improve education, you have to put money and time into it.

JM: I don't know about you, but I'm a little worried because I think medicine, I don't know even though I'm an optimist, I think, but maybe I'm changing a little bit. But you're obviously vocational, Anna. And I think the majority of surgeons and doctors, good surgeons and doctors of your, of our generation are vocational. Do you think that this is the same now?

AP: Well, I think. I think they are vocational because as you know, to reach medical school in Spain it is very, very difficult. You have to have a good mark before university you have to do an exam so it's very, very difficult. You have to be vocational. But then they arrive to hospital and they're not treated very well. They're not well treated. I mean, they are unpaid. They're not very well paid doctors. I mean, doctors. I mean, in the UK, you are well paid, in copmarison. They could live in hospital; they have rooms in hospital but here in Spain they don't have this. They have to look for flats. They're not very well looked after. So, for us, we were proud of working for our society and I think we are quite well treated now. Young doctors are very badly treated by the health authorities.

JM: But this is not only in Spain, but this is also more of an international, global problem, wouldn't you think?

AP: I think so. Nobody, at least in Spain, nobody wants to become a doctor, especially GPs, because they have to see 50 patients in the morning. We have to see too many patients. We have no time to spend with patients. And the resident doctors should be there to learn, and they are there as workers. They are workers from day one, so. And then they get terrible contracts when they qualify. So, they say what we're not able to say to the health authorities that if you don't look after me, I'm going away. And they can do this.

JM: No, no, they're not well looked after. I think. I don't disagree. I think I agree with you. There's something called the third-year syndrome in the medical degree because normally students enter the first and second years with a lot of illusion, with a lot of desire to change the world, but like you, with this desire to become a great doctor, a great surgeon.

AP: Yes, that is true.

JM: And then this, let's say this illusion gets drained, or squeezed out of them.

AP: Yes, yes They are tired, they spend many, many hours; for instance, they should have the day after a duty off. But they don't or they cannot. They stay in the hospital and they have to pay for their training, they have to pay for their courses. It's quite difficult in Spain at least, to be a junior doctor. It's quite difficult and I don't know why, but junior doctors are treated badly by everybody, although they are very well qualified, but few treat them them nicely and they should be treated nicely because **they are the future of medicine**.

JM: You know, this is critical. The future of medicine are the medical students who are coming through the ranks and the young doctors. What would you change, Anna? What would you change in medical education?

AP: Well, I think in Spain, medical education is very theoretical. They spend hours in university learning, learning or watching slides. And it has to be more practical. You have to look after your people better. At university, they need to be taught humanization, communication, giving bad news, you know, they have to teach them the critical importance of communication between patients and doctors. They have to teach them properly how to examine patients. You know, they have to go to your conference in Barcelona. [Medicine and the Arts: Exploring the Healing Relationships, UPF, Barcelona, 19–21 October 2023]. **The relationship between doctors and nurses, between doctors and patients is the basis of medicine**.

JM: And is it changing?

AP: No, it's not changing.

JM: Is it still the center of medicine? Is the doctor patient or the surgeon patient relationship?

AP: I always tell the resident, listen, **the patient is giving you a diagnosis**, talking to him, the patient gives his diagnosis. **But no, people don't use their hands, don't use their eyes, their ears to listen to the history. We don't take medical histories anymore, we don't examine the patients, we ask for an MRI, for a CT scan**. I think the managers are responsible for that because the patient wants speed, you know, when patient wants speed, they want to be seen quickly by a doctor. Yeah. So, the manager said, well, you know, you have 1 min per patient. They give us the time per patients, so we have no time. Ridiculous. And the patients realize they have the speed, but not the time. They wanted time for quality. And quality and lack of time do not go together.

In medicine you cannot go fast and have good quality. You have to go slowly. Yes. You know, in Spain, doctors in the outpatient's clinic have a bell, or we call the patient inside. The patient comes in, you get the history, medical history, and then the patient takes their clothes off, you examine the patient, they put their clothes on, and then you explain to them what it is. You ask for the MRI, you do everything in 10 min. You have to do all of that. And that was managed by politicians, because, you know what I think is when the politician realized they could get votes from education, from medicine, they went into medicine, you know. So, they went into health and got the patient on their side, you know, you give them the medication. I think this is when health or medicine began to go down.

JM: This is a general problem and is extremely distressing to hear.

There must be some hope at the end of the tunnel.

AP: I think while we have politicians who are not doctors leading health, we won't get anywhere, you know, we won't get anywhere. Now in Spain, we have economists, lawyers.

JM: Once a philosopher, do you remember?

AP: Yeah. Salvador Illa.

JM: Ah, yes, I remember.

AP: He's a philosopher and he was the Minister of Health.

JM: But maybe a philosopher would be better than an Economist as a Minister for Health? Could be? The idea of philosophy and medicine is something which is very important; philosophy for medicine. The philosophers maybe have a more open mind and are more open to new ideas while economists only look at the money, but a philosopher is looking at the ideas.

AP: We have changed the fashion of teaching medicine at a medical school. I think the doctor, the student should come to the hospital sooner and work with that. You should have students that are attached to a doctor.

JM: There is the term, Anna, "Shadowing," which I love that idea. I mean, it's when you shadow a senior doctor. This is, I think is a very strong way of learning.

AP: Yes. Yeah. You will be surprised. I'll do it with students, my daughter went to a school called Maristas, and every year I have students who come with me, and they spend a day shadowing me and I take them all around the hospital. So, we have that. But there was a student baccalaureate.

JM: Yeah. So in sixth form, in the equivalent of sixth form. So 16, 17, 18 that age?

AP: Yeah. Before going to university, they come and rotate with us. We do that in Orense. Yes. We call it **shadowing**, actually.

JM: Yes. And they must be fascinated. This must be an opening up of a new world for these children.

AP: Many of them become doctors after rotating with us. Many of them become doctors. Yeah, yeah.

JM: So you are a mentor to many.

AP: Yes. Yeah.

JM: This is beautiful. Because my next question moves on to this; you are the first woman Head of Neurosurgery in Spain. And hopefully other women neurosurgeons will follow. I don't know if there are many.

AP: Other women surgeons who are Heads of Neurosurgery? We are nine. Yes, there are 90 hospitals with Neurosurgery in Spain and nine of us are women now.

JM: Do you think the fact that women, women in surgery now, there are probably more women surgeons than male surgeons? I don't know. Probably in General, not in Neurosurgery, but maybe even Orthopedics, Anna, which has always been the male bastion of surgery. There are women surgeons, Orthopedic surgeons. Do you think this is benefiting the profession?

AP: I think so, because I think we are different; men and women. We are different genetically, by education. We are different and we see things differently. Yes. So, bringing professionals who see differently, who see medicine, life, human being differently is good because you bring different approaches from a human being, from a human point of view, you see different approaches, Yes, I think it's very important. It is. I think it's good that we are here, but I think we shouldn't be here because we are women. I think we should be like men. I think we should be here because of how professional we are, not because we are women. You know, nobody agrees. Nobody should be there because they're women. Because based on the race, based on the religion. No, it should be out. There should be out.

JM: No, but this is because there are more girls, more women going into medical education. The ratio has changed considerably, but I'm wondering whether this could be a trigger for a more humane approach to surgery.

AP: I think at the beginning, women, we had to be very strong and very hard to be respected. We had to be hard with our colleague, hard with the nurses, hard with the patient, because male doctor didn't want to leave us space. To me, the biggest revolution in work was done by the woman, because if you realize 100 years ago there was no female employed in anything. We're all, you know, we're all like married women.

JM: Housewives.

AP: Housewives. So in 100 years, we have arrived, you know, there's a bigger revolution in the employment system, you know, but so at the beginning, when we became doctors or surgeons, we had to be hard with our female colleague because they didn't want us there. They didn't want us with nurses who were used to being with male doctors. So nobody wanted us. So it's why we had to shout to be heard, you know, I love that. Now we can be heard being ourselves.

JM: I love that. That's beautiful. That's beautiful because that's really, really interesting. I don't know if you remember, but maybe a long time ago, 2004, 2007, they had in the British Medical Journal (BMJ), they had a list of milestones since the beginning of the journal, which started publishing what, about 1800 or something like that. I can't remember exactly. And one of the milestones proposed was the pill. For this reason.
Well, in the end, sanitation was the winner, I think. Yes, if you can talk about a winner, but what you're saying is very, very interesting. Very interesting.

AP: But now we are more accepted now women, we are accepted.

JM: You know, how it should be. I'll always remember Anna, a beautiful comment you made, and I think it was in Santiago de Compostela when you started a talk by saying a patient came in, into my consultation with an MRI or with an image and showed me the image and you said, 'I don't want to see the image. I want to see you'.

AP: Yes.

JM: You're a great believer in a humanistic approach to surgery. Can you explain this? Can you further this?

AP: Well, I think medicine and surgery is a philosophy of life, you know? Is a philosophy of life. It's the way you have chosen to live. You have chosen to be a surgeon, a doctor to help, to help people. And if you want to help, you have to be a human being. **First of all, you have to be human**. Yes. Me, I prefer to have a human person as a colleague, who is a normal surgeon, than to have a genius as a surgeon who is a not a very nice person. That's it. You know, so I think medicine is not an art nor a job, but it is a philosophy of life in giving what you know to somebody without asking for anything in return. You know what I mean?

AP: I know.

JM: So it's why humanity, you have to be human being to be a doctor. Otherwise you should not be a doctor. If you cannot feel, what? When somebody cries, if you can't feel, live and go away.

AP: And this is happening, the fact now that more and more doctors maybe they can't feel or can't have this empathy with the other person.

JM: I don't know, in the UK, but here at the moment,

AP: Yeah. So many people don't have empathy. Sometimes you don't really know what the patient wants. Many people who are not very well, who are very unwell, come to us with other objectives. That means, you know, so at the moment, we are very unprotected by everybody, by the politicians, by the health authorities.

JM: By the directors of the hospitals?

AP: Yes. So, you know, many people want to get money through health now. So, I think we need a rehumanization of everybody, really, you know, of everybody Of everybody. Yes, we have lost empathy because we have no time. We have no time to be empathic. And neurosurgery is no different. We are between 20 minutes per new patient, but for revision it's 10 min. We have 10 minutes. You know, GPs have 3 or 4 minutes. You cannot be a doctor. You have to write in the computer, you have to undress the patient, you have to dress the patient, you have to explain to the patient. So when can you be empathic?

JM: Yes, I see your point completely. And you touched on something which I think is very interesting. The other day we had Gavin Francis speaking to students and he said that all medical students, you should read as much literature as possible, because literature opens up different worlds to you, opens up worlds that you don't know about. Opens you up to different backgrounds, multicultural, multi-lingual, and this teaches you a lot. So, for those who don't have that, literature can do that. And literature maybe the problem is not in medical education. Maybe the humanities have been pushed aside completely.

AP: Totally. Yes. Yeah. What I can understand, Jonathan, is why it happens so quickly, you know, I mean, in Spain, if you look at this, we have changed so quickly. You know, people don't say 'good morning' anymore. You go into the lift, where there are twenty persons, and say, "Buenos dias." Nobody says anything. You know, as though we're transparent, you know. Like if we're invisible.

JM: But I always **insist**, if I say good morning to somebody and they don't answer, I insist. I say good morning again !!!!

AP: But, you know, I don't know what has happened and so quickly.

JM: Very quickly. There's a beautiful saying by, I think it's Professor Roger Kneebone who did something incredible. He went from becoming a surgeon to a GP, which you don't normally do. It is very, very interesting. But now he's Professor of Academic Surgery at Imperial College in London. He wrote a beautiful book called *Expert*. And he said medicine is neither a science, nor an art, nor a craft, but a combination of the three. Is this true of surgery?

AP: Yes. Surgery is not. I forgot to resume here what I think here. Surgeries, humanities. **Art is magic**. It is a miracle. His life is dead. Surgery is everything. It is everything. There are no definitions for surgery.

JM: I love it.

AP: Everything is everything to me.

JM: Surgery is life.

AP: Life is life is what it is, you know, dynamic. Dynamic. Some people come very ill, then you operate, and then perhaps they get better, perhaps worse. It's dynamic. I don't know. It's wonderful.

JM: Surgery is wonderful. I mean, I love that because we've come from a little bit of a dark area when we're talking about the way things are moving. And then you say surgery is wonderful, is everything, is life. And I remember in Barcelona you said that, um, **the art of medicine is the patient**.

AP: Yes, it is. And our relationship with him and the relation between patients and doctors is what it is to me anyway.

You know, we don't have to look. We only have to look back. Back the way, you know, people want a doctor to hold their hands. People now realize they don't only want an MRI. They want to be listened to. They want to be loved by a doctor, you know, I know they want to be with you. They want to decide their own life, but they still want to have a doctor like we have always been, you know, like the old GP where they were like their fathers. I know we are against that type of medicine, but patients want that. They ask me what should I do. What should you do? And we don't say that anymore. We're not allowed to say that.

JM: But it's not. It's not only the patient who wants that. It's the doctor who needs that relationship as well.

AP: Yes,

JM: And yeah, sorry.

AP: I want to see a patient as a friend. I don't want to see them as an enemy. We are not enemies. We didn't do it deliberately. You know, that happened. So, they see us very often as an enemy. And we, sometimes we see them as an enemy because we're scared they might sue us, you know. So that love; that relationship is sometimes very delicate. Be careful.

JM: You know. You've used a word which is very, very important. You use the word love.

AP: Yes.

JM: In surgery. And some people might find this a little strange, but I don't. But can you explain that a little further?

AP: Love, meaning surgery.

JM: Love in surgery. Love. The word love coming from a neurosurgeon, for me, is fabulous.

AP: Yeah. Well, love, I think we're in love. The different aspects of. We can apply love in many aspects. We're in love. We have a job, you know, I mean, neurosurgery is our companion, which could be a good companion or a bad companion. You know, you always remember, you only remember when he's a bad companion, like a, you know, Henry Marsh said, you have a cemetery in your head.

JM: Yeah, yeah, yeah, that was Marsh. But I think that he was quoting from Rene Leriche.

AP: Yes, that's it. It is. It is. So. We are in love with our job. We are in love. We are also in love with patients, we also love patients. We want them to get better. We want that without knowing them because, you know, I don't know, in the UK, but here in Spain, a patient comes to the hospital, and they put their life in your hands. So, there is. We're in love with our job. We are in love with patients. You know, as well, it's what we should do. Anyway, you know.

JM: I'm kind of in awe of what you say, Anna. You know, I remember we had a very short conversation in Santiago when we were going on the roundtable, and I was impressed straight away. But the words you say now touch a real chord with me. And I'm saying touch for another reason, because I'd like you to explain the importance of touch. And I know there are many kinds of touch, and for a surgeon, touch is exceptionally important.

AP: Well, in surgery, there are two ways of touching. There's a touch for diagnosis, examination, and then there's a touch or communication. You know, mind you, now, before I always used to use the patient to tap the shoulder. And now I'm a bit scared because you have to be careful. No, no. Spanish people love touching. There is a way we express our feelings. So, we have two ways of touching. Touching using our hands. Hands are wonderful to explore the patient, to reach a diagnosis. And then we have touching for showing the way we feel at that moment with the patient. You know, when I give bad news, I always come and hold the hands because they feel a connection, you know, they don't feel lonely. They feel that somebody is with them at the moment, you know, they don't feel lonely. So that way of touching is telling the patient, listen, you're not alone. I'm here to help you.

JM: And this you're talking about like cognitive and therapeutic touch. And therapeutic touch is scientifically proven to help patients.

AP: Oh, yes, yes, yes. I was watching, somebody in a meeting recently and they were doing some study on patients with brain injuries and where they were only telling the name. You know, so it was not touching, it was saying the name, you know, so because the patient could feel somebody was caring for them.

JM: So, in reality, if the politicians or the policymakers, let's say, or everybody who has the money to spend in improving the medical systems, they could, they could do it. They could do it very easily just by simple things like giving more time to the doctor. This would reduce the money because you would have more time to touch, to speak, to listen. It's obvious. It seems obvious to us, Anna, but maybe we're more philosophical in approach than economically inclined. I don't know, but it seems obvious.

AP: Well, they have different interests. They have political interests. We don't have. As they have quantitative objectives, as we have qualitative objectives. We want patients to live. So, we are led by people who lead us with different objectives. So, it can't work. It cannot work. It's impossible. You know, it's very important to remind the people not to go to A&E if they don't need to.

JM: We're at a loggerheads. We're kind of clashing at the beginning of this fascinating interview. I'm really loving it. At the beginning, you said that you went into surgery and neurosurgery because you wanted to help and you saw that you can, in surgery, you can see the results.

AP: Yes.

JM: My father, who was a surgeon, and he was vocational like you. And when he retired, he said, "I think if I studied medicine again, I would go into preventive medicine; you can help more people or education."

AP: Yes. Me, I would become, I think, an anesthetist or surgeon, because anesthetists are very good doctors, and they can help anywhere, you know, in every field, pain, cardiac arrests. You know, I would become also a neurosurgeon. But I think the bad thing about neurosurgery is that it is a specialty for rich countries, not for poor countries. In poor countries, they don't need neurosurgeons but they need over kinds of doctors: surgeons, orthopedic surgeons, physicians. So, neurosurgery is for rich countries, really, because who has a hernia operated on in Africa? Nobody.

JM: This brings me to another topic of great importance. Have you worked or are you working in any humanitarian projects in poor countries or developing countries?

AP: Yeah, I went a few times now six, seven times with the Spanish government to Niger. And we stopped because there was a coup d'etat. And it was a wonderful experience. Wonderful experience. And I'm proud that Spain helps other countries, but I'm very proud that Spain, despite not being a rich country, we are thinking of people who are worse than we are. And I think not with politics. I don't think Spain is looking for getting money from there. You know what I mean? Like all the countries, you know, it's only to help. So, yes, I went, and it made me realize how much we have. It made me realize how stupid we are, complaining about things every day, all day, you know, how stupid we are, losing time complaining. "I don't have that." "I don't have that." "I want that." I mean, in Niger, there are 42 anesthetists for the whole country. People have to travel 5 or 6 hours. Last time I went there, I went to the casualty department, and there was a patient with a knife in the sternum after traveling for days. I came from the city and there was a girl with an amputee arm. I mean, amazing, you know. So, I realized. So few people have access to healthcare.

JM: So, you know, did you, did you take those experiences back to you, back to Ourense? To teach them to your residents, to your students?

AP: Yeah. Well, I gave a few talks in Ourense. In schools they invite me to speak in schools. Yeah, in schools to speak to kids and to teachers about my experience with my slides and soon. And since then, many people, even in the hospital, for example, now we, we change all the theater tables. So, it's good. Very good. Yeah.

JM: So is there any chance of you restarting in Niger or would you consider going to another project?

AP: Yes, I think the Spanish government has made an announcement for doctors to give their name, the one who wanted to go to countries, and I told them that I don't mind going to any country because what we do in Niger is teaching, for example, to put a cervical collar. We don't need MRI or CT scans. We need to teach them how to carry a patient with a spinal injury or, you know, is what we do there, you know.

JM: So, you don't operate or do you operate? You don't operate?

AP: No. Because I don't think if you go there and operate them with navigation instrument and then you go back to the country, and you take your navigation instrument back with or you take them some technically advanced instrument and then they don't have the tools to make it work. So, it's ridiculous. So, I don't think you should but if you do go there to operate on, you should leave everything there, but they should be able to use it again, you know. Yeah. You need a follow up.

AP: That's it.

JM: You need a follow up.

AP: Yes.

JM: So you are, you are a doctor when you go to Nigeria. **But all surgeons are doctors**.

AP: Yes. Yes. first of all, we are doctors. Yeah, yeah.

JM: Do some surgeons forget that?

AP: Well, we are becoming very specialized. Amongst all the surgeons, general surgeons are still very good doctors, you know, because their patients can have complication with electrolytes, with fluid or with sepsis after the operation. So, general surgeons are still very good. Others? Neurosurgeons? we see a doctor because our patient can have lung problem or, you know, or you lose sodium or have had an epileptic fit. Others are different. Others specialties have forgotten to be doctors.

JM: Yeah, yeah, yeah. It's a fascinating. No, there was always, there was also in the BMJ, there was a question many years ago, "Do you need to be a good person to be a good doctor?" Yes. And my answer is pretty obvious. But I want. I think you would agree with me. No?

AP: Yes. Yes, I do. They're saying young doctors have no vocation. I would say no because many young doctors are wonderful persons. I'm in a hospital, my hospital here in Ourense, the residents are wonderful persons, you know, they smile and despite working for countless hours, you know, you call them, and they never say no. They always say yes, you know. So, I see the resident doctors at my hospital. They all very nice persons.

JM: Well, maybe this is because of the atmosphere but this is positive. And I'm very happy because my next question comes to AI and whether this, how much this will change medicine and how much it will change surgery and neurosurgery with, with things like the Da Vinci. Because you don't touch anymore.

AP: No, but you still have to be in theater. Somebody directing from the machine by a surgeon on the ground. But I think we navigate now in the brain, we have navigation. We have, neurophysiological monitoring. But I think artificial intelligence will improve, and will decrease complications. But a robot will never give you a hug. A robot never will give you or will never, you know, never give you a kiss. Fantastic. So, will AI take it away? I mean, they say that, that the machine will replace the radiologist. No, I think, as I told you, no machine will hug or kiss a patient. Human beings will do that. Yeah, you're going back to the idea of love, the idea of the relationship-based medicine. Yes. Definitely, yes. So, will AI take the humanization away? But we shouldn't allow that. We have to learn to live with machines, with technology, because it's good for the patient because it gives you security, but it cannot replace the figure of a doctor or a nurse, you know.

JM: Yeah, no, this is. This is magic to my ears. Oh, no, this is magic to my ears because it's a big debate. Maybe I think it's being pushed as well. It's being pushed. There are, let's say, big interests behind.

AP: Yes. I mean, we need technology. Technology has been wonderful for us in neurosurgery. We can navigate in the brain. Before, when we opened the brain, we were not too sure where the tumor was but now, we can navigate the craniotomy. We go inside the brain. We know where the tumor is. Technology has improved a lot, you feel more secure, but the technology, when the patient wakes up in the theater and, for example, he has a hemiplegia, or he's not talking, the patient still needs somebody to talk to them, to explain to him, and he cannot be with a robot. No way. No.

JM: This is fabulous. I had the privilege with my daughter to go and see a neurosurgical operation, it was a biopsy of a glioblastoma. But I was really impressed. Not only by the technical side but I was really impressed by the love that the neurosurgeons showed, when they held the head of the patient in their hands, and then after the operation, They were stroking the head of the patient after they had finished the procedure, and this is what I took away.

AP: Yes, it is. Do you know, for a surgeon, for a neurosurgeon, the worst moment is waiting for the patient to wake up to see if he's talking. Is he moving? You know, to me, waiting for the patient to wake up is terrible. Because if he doesn't talk, it's your fault. If the doesn't move, it's your fault. You know, you are responsible for it, and you cannot do anything because often it is irreversible. I mean, you condemn somebody to be in a bed.

JM: You carry this with you?

AP: You follow up. You do the war drum the following day, and you see the patient there, and then you follow up. You see them in the outpatient's clinic. The only patients who disappear are the ones who dies. The one who has a complication stays with you for the rest of your life. Sorry.

JM: How can you manage this responsibility?

AP: Well, at the beginning, it's terrible. You feel terrible. Well, every time you have a big complication, you feel terrible. You don't learn how to get over it. And I think you shouldn't. Because if you, if you try, if you don't feel anything that is terrible, you, you don't, learn how to live with it. Every time you have a bad complication, it's terrible. Terrible. There's no way. You don't. There is no, there are no tools to help you. It affects you. Deeply.

JM: Nobody helps you.

AP: Even the psychologist tries to help you. You feel it is your responsibility. That man is hemiplegic because of my operation, you know. And what you have to do is know, is you have to go. I've learned that what you have to learn is to go and talk to a patient and apologize, you know, not to run away because some doctors don't go to see the patient after that. You know, you have to, you have to go with him and to tell him what happened and that you have to learn to do it. You have to learn how to put your face in front of the patient and say, 'well, I'm very sorry what happened.' And you explain to him, and if you explain to the patient and you apologize, the relationship between you and the patient is great.

Yes, it continues. If you escape from the patient and if you don't go, it's terrible. The patient feels abandoned. You can't abandon the patient in the worst moment of his life. It's when you have to be present, with him, next to him, spend more time with him, and try and understand his sadness, you know, it's when you have to be with him more. More than ever. He's in the worst moment.

JM: So I always think that humility is an important quality for a good surgeon. Would you agree?

AP: Humanity?

JM: Humility.

AP: Humility. Yes, it is. Oh, yes. It is something which, when you are young, you don't know what it is. The older you are, the more humble you become. You are, you know, I love it. Oh, yes. When you are young, you think you can eat the world and then the world eats you. You know.

JM: This is. I don't really want to finish this, but it's a Sunday evening and tomorrow you have to get up. I have to get up early. But I have one last question.

AP: Yes.

JM: And what advice would you give to a young student if they wanted to go into surgery?

AP: Well, I would definitely tell them to go ahead. It is wonderful. I don't like to say, job, it is a wonderful way of life, you know, it's not a job, it's a way of life.

JM: To know how to take a medical history, to examine patients, to study, to be up to date. And then maybe I should not say that; not to listen to the managers.

AP: I just told you, definitely. But I also tell them, it's a hard life, a very hard life, full of responsibility. They have to accept responsibility, but it's a wonderful way of living because you give life and you save life. Life is a friend. Our enemy is death, and we always have to fight against death. You have to be with the patient in the best moments and in the worst moments. But it is very hard. Life is a very bad companion sometimes, and you don't have to when it's a bad companion. Don't hate it, you know as it makes you stronger because the one who has the complications is not you but somebody else, you know? And what I definitely say is we have to change the way we work because it's not working at the moment. Healthcare is going in the wrong direction because it's politicized. We are managed by politicians; we are managed by people who don't know what medicine is about. We only look at numbers. We have to look about quality, about humanity. But I would definitely tell them, go ahead, it's a wonderful way of living.

Chapter 23
Humanism in Surgery

Patrick C. Walsh

Thank you for giving me the privilege of speaking to you today. I'm going to begin by telling you a few things about myself that are very personal. I was born in Akron, Ohio, in February 1938, into a relatively poor family. From the time I was 3 years old through high school at age 18, I was taught by Dominican nuns. As I reflect on the factors that most influenced my career, it was my Catholic education, and the example set by my parents. Throughout my life, I have been surrounded by contemporaries who had a better, more elite education, were more intelligent and talented, and possibly worked harder. Yet many of them lost focus and changed direction, losing the momentum necessary to make a sustained contribution. On the other hand, from the time I was very small, I was constantly reminded by the Dominican nuns and my parents why I was on this earth—to know, love, and serve God and to use the gifts that I had been given to help my fellow man—literally to give the gifts away. I always wanted to be a doctor and the pathway for my future seemed very clear and relatively uncomplicated. For those reasons, I never seemed to lose my way and when the future was unclear, all I did was ask for God's help.

It is my belief that the first responsibility of surgeons is to know their patients well. My core belief is "The secret in the care of the patient is in caring for the patient." This statement is taken from a talk given by a Boston physician, Francis Peabody, who was a professor at Harvard. In 1927, he developed terminal cancer and before he died, he gave a lecture to the Harvard Medical School class. The title of this talk was "the care of the patient" and it was based on his experience as a patient while he was dying from cancer. The final sentence in this talk was "the secret in the care of the patient is in caring for the patient." The humanism I practice is based on my Catholic faith and as Jesus said, "we should love one another as I have loved you." To accomplish this, before operating on a patient I spend time

P. C. Walsh (✉)
Johns Hopkins School of Medicine Faculty, Baltimore, MD, USA
e-mail: pwalsh@jhmi.edu

J. McFarland et al. (eds.), *Humanism in Surgery*, New Paradigms in Healthcare,
https://doi.org/10.1007/978-3-031-86018-8_23

getting to know them and showing them that I care for them. I believe that the healing begins that day.

Being a surgeon at times can be a great challenge—indeed, a dramatic challenge in which life and death are literally in your hands. As a young man I worried that I would not be able to do this and wondered about how I would feel if something went wrong. But, as I got older I realized that God would be there to help. He would be present in the operating room but only if I asked for him. After all, patients pray to God for help. But how is this help delivered? Sometimes, rarely, it is in the form of a miracle. More often, I believe the help is through their physician and other health care givers. However, for God's influence to be maximized we *must be receptive to it*, we must *ask for His help* and we must *understand* that we are *God's instrument—quite literally surgeons have the responsibility to be the hands of God*. Patients must also understand that we have been given a talent that comes from God and that our ability to cure them can only be successful with His help. Whenever possible, I try to make this point when I first evaluate a patient and give advice on treatment. I tell them that I work for God, that we are all given gifts, and it is our responsibility to share them. Then, I repeat this message at several pivotal times in their subsequent care. At the end of every operation when it has gone well, I am eager to give God the credit and I openly declare so in the operating room for all to hear. If the case is difficult, I find it easy to tell everyone in the operating room that right now we need to ask for God's help. And when I come out of the operating room and talk to the family, and later to the patient, I again make it clear that the operation went well because of that help. The next time I repeat this theme is when the pathology report comes back. This is a tense moment. Has all the cancer been removed? If it has and the patient tries to thank me, I remind them that this is not in my hands but in the hands of God. I am only His messenger and cannot make a good pathology report. They need to thank Him for being cured.

The process I am describing is not an act nor a script that I've rehearsed, but it is an honest admission of the limits of what I can do. In fact, I am often not aware of what I have said. However, I did have a wonderful reminder a number of years ago. We were in the process of building a new church and I was very active in raising the money to make this possible. Because I enjoy talking to patients so that they can get to know me, I'm sure I must have mentioned this. One Sunday at Mass our Pastor read a letter from a patient without mentioning my name. This letter was accompanied by a generous check for construction of the new church and by the following comments. "My doctor does not realize it but he has saved my life twice. Not only did he cure my cancer but he has also brought me back to the church. Although I don't think he realized it, many times when we spoke he gently, ever so gently mentioned the role that God played in his own life. What he did notknow is that I had not been to church in 30 years but now I am reunited with my faith."

In addition to patient care, God can be a powerful ally in the field of discovery. Francis Collins, the great geneticist, is fond of saying every time he makes a new discovery he realizes he now knows something that only God knew previously. Patients are constantly praying to God for help and often for that help to occur there must be progress in scientific discovery. I have been very lucky in my life to have made some important discoveries that have improved the care of men with prostate cancer. In retrospect, some of these discoveries actually turned out to be something that should have been relatively obvious. How did this happen? I asked for God's help and then did something else. I listened to my patients. If a patient asks you a question and you cannot find the answer or tells you something that sounds incorrect, this may be your opportunity to make an important discovery.

Here are 2 examples.

In the 1980s, because all men were impotent following surgery for prostate cancer, radical prostatectomies were rarely performed and because radiation therapy at that time was underpowered to cure, essentially no one was being treated with curative intent. At that time everyone believed that the nerves responsible for erectile function ran through the prostate and it would be impossible to preserve potency if the prostate was removed. However, when a patient of mine returned following surgery and told me that he was fully potent, I knew that was not true. But where were the nerves? This initiated anatomical studies that dramatically transformed our understanding and made surgery at that time the most common form of treatment for the disease. The second example was a patient whose father, his father's 3 brothers, and his grandfather had all died from prostate cancer. He asked me if prostate cancer was hereditary. I could not find the answer, and this initiated a study that has gone on for 3 decades unraveling the mystery of prostate cancer genetics.

Up to this point, I have talked about how health care givers must be aware of the role that God plays in our lives. However, we also have another responsibility to reawaken the same spirituality in our patients. At the appropriate time, it is important to ask patients if they have a personal relationship with God or a religious belief and to remind them that this is an important bonus in the healing process. An illness is an important wake-up call—a reminder of an individual's mortality and an ideal opportunity to reawaken religious feelings, like the patient I described above. Also, for some patients today there is no way to cure their disease and here it is important to encourage them to rely on God's help.

I have just recited stories where I was successful in using God's help. Let me tell you of a case, early in my career, where I was not successful, a case that taught me a lot. I came to Johns Hopkins in July 1974 and on *February 28, 1975*, I saw the brilliant 54-year-old Director of the Smithsonian Institutions. His wife has given me permission to tell this story and to use his name—Robert Brooks. Unfortunately, when he came to see me he had an inoperable cancer. Although I had been schooled in delivering this diagnosis with compassion, the patient was very direct—"Am I a candidate for surgery"—unfortunately no. "What else is available"—radiationtherapy. "What if it doesn't work—is there chemotherapy?" Unfortunately, at this time no. "If that happens how long do I have to live"—probably no more than 2 years.

Eighteen months later I received a letter from his wife who was typing this poem for inclusion in a book of all his poems. She told me that she thought I ought to have a copy since few doctors, and especially those in my special position, had a poem written especially for and to them. It was entitled "Consultation February 28, 1975."

I'll never forget the July evening I received that poem and I've tried never to make that mistake again. At a moment like this, patients need to have hope by understanding the multiple ways in which God will help them if they place themselves in His hands. I tell this story and read this poem to every student and resident who works with me in clinic so that they will learn this lesson early in their careers. But the story doesn't end there. Seven years ago, 40 years after that episode, I was alone in clinic on a Friday afternoon when an elderly man and his wife stopped in to see me. He was a neighbor who just had a CT scan of his abdomen and he asked me to look at it. He had a large bladder cancer extending outside the bladder to the pelvic sidewall associated with large lymph node metastases. Doesn't this sound familiar? When he asked me what I saw, I told him that I thought he may have a bladder tumor. "That's what Dr. Carter thought when I saw him last week because I was having blood in my urine. What do you think they will do?" I told him that "in most cases like this we remove the bladder but it looked like the tumor may have spread to lymph nodes and in cases like this we begin with chemotherapy and if the lymph nodes shrink sometimes all we need to do is radiate the bladder." Every word of that was true but I left out one statement—I had never seen anyone cured with that treatment. But he was! And he is alive today cancer free. The moral of this story is to never take away hope. 45 years ago that was not possible but it is today even though the chance of success may be marginal. Never take away hope.

In closing, as I put this talk together, I thought I should retitle it using the title of the autobiography of Francis Moore, the famous Harvard surgeon, "Medicine, Is a Miracle and a Privilege."

Thank you for the honor of addressing you on this special occasion.

Chapter 24
Conversation with Surgeon 12—John Varallo

René Génadry

Recorded online on May 16th, 2024, by René Génadry.

Abbreviations that follow

JV: John Varallo
RG: René Génadry
Jhpiego: Johns Hopkins program for international education in Gyn/Ob

RG: Hi John and thank you so much for taking the time to talk to me. I would like to get an idea of your journey and get some insight on what it takes to be a humanitarian physician and surgeon. It really has been quite a journey, how did it all start?

JV: Well, I would say that one the biggest, early influence for me was my undergraduate education going to Georgetown University. I was pretty isolated, growing up in a pretty small town in NJ and, like a lot of people around there, I did not have the most expansive worldview. Then being at Georgetown, and I'm not a particularly religious person, but the Jesuit approach, their worldview around social justice really struck me; and I think that was one of my earliest influences that got me interested in medicine and in trying to address social injustices. I went to medical school at Georgetown, on a scholarship, and then specialized in Obstetrics and Gynecology. What drew me to that specialty was a combination of things: one was personal, my mother for example—it was not a great family situation. And I just felt like she was really marginalized—in the community, in the marriage, and both sides of the families for various reasons, but that made me think more about women, the importance of women and how they are often marginalized and vulnerable in many societies. I went to

R. Génadry (✉)
Carver College of Medicine, University of Iowa, Iowa City, IA, USA

J. McFarland et al. (eds.), *Humanism in Surgery*, New Paradigms in Healthcare,
https://doi.org/10.1007/978-3-031-86018-8_24

Georgetown medical school on a Navy scholarship, so they paid for that and then I did my residency with them. I was also involved with various teaching programs… another big influence for me was going to Australia and my first true work with indigenous communities. This occurred about 1 year after getting out of the Navy. I was working with a large health care delivery system that I didn't particularly like because I just felt like I was on a treadmill, and to be honest, I was a bit disillusioned by medicine after getting out of the military, which was like socialized medicine, but I did like working in the inner city and in the urban areas. Then I went to Australia for a year and a half off and on, which is when I got interested in global health and public health. We were a referral hospital for and doing outreach clinics to Aboriginal Australian communities in Far North Queensland. And that experience struck me and stuck with me—just looking at the injustices, the inequitable burden of disease among the population. And it's obviously happening in the US, but maybe it was just looking at different populations and different contexts. Later, I worked with the Indian Health Service on various reservations in Montana and Arizona and saw how marginalized the Native American communities are. Around this time, I started doing volunteer work, going to Guyana in South America. The first day I was on the wards, and you have indigenous women, Amerindians from the interior, who are in their 30 s or early 40 s just waiting to die from advanced cervical cancer—it was just awful. So, all those things influenced me to want to do more global health work. That's when I shifted my career, and I went back and got my master's degree in global health at GW (George Washington). I continued working in Guyana and that's how I got connected with Jhpiego, around some of the work I was doing with cervical cancer prevention there. I joined Jhpiego about 2 years now over 12 years ago and was senior technical advisor with them, working on maternal and newborn health, cervical cancer prevention, and then the last 6 years as a global director for safe surgery: I've worked in over 20 different countries experiencing the different contexts and the inequitable burden of disease and the conditions that people are living in. Connecting with the communities and with the teams on the ground is just awesome: I mean it was just really it was like a calling, and it was like this is it, this is what I want to do for the rest of my life. I've been very fortunate to be able to follow that path and to have that kind of rewarding experience. This is a quick overview: I can go into great details if you have questions about certain things; wherever you want to take this is fine with me.

RG: You've seen it from both ends from a caring physician to a programmatic administrator, so you really have a unique perspective on how humanitarian work is really planned and delivered. John, was there in growing up any person besides your mother that has made an impact and directed you along the path that you've taken?

JV: So, as I mentioned the Jesuits, surprisingly, and I'm an atheist, but their worldview and that kind of philosophy and social justice thinking was really important to me. The other was during my training, my chief residents were influential as great role models.

RG: For example?

JV: Just to see how caring someone is. Not just that you're going through it, trying to do your work—it's all very technical type of thing—but seeing them sitting down and listening to a patient: you can see the empathy and you see that connection but also seeing it and understanding it, because you can get overwhelmed by work and it's just all about getting the work done, but that connection is really powerful. The other part is working with nurses and midwives and seeing how they are—their empathy and how their compassionate care can make a difference; and you continue to see this. I think about this with my mother-in-law who recently died from pancreatic cancer and others that you know and that go through health crises. If you're there with them, now you're on the other side, and experiencing how things are from that perspective, and how people communicate is really important. Another influence was when I went to Australia and saw how the team I was working with approached life and approached medicine; and working with the indigenous population, those are just powerful moments for me. And honestly, I could share examples in almost every place I go to, I get that kind of inspiration from people that are on the ground doing the work and developing those relationships with them. It is one of the beautiful things about the work I do.

RG: Is your impression that the tendency to be a humanistic physician is innate or is it something that's teachable?

JV: It's a good question. I think it's innate. I think you can teach it to a degree and some people will do OK with it for a while: I've seen people turn it around, improve, but I think a lot of it is innate. It's interesting I'm thinking about this one doc in Kenya, and this was recently. We did a training with them, that included non-technical skills such as teamwork and communication. She came across as a very stern person that didn't really communicate very well: her teaching approach was close to, I'm telling you what to do, you do it, and things like that. But in our approach, we focus a lot on teams coming together, breaking down professional hierarchies, a lot of focus on teamwork and communication, and you saw the light bulb go off for her and she became a totally different person. People on the ground were saying it's unbelievable what she is like now because before she was this very stern person, you couldn't break through this exterior and she is now the model coach and teacher. So, I think you can teach some of it, it's a rare thing that we have that kind of turn around, but something must be innate. Maybe that's where talking about the humanities could cause someone to open up and they're going to be much more responsive to it.

RG: So, you need a trigger besides the environment, and do you think such education could be a trigger?

JV: I do. I do and I think a different way of doing medical education can attract people that have that innate ability, and they're going to be the ones that are going to be more receptive and will respond to that kind of teaching better; and I think for those who don't have that, it can help soften some of those rough edges,

RG: I'm again impressed by your background and I'm surprised that the Jesuits had let you off, but do you think one has to be religious to be humanitarian?

JV: Ohh God no, not at all.

RG: Can you expand on that.

JV: Being humane doesn't mean you don't need a God or a spiritual being to help you with that. If you want to call it spiritual that's fine but it's not a supreme being or some religious entity that is needed. For me honestly part of what drove me away from religion is just my mother's experience and the hypocrisy that I witnessed.

RG: So, I guess if you went back, you would be a reformer (Laugh). John, you've had a lot of experience dealing with patients in Guyana and Africa, how would advise somebody who wants to get into a humanitarian career in dealing with a patient in a different environment?

JV: I would say that you need to be flexible, and you need to be humble. That's the huge thing, not this "cultural competency," but cultural humility. That's the main thing, and not coming in with preconceived notions, and not coming in with the notion that you're a savior. It's working in true solidarity. There are going to be many things that you can't control and you're going to see a lot of terrible things and you know you need to be able to manage that. To me, it's really a calling and you know it's not for the experience, you're not doing this health volunteerism type of thing but it's really about a calling. You think about working with the communities but it's also individuals and being able to connect on that individual level and being empathetic. As they're getting into that field, people need to be aware of and realize as well that there's going to be sacrifices on your own time, on your personal life, on your family life from the travel and from the stresses, but that that's the tradeoff for the work that you're doing.

RG: John, do you have a family.

JV: I have a wife, no kids by choice. She's a biological archaeologist. We met when she was a nurse in the Navy and she continued to do nursing, but then she went back and got her anthropology degree, master's then her PhD and she's working for the Smithsonian.

RG: Does she go with you?

JV: She's only gone a couple of times. When I'm working it tends to be in more remote areas and it can be difficult for her to get the time off and to coordinate schedules. But she joined me on a few trips.

RG: It sounds like when you started out, you started out individually: you weren't part of an established organization. So, you really made it happen for you is that correct?

JV: Yeah, are you talking about within public health?

RG: No, I'm talking about the humanitarian work that you started out with in Australia you went on your own and in South America you were going as a as an individual physician or were you going with some colleagues?

JV: For Australia I was by myself, and then Guyana at first it was volunteer work with a very small NGO. Then I got connected with Jhpiego and started doing consultancy work with them.

RG: So Jhpiego was the largest organization you've been working with. And this was circumstantial because of what you were involved with that coincided with their interest. Was there any other personal or any other factor that moved you from delivering individual care to getting involved in more programmatic global view?

JV: This was in Guyana in South America. I was doing my master's in public health at that time and for my thesis I did a poster on some work we did for an outreach to the indigenous community deep in the interior where we're taking cervical cancer prevention work in mobile clinics. And so, I just developed a poster that got accepted at a conference in Boston. Just happenstance you know Jhpiego walks by, and they're interested; so, we start talking, and I started using some of their materials and I helped develop the national cervical cancer program in Guyana. USAID heard of this (they were in Guyana, and we met) and they wanted to fund it, but they couldn't fund me as an individual, so that's where Jhpiego came in developed that kind of relationships.

RG: OK. Are you still involved in individual care or you're just not doing it as much you're basically just in training and developing programs?

JV: Yeah, so now I'm with the Global Surgery Foundation. I've been with them for a year. I'm the team lead for Women's Health programs. I still develop programs and manage programs, but I also still go and do training. I was just in India for example, we have a Nepal project coming up, and I also still go to Alaska for clinical work every 3 months or so for a couple of weeks at a time.

RG: You're keeping your hands wet; I mean you're not just sitting behind the desk and developing programs.

JV: No. This is OK, sitting at a desk, but after a while I start getting antsy, I need to be in the field. Well, it's a little bit better now since I left Jhpiego because I was traveling close to 50% of the time, and it just takes a lot of wear and tear on you personally and on your relationships.

RG: Well from your perspective do you think that insisting upon exposing physicians to the humanities is critical and at what level if you think so.

JV: Yeah, I don't know at what level. I think the principle of it is important because it can help inform a person's worldview. I think it makes you a better person all around because, for me, medicine isn't just technical. There's a lot of non-technical aspects to it—the more you can bring that into medicine the better for everyone. You're able to have more compassion, you're able to connect better and with a more diverse group of people. I think the older generation tend to be more technical and with very limited humanities type of background. I think you can see that in the quality of care that's provided, not from a technical standpoint, but from a holistic approach and being able to understand and to connect with patients: that's the beauty of it when you're able to connect on different levels, it just brings a richness to the experience and to the care.

RG: So, do you think the newer generation seems to be more humanistic than the older generation?

JV: I don't know necessarily about the generation, but I think we are attracting a different type of person to medicine now, whereas before it was very scientific-focused. Now we are attracting people with different backgrounds and different approaches more of that humanistic element.

RG: Yeah, are you talking primarily about the people that are getting involved in humanitarian work?

JV: No. I think across the board actually.

RG: So, what you're saying is that there certainly is some material there that is very receptive or would be receptive to the humanities because of where they're coming from.

JV: Yeah, yeah yeah definitely.

RG: So that would be encouraging to capitalize on that tendency.

JV: Absolutely and I mean even thinking about my pathway, I regret a little bit that my undergraduate studies were pre-med biology major; and even with our medical school, anyone who wasn't a biology major was very rare. But now it is less so, and I think we would have been a better kind of class, more diverse class if the humanities had a greater presence.

RG: With all the science that is required in medical school, maybe pre-Med should be where humanities is insisted upon.

JV: I think that's a really good point because there's so much that needs to be covered from the science perspective, but I still think that could be improved: you sprinkle in these different pieces, and I think it would make the learning more enjoyable, and lead to a better-rounded person. For example, I felt I grew quite a bit during my undergrad years, I moved from a small town in South Jersey, and I wasn't really exposed to the world. It was in Washington DC, with the politics and urban life—I got involved working with urban youth—and my roommate was very liberal and open minded, so I think that helped. Then you got the crush of medical school and all the focus on studying, and you feel like you get a bit narrow, which isn't good. So, I think just being able to bring the humanities in a little bit more. But I think your point about catching early helps. And that goes back to the point with the older generation of physicians where it's difficult to bring that back, but it could soften those edges.

RG: Yeah, sometimes it gets too late. So pre-Med, Med and post Med I think it's just the whole spectrum right, it's a philosophy.

JV: Even before, maybe it's possible through all of education, just better exposure to humanities is going to pique your interest in them and make you a more well-rounded person.

RG: Do you think it's possible to identify somebody who's going to be humanistic, or do you think you just see how they go and let them find themselves.

JV: It's a good question. A lot of it is that you can identify some characteristics in a person, and you think that there is some potential, that you might be able to facilitate some of the growth.

RG: So, you need to basically expose every individual and see who flourishes and who doesn't. OK, so there is a point to be made for exposing everybody and not being selective in who gets exposed.

JV: So, what do you think?

RG: I think you're absolutely right. As the tendency is innate, those that have it will certainly declare themselves very early, but there are still those like the doctor from Kenya that you mentioned that are very reserved and they really need to be given the opportunity and it's hard to tell what that trigger is going to be: sometimes it's being exposed, and sometimes it's finding your calling, whether it's a teamwork, whether it's a project or whatever it is but those that have it will declare themselves I think.

JV: Yeah, and also the idea of a role model. I think it's also something that can be a real trigger.

RG: Yeah, you made that point with the chief residents that you mentioned. Did you get any support when going through medical school when you first started being interested in humanitarian work, any faculty support, any institutional support, any family support?

JV: I have to say no. When I think about that, and I wonder how that happened. People say that to me as well, but I say that's not the usual path. I think that someone may have that support and that kind of enabling environment and then people are able to rise and flourish in that environment, and then you have others that don't have that enabling environment but somehow, they're able to overcome that and you just feel very fortunate that you're able to do it.

RG: Now John what proportion of people you train in the field present the humanitarian trait as compared to what you remember in medical school and your colleagues?

JV: Yeah, it's difficult to know people's backgrounds and where they're coming from and often in many settings some of it is language: people tend to be very reserved initially, and you think that they're reserved and they may be focused on their work, but when you get to know them, you see that there's a lot more depth to them. I would say compared to the US, or at least through my training, I think that those on the ground in other countries that have worked in low- and middle-income countries tend to have more of that humanistic tendency and that may be because of their exposures and the stresses that they have may bring that out and then more.

RG: Yeah so, the human factor is very predominant there. You were mentioning cultural sensitivity, how do you deal when you go to a different environment and what would you recommend to a medical student who wants to go there?

JV: What I would do is say you know keep your mouth shut, listen and observe and just be humble. Try to learn about the culture that you're going to beforehand, be informed, but be humble: you're not a savior, you're going there to listen, to observe and to learn from them. Be as humble as possible, and thankful for them and, you know, just learn from them.

RG: Empathy, humility is what I completely get and yeah charity if you will in just being humble to give what you can, but not to have the pride of giving.

JV: Right and especially if it's a longer-term activity, you should think of it as you are working in solidarity with them on a common purpose. And not that you're going to come in and save the world; and don't go back and pat yourself on the back and show all these photos. I would say put the camera down! Honestly just go in and immerse yourself, listen, observe and just be as humble as you can and then your experience is going to be so much richer as people open up to you and are going to share their experiences. You need to go a little bit outside of your comfort zone, don't be afraid, do it and take the opportunity to also socialize outside of the workplace so you see people in different situations because it's interesting. Especially when they're with friends, and they're with family, now you're seeing these different roles. You need to get immersed and basically get into that society and not stay apart. That's the best reward, this connection, feeling a part of the community.

RG: Do you recall any experience that really impressed you during all the years that you have worked on in low- and middle-income countries? Some event or some happening either with a patient or with a program or with something that was quite impressive for you.

JV: Honestly, I find it difficult to settle on individual events. A lot of them are popping up in my head but to me it is just thinking about the relationships, and the number of friendships that I've developed and these connections with providers and with patients. To me that's the overwhelming thing that comes to my mind when I think about it. It's not anything in particular. I can think of certain cases but that's more from the medical side of things, but to me it's just the depth of the relationships that I've been able to develop across. I'm serious there are times when I'm leaving, I get tears thinking Oh my God now I will miss them so much. Yeah, and so that, to me, is the beauty of it.

RG: Yeah, John you might not be religious but you're very spiritual. Can you tell me of the best program that you have developed the one that you're most proud of anywhere in the world? Or is each one of them unique?

JV: It is really tough to single any one out. Though, I would say because of it being recent, the work in Kenya and that doctor that I was telling you about. It's a safe surgery program where we were working in Makueni county, Kenya. This is a very much a team-based approach using multidisciplinary teams of 5 to 6 from each facility—from the higher-level facilities and the lower-level facilities. Our approach aims to build the technical aspects of surgery—techniques, evidence based best practices, but importantly, a lot around teamwork and communication and breaking down those professional hierarchies. It was interesting—we had five different hospitals, five different teams together. And the first day or so was very quiet, or one-sided, with the doctors answering, responding right away, dominating discussions. But we try to encourage others to speak up, to contribute. Eventually, especially when we're doing group work, that things turned at some point, and everyone just opened up. It felt like we were becoming a team. Over the years I developed these strong relationships with all of them with all the teams and the fantastic work that they were doing. I mean we're really making a difference, and they were we're talking about this as a game changer—the approach and things like that. I think the relationships and the depth of relationships that came out of that and the connection that continues. You're connected via WhatsApp, individually and groups. Then when you come back, everyone is excited to see each other again in person. It's just beautiful, you know, and that's the thing. They're also sharing their challenges on what they're trying to do, and that gets to solidarity part. You feel like a part you know of the team and of the family and how you're trying to move things forward.

RG: Yeah, well that's wonderful. It sounds like you're having fun doing what you're doing. So, you're training the trainers of sorts, or are you having multiple repetitive sessions?

JV: That's the beauty of it as well. You build sustainability and scalability. And when you see how people grow over time and take on these different roles, yeah, and seeing them being really effective in those roles yeah, it's just so cool.

RG: Seeing the results is really what justifies everything. John who are you? How would you define yourself.

JV: Who am I? I don't know how to describe myself honestly. The only way I describe myself is that I would say that I'm an introvert except

RG: Except when you're in the field!

JV: Well, that's true I don't know what it is, it's strange.

RG: That's your trigger you need to go away to be yourself. Well, anything I didn't ask you about, John that you'd like to share with me. I really enjoyed our conversation very much.

JV: I'm laughing. That's right. But no, I don't have any questions but if you go back and if you want to follow up on anything I'm glad to do that.

RG: Thank you very much.

Chapter 25
Learning from the Human Experience of Patients and Practitioners

Jacek Mostwin

25.1 "I Never Understood It Until Now"

When in the fall of 1982 I was in the final year of my urology residency in Baltimore, it fell to me to drive Dr. Hugh Judge Jewett to the Mid-Atlantic sectional meeting of the American Urological Association. Dr. Jewett had been one of the earliest urology residents at Hopkins. He had entered the medical school there in 1926 and completed his urology residency in 1936. He was classically educated and came from a privileged background, rarely hesitating to correct speakers in conference for using incorrect pronoun cases in their presentation or criticizing peers for their limited contributions to the profession. He dressed immaculately in shirts imported from London and always wore a suit. He did not, as they say, suffer fools gladly. During his many years at Hopkins, he had become a highly sought surgeon who was an expert in perineal prostatectomy for both benign and malignant diseases. By virtue of his experience treating many patients who had developed bladder cancer while working at the DuPont chemical plant in nearby Delaware, he created a system of classification that showed the predictive value of tumor depth penetration into bladder muscle for prognosis. He held editorial positions for the Journal of Urology and Investigative Urology and was at one time the president of the American Urological Association.

Now he was approaching 80 and knew that he had prostate cancer [1]. At his request, I drove him in his car to the meeting, several hours away. We arrived a day early and had dinner together in the Old World dining room of the Greenbrier, a West Virginia resort near underground sources of hot springs, characterized by Southern charm and hospitality, as sentimental residents of that region might refer to it, tables set with linen, crystal, heavy silverware, flowers and all the refined, older privileges of the elite professional group that I thought I was becoming part of.

J. Mostwin (✉)
Department of Urology, Johns Hopkins Medical Institutions, Baltimore, MD, USA

J. McFarland et al. (eds.), *Humanism in Surgery*, New Paradigms in Healthcare,
https://doi.org/10.1007/978-3-031-86018-8_25

It was a quiet dinner, mostly filled with Dr. Jewett's reminiscences, at the end of which he said, "It's been a good life, after all." Over the next few days of the meeting, he began to develop bone pain from metastases from the prostate cancer. I searched around the local pharmacies to find a synthetic opiate to ease his pain and also to obtain a supply of the recently released ketoconazole, an androgen deprivation medication that would immediately block the effect of his testosterone on the tumor to provide rapid relief of the pain caused by the expanding metastases in his spine. The following day, we drove back to Baltimore in relative silence. As we neared his apartment, he said to me, "All my life I've treated this disease, but I never understood it until now."

For all the thousands of men he had treated for prostate cancer, he "never understood the disease until now". It took his personal experience with the disease to bring the understanding to full realization, completing the journey which he had started earlier in his life as a surgeon and an investigator.

I remember many things about Dr. Jewett. How he would sit distantly and thoughtfully in conference, always in the same seat, choosing when or when not to comment on a presentation. I remember his secretary phoning us at Christmastime: "Come down to the office to get your Christmas present from Dr. Jewett". On arrival at his desk, she would reach into a case of Maryland Rye Whiskey and pull out a fifth (750 ml) that she would unceremoniously hand to us without card or wrapper, just a plain white label identifying the amber liquid as "Pikesville Rye". And when I had started my residency at Hopkins, and Dr. Jewett had just stepped away from his clinical work, as I have recently done, I inherited his locker in the changing room just above the now closed Blalock operating rooms. Inside the locker were his crusty old cordovan penny loafers, stiffened by the sticky sorbitol that was used to irrigate the bladder during transurethral operations. I kept them there for several years, eventually discarding them, though perhaps I should have had them bronzed and placed in the American Urological Association's museum alongside the instruments he had used for his procedures. But among these many memories I have of Dr. Jewett, his comment to me about understanding prostate cancer now that he had it has resurfaced during my own advanced stage in the profession and after many years of my own clinical experience. Perhaps that one phrase that I remember from our trip back to Baltimore in his elegant automobile summarizes the entire goal of this essay, which is to make it clear that knowing about the disease is not the same as understanding it.

Shortly after 2005 when I became director of the preclinical course entitled "Patient, Physician and Society" (PPS) at the medical school, one of the members of our faculty, a young mother of several children whom I'll call Dr. B, rose to speak about her recent episode of severe pancreatitis for which she had been hospitalized for a month. In a quivering, emotional voice she spoke about finding herself in a situation after a long period of abdominal pain that led her to our emergency room, at which point a diagnosis of pancreatitis was made, and at which point she was told she had a 50% chance of dying. She was admitted to the hospital and placed in a gown, rolled on stretchers from one place to another for imaging studies and to other treatment venues but otherwise left alone. She spoke of situations when she lay on the stretcher in which she would be passed in the hall by people with whom she worked every day but who did not recognize her, given that she was now dressed in a hospital gown and probably without her white coat, her makeup, her badge, or her more familiar, upright, ambulatory position. When she finally recovered from her illness, and although she was deeply grateful for the expert medical care she received, she was determined that every medical student should understand what it means to be sick. She created a program called Adopt-a-Patient, which we incorporated into the PPS curriculum. At first it was just to be a limited elective for a few students who wanted the experience, but very quickly it became a required exercise for all students that would be repeated annually for several years. Students would be assigned to patients selected by nurses in various hospital units to spend two to three hours simply being with them, speaking with them or observing what happens to them while they're in the hospital. After the experience, they were required to write a short essay about it. It was not a course without its difficulties. Very often conversations would trend towards a clinical discussion, and patients would revert to a familiar pattern of describing symptoms. Some students would complain that their patients were not "interesting" enough. Occasionally, however, students would convey remarkable insights about the human condition that the patients found themselves in, and the student's own reactions and memories elicited by the encounter. Eventually, however, student interest drifted elsewhere and the course underwent significant changes with the advent of a new curriculum. Adoptions were eliminated. Adopt-a-Patient fell by the wayside as do other such programs that come and go in medical curricula.

Our young faculty member's experience with pancreatitis was not very different from the experience depicted in the 1991 film "The Doctor," [2] adapted (very loosely, I might add) from the 1988 memoir by Dr. Edward E Rosenbaum entitled "A Taste of My Own Medicine, When the Doctor Becomes the Patient" [3]. The film, which I saw before reading Dr. Rosenbaum's memoir, was surprisingly well crafted, well acted, and quite moving. It presented the story of a somewhat arrogant and self-assured thoracic surgeon (Dr. Rosenbaum appeared to be none of these in real life) who discovers he has a pharyngeal cancer for which he will need to undergo radiotherapy and suspend his practice for the duration of the treatment. While undergoing radiotherapy he meets a young woman with a brain tumor who is vivacious and lively and would appear to have everything to live for, but she dies before she can manage to do so, although not before she introduces "The Doctor" to some of the depth and beauty of the lives he has been working on all this time by allowing him to see her own beauty as a person. He is deeply affected by the relationship, and his approach to medicine is transformed by it after her death. At the end of the film, we see him returning to a hospital unit before a group of students waiting for him among beds partially enclosed by drapes. He then tells them that today's lesson will consist of removing their lower garment and preparing to undergo a barium enema so they can get a sense of "what it's really like to be a patient".

Dr. Jewett, at the end of this career, our Adopt-a-Patient faculty member at the beginning of hers, and "The Doctor," powerful, successful, and seemingly untouchable as portrayed by William Hurt in the film, had all become characters in stories unfolding before us. These were stories from Lives in Medicine, presented as personal accounts, filled with emotion or insight, learned through experience rather than as part of medical training, opening our eyes to another dimension of the medical experience, the experience of illness as opposed to knowledge about diseases. These three represented a special category of knowing, because they were all physicians, people whom we think understand illness, yet in their stories and in the film, it was clear that they had only partially understood the diseases which they treated. These physicians, who had lived primarily within the culture of medicine, whose stated goal was to help the sick, had been brought by events to enter the world of the sick, the actual world inhabited by those who lived with illness, two overlapping domains of life, yet until they were personally affected, they did not "understand the disease until now."

25.2 Reconstructing Illness from Patient Experience

Thirty some years ago, Anne Hunsacker Hawkins was an anthropologist working on a doctoral dissertation about religious conversion narratives. At the time, her father suffered a stroke. She observed and monitored his recovery, noting similarities between his experience and the conversion narratives that she had been studying. She became interested in the ways by which patients made sense of their illness, changing the direction of her research to study published accounts by patients of their illnesses, which she named "pathographies" [4]. In a way, she was echoing the approach used by William James in his study of *The Varieties of Religious Experience* [5], directing her attention to what could be called the Varieties of the Illness Experience. In her monograph on the subject, she wrote the following:

> "Robinson Crusoe – that is what I think of. Surviving a terrible storm at sea; then being shipwrecked; waking from catastrophe and finding oneself alone in a new, alien and dangerous world." This was written not by the survivor of a shipwreck but by a woman who suffered a brain tumor and the operation that removed it. Her book, entitled Surviving, is an example of what I call *pathography*, a form of autobiography or biography that describes personal experience of illness, treatment, and sometimes death [4].

The novelist Joseph Conrad would agree. After suffering a stroke, he wrote: "the memory of an illness is very much like the memory of a nightmare" (Preface [6]).

This is how it must have seemed to Jean-Dominique Bauby when at age 40 he sustained a thalamic stroke that left him with a locked-in syndrome limiting him to communicate only with the blink of one eye using a code he had developed with his secretary. Over the course of a year he composed a brief but lyrical collection of vignettes that he entitled "The Diving Bell and the Butterfly" to reflect the imprisonment of his butterfly soul in the deep diving bell of his motionless body. In one of the early anecdotes entitled "The Wheelchair" he described an encounter with the staff at the rehabilitation center where he has gone after surviving the acute stages of his stroke. The contrast between his understanding of the disease and the staff's understanding could not be more striking:

> When I was finally dressed, the ritual could begin. Two attendants seized me by the shoulders and feet, lifted me off the bed, and dumped me unceremoniously into the wheelchair. I had graduated from being a patient whose prognosis was uncertain to an official paraplegic… They had to place a special cushion behind my head: it was wobbling about like the head of one of those African women upon removal of the stacks of rings that has been stretching her neck for years. "You can handle the wheelchair," said the occupational therapist, with a smile intended to make the remark somewhat good news, whereas to my ears it had the ring of a life sentence. In one flash I saw the frightening truth. It was as blinding as an atomic explosion and keener than a guillotine blade. They all left [7].

Virginia Woolf, who suffered from migraine and depression for much of her life, had written: "Considering how common illness is […] it becomes strange indeed that [it] has not taken its place with love and battle and jealousy among the prime themes of literature" [8].

Hawkins would agree. She collected some 240 pathographies and sorted them, not just according to disease categories, which is how medical libraries might have sorted them at that time, but also according to the underlying myths and assumptions that characterized these memoirs. Some were presented as athletic contests, religious or spiritual journeys, others likened to military challenges or images of war. Patients would use what was most readily at hand to serve as a metaphor for framing and presenting their experience. She described also what she saw as general differences between pathographies and clinical case reports.

> The subject of a case report is a particular biomedical condition, the individual reduced to a body and the body reduced to its biophysical components ("the disease in the body in the bed"), while the true subject of the pathography is illness and treatment as experienced and understood by the person who is its author. The purpose of the case report is to record diagnosis and treatment; the purpose of the pathography is to draw out the meaning of the author's experience. The medical report is usually composed of brief factual statements about present symptoms and body chemistry, whereas a pathography is an extended narrative situating the illness experience with the author's life and the meaning of that life. / The ideal medical report disavows any authorship at all (the first person pronoun is almost never used); on the other hand, the authorship of a pathography is never in question. / Moreover the ideal case report omits any reference to the emotions either of physician or of patient…. Pathography, at the other extreme, tends to focus on the emotional components of a medical experience, sometimes with unavoidable theatrical results [4].
>
> …..another way to look at the popularity of pathography today is to see it as a reaction to our contemporary medical model, one so dominated by a biophysical understanding of illness that its experiential aspects are virtually ignored. Medicine today has been criticized for its narrow focus on disease and its disregard for the experiencing patient. / The patient, observes Richard Baron, is in a sense "subtracted out" of the medical paradigm: "One obtains the idea of pure disease which is, ideally, distinct from any particular patient. The disease manifests itself through the patient and the patient comes to function as a kind of translucent screen on which the disease is projected." / Pathography restores the person ignored or cancelled out in the medical enterprise, and it places that person at the very center. Moreover, it gives that ill person a voice [4].

The realization that the patient's voice should be restored would later be repeated by Rita Charon, whose programs in Narrative Medicine have developed within structured medical curricula. She wrote:

> In all of medical practice the narrating of the patient's story is a therapeutically central act, because to find the words to contain the disorder and its attendant worries gives shape to and control over the chaos of illness. / As the physician listens…in some way enters and is moved by the narrative world of the patient. /. A medicine practiced with narrative competence enables the physician with empathy, reflection, professionalism and trustworthiness. Such a medicine can be called a narrative medicine. [9]

Roy Porter, former director of the Wellcome Institute for the History of Medicine at University College London, had advocated for a patient centered history of medicine, arguing that historians should look more carefully at the personal experience of patients rather than limiting their studies to the achievement and progress of medicine as a field:

> … the sufferers' role in the history of healing – in both its social and cognitive dimensions – has been routinely ignored by scholars.
>
> At present, we remain so profoundly ignorant of how ordinary people in the past have actually regarded health and sickness, and managed their encounters with medical men, that our initial priority should be to "defamiliarize" ourselves with the assumptions of modern physician-focused history and sociology of medicine, and hack our way into the empirical forests of the past in all their strangeness and diversity.
>
> My point, in fact, is that we don't know what to make of all this; we don't know what is typical, what exceptional; we lack a historical atlas of sickness experience and response, graduated by age, gender, class, religious faith, and other significant variables. It's *terra incognita*, partly because it has been discussed so little in histories of medicine.
>
> And … the testimony of the doctors themselves. Suitably interrogated, what the doctors recorded can often be decoded to reveal what the sufferers dreaded or demanded…
>
> A people's history of suffering might restore to the history of medicine its human face [10].

Yet many years after Porter's argument for the study of patient accounts, Flurin Condrau noted that not much had been done:

> It is surprising to note that after more than 20 years, Porter's article remains the main source of inspiration for the history of patients and is still so widely quoted. Conceptually, it appears to this author, that the history of the patient's view is as undeveloped now as it was back in the mid-1980s when it seemed that patients' history could turn into the new paradigm for writing history of medicine. While it is true that the patient has been getting more attention since Porter, it is also undoubtedly true that mainstream historiography has not incorporated the radical change of perspective for which Porter argued [11].

At about the same time, nonetheless, patient's stories were being treated seriously. The medical historian Guenter Risse argued that patients were very capable of writing about their experiences and providing insight into medical care as they saw it. In *Mending Bodies Savings Souls: A History of Hospitals*, Risse began the analysis of each of his various historical stages of hospital development by citing the experiences of patients from that era. He wrote:

> Whether expressing themselves orally or in writing, sick individuals in the past as well as the present have been quite capable of articulating their experiences, presenting them as dramatic stories of suffering and redemption.
>
> In a world increasingly distrustful of experts and professionals, recent patient narratives constitute a complementary source of empirical knowledge. However crafted, the stories provide valuable insights into the universe of meanings and emotions surrounding patienthood.
>
> For those sufferers who talk or write about their experiences, their sharing often has a healing quality that contributes to the recovery of others [12].

Risse noted that patients writing about their own conditions experienced a cathartic quality of their work but also showed a desire to help others. Such a goal had earlier been described by the sociologist Arthur Frank in his personal and sociological account *The Wounded Storyteller*, someone who has been through the experience of illness and could now share that story with others to help them [13].

25.3 Lives in Medicine as a Sub-Genre of Life-Writing

These stories, or narratives, or personal accounts can be subsumed under a broader category of literature now called Life-Writing, a genre that has been identified since World War II, consistent with the greater social understanding of the plight of individuals as reflected in the Nuremberg trials after World War II and the French *Annales School* of history that created the multi-volume *History of Private Life* [14]. The highly regarded report on Hiroshima by John Hersey took a similar approach, but its structure was accidental. Hersey had been sent by the New Yorker to report on the aftermath of the bombing. On the way to Japan, he became ill and required a period of convalescence. As reported by the BBC on the 70th anniversary of the bombing:

> On the voyage out he fell ill and was given a copy of Thornton Wilders's *The Bridge of San Luis Rey*. Inspired by Wilder's narrative of the five people who crossed the bridge as it collapsed he decided he would write about people not buildings. And it was that simple decision that marks Hiroshima out from other pieces of the time [15].

Hersey decided to write about people not buildings, much as Plutarch had chosen to write about men's lives rather than the history of wars and great political movements In *Lives of the Noble Greeks and Romans*, he wrote:

> It is not histories I am writing, but lives; and in the most glorious deeds there is not always an indication of virtue or vice, indeed a small thing like a phrase or a jest often makes a greater revelation of a character than battles where thousands die….The world of man is best captured through the lives of the men who created history [16].

Life-writing may be a new term, but the realization that events and circumstances can be viewed through the eyes of personal experience and that experience is both valid and compelling is ancient.

The Center for Life-Writing at Wolfson College, Oxford University defines Life-Writing thus:

> Life-writing goes beyond and encompasses biography. It encompasses everything from the complete life to the to the day-in-the-life, from the fictional to the factional. It embrace the lives of objects and institutions as well as the lives of individuals, families and groups. Life-writing includes autobiographies, memoirs, letters, diaries, journals (written and documentary), anthropological data, oral testimony and eyewitness accounts. It is not only a literary or historical specialism, but is relevant across the arts and sciences, and can involve philosophers, psychologists, sociologists, ethnographers and anthropologists [17].

Within such a broad category as life-writing, the published memoirs of patients offer not only the patient's perspective on "Lives in Medicine" as I choose to call it, but "…for those sufferers," as Risse indicated "who talk or write about their experiences, their *sharing often has a healing quality* that contributes to the recovery of others."

The writer and literary editor Robert McCrum experienced a stroke at the age of 40. He required a year-long period of convalescence and then wrote about it in his memoir *My Year Off (1998)* in which he described the monumental significance of the event in his life, how writing helped him respond to it, and how he sought to provide help to others:

> When I was seriously ill in hospital, I longed to read a book that would tell me what I might expect in convalescence and also give me something to think about. There are many books about stroke in old age, but I was young and had been vigorous and there was nothing that spoke to me in my distress.
>
> I have written this book to help those who have suffered as I did, and indeed for anyone recovering from what doctors call "an insult to the brain". I've also written for families and loved ones who, sucked into the vortex of catastrophic illness, find themselves searching for words of encouragement and explanation.
>
> The other audience for this book is, of course, myself. The consequences of my stroke were simply too colossal to be ignored or shut away in some mental pigeonhole. Writing the book has been a way to make sense of an extraordinary personal upheaval, whose consequences will be with me until I died. Besides, I am a writer. Communicating experience is what I do, and quite soon after I realized I was going to survive the initial crisis I also realized that I'd been given a story that made most of what I've written previously pale and uninteresting by comparison [18].

McCrum not only underscored the catharsis and the information, but also professed an awareness of the power of his personal narrative, describing it as the story he'd been "given, making all others pale and uninteresting in comparison". Virginia Woolf's question, mentioned earlier, it seemed, was begin reconsidered.

Robert Murphy, an anthropologist at Columbia University, expressed similar sentiments in his memoir entitled *The Body Silent (1987)*:

> I am an academic person who has published a dozen books in the field of anthropology, most of which have been greeted with interest by the scholarly community, but never with the kind of enthusiasm shown by my disabled readers. This was my first attempt to reach out to the general public, and I was totally unprepared, however much delighted, by the response.
>
> There has been a consistent theme in these letters from disabled readers, and phone calls as well, that I have given shape, form, and meaning to thoughts and emotions that have turned in their minds but had remained inchoate and disconnected. My interpretation of the inner life of the disabled has allowed them, through identification with me, to connect all of their own free – floating fragments and snippets of experience, all the litany of their hurts and rages, into patterns of meaning applicable to themselves. And out of the self – knowl-

> edge comes liberation. In a way, reading the book has been almost as therapeutic for many people as ... writing has been for me. [19]

Surgical patients also have written dramatic and deeply personal memoirs. Some are published in traditional ways, others self-published.

Lucy Grealy was nine years old when she discovered she had a lump in her jaw that on biopsy turned out to be an osteosarcoma, a malignant bone cancer. She required excision, radiotherapy, chemotherapy and multiple reconstructive operations to attempt grafting and reshaping of her face. Most of these reconstructive attempts failed due to limited blood supply to the host site after her radiotherapy. The book follows the chronology of events: the discovery of the tumor, its treatment, and her eventual adaptation to a complex question of identity in which the question "Who Am I?" can only partially be answered by looking into a mirror. For Grealy, the face became an all too realistic representation of her entire identity for many years of her early life, as she poetically recalled many scenes of her journey, sometimes with lyrical if heart wrenching candor.

In her early years, living with the initial deformities her treatments created, she described one Halloween, dressing up in costumes.

> The school year progressed slowly. I felt as if I had been in the sixth grade for years, yet it was only October. Halloween was approaching. Coming from Ireland, we had never thought of it as a big holiday, though Sarah and I usually went out trick-or-treating. For the last couple of years I had been too sick to get out, but this year Halloween fell on a day when I felt quite fine. My mother was the one who came up with the Eskimo idea. I put on a winter coat, made a fish out of paper, which I hung on the end of a stick, and wrapped my face up in a scarf. My hair was growing in, and I loved the way the top of the hood rubbed against it. By this time my hat had become part of me. I took it off only at home. Sometimes kids would make fun of me, run past me, knock my hat off, and call me "baldy." I hated this, but I assumed that one day my hair would grow in, and on that day the teasing would end. We walked around the neighborhood with our pillowcase sacks, running into other groups of kids and comparing notes. The house three doors down gave whole candy bars, while the house next to that gave only cheap mints. I felt wonderful. It was only as the night wore on, and the moon came out, and the older kids, the big kids, went on their rounds, that I began to realize why I felt so good. No one could see me clearly. No one could see my face [20].

She describes in haunting terms the isolation and misery of undergoing chemotherapy at the hands of a cold, impersonal oncologist whom she appropriately names "Dr Woolf". In recalling her experiences, she makes reference to a book that was popular at the time entitled "Be Here Now" by Baba Ram Das, the pen name of Richard Alpert, a colleague of Timothy Leary who became well known during the era of transcendental meditation, personal gurus and psychedelic exploration with drugs for everyone else, it seems, except Lucy herself:

> It was an old bathroom with only two stalls. Each stall door was wooden and closed on the inside with a silvery metal latch. There was no graffiti anywhere in the bathroom except on these latches. Someone, certainly the same person, had scratched onto each rectangular piece of metal a message sitting on the toilet. In the first stall you could read "God Is Near" and on the second "Be Here Now". I always pictured the person who wrote these messages sitting on the same porcelain as myself, bending forward, one arm raised up and resting against the warping wood of the door, a nail file in the other hand. I sensed that it had been done a long time ago, before my time. What was wrong with them? I wondered. Why were

they here? I never asked myself what might have happened to them. Still spending my private moments trying to engage God in conversation, alternately attempting to barter him into answering my questions and silently trying to listen to the answer. These bathroom communications seemed important to me. Each Friday I'd plod down to this bathroom, killing time before the inevitable, and I'd pause for a moment before the two doors, trying to decide which message I wanted to read. "God is near." Well, okay, how near? Did this mean he was near in the way someone is near when they're coming toward you, moving closer and closer, not yet here but expected sooner or later? Or did it mean he was near but not showing his face, present but unseeable, someone breathing quietly in a closet? "Be here now." I didn't want to be here now. My wanting was inconsequential. I was here now, whether I liked it or not. But something about the saying attracted me, either despite or because of its seeming simplicity, and two out of three times I went for door number two. / Some weeks I stared at it dumbly, thinking only of what was happening back in the waiting room with my mother. How many more rows of knitting she'd finished. Some weeks I thought of the impending injection. Or I simply continued with my fantasy life. The pony express rider seeks relief in the town's saloon. The alien ponders the wonders of waste disposal. Some weeks, especially when it was hot, I thought of nothing, and only listened to my urine hiss into the water below my legs as I leaned forward, pressing the coolness of the inscribed medal against my forehead and wept [20].

The placement of the final sentence, the preparation with the young philosophical meditation so far apart from the two conventional mantras of "God is Near" and "Be Here Now" are used artistically to prepare for the delivery of the final verbal *coup de grace*, the final description of the inevitable weeping in the face of "being here now".

Lucy Grealy became recognized as a poet, she came to terms with her many operations and treatments, she came to terms with her identity, or so it would seem, and she was interviewed on national radio. Then her life ended prematurely, possibly from painkillers, something that must have been a regular feature in her life. The power and poignancy of her memoir cannot be overstated. It must be read in its entirety to even begin to get an idea of what it might be like to undergo so many operations, so many treatments to have such a disruption of childhood. While other children are attending pony rides, dances and parties, playing games with each other, Lucy relates again and again that she can never be loved because of how she is, because of how she looks. From the surgeon's perspective, helping such a person would seem foremost in mind even as one has to concentrate on the technical demands of the operations, yet as Lucy relates, surgeons can become so enamored of the technical wonders of their proposed operations, fully expecting that patients will share their enthusiasm with them, that they completely miss the chance to see the situation from the patient's point of view.

Dr. Baker and I decided to try another soft tissue free flap. So much of the original irradiated tissue had been replaced with non-radiated tissue that he felt there was a good chance this graft would stick. But a few months before the operation, I discovered that Medicaid would not pay my hospital bills. The accumulated reasons ranged from my not living in the state where the operation was to be performed to my being a full-time student with the teaching fellowship. I had to put off the operation until the following summer.

Dr. Baker suggested I go to the University of Iowa Hospital for a consultation with the head of plastic surgery, who was an old friend of his. Perhaps there was a way for him to do the operation. Because Iowa's Medicaid system was on a first-come-first-served basis, I

> could not apply for funding before the operation. I had to have it, submit the bills, and wait to see if there was enough left in the budget to pay for it. I wasn't very optimistic when I went for my appointments.
>
> The surgeon was from the old school. Of course my free flaps had shrunk, he told me. They always did. He suggested sticking with the pedestal method that Dr. Conley had outlined for me so many years ago. He was very enthusiastic, explaining in far greater detail than Conley had about all the different incisions he'd make. He described how I could stay in the hospital for the six weeks when my hand was sewn to my stomach and then to my face. While my hand was sewn to my face, he would rig up a special cast to hold everything in place. He even introduced me to a patient of his who was having a pedestal to rebuild his nose. This patient's nose had been shot off with a gun and he was sporting a very complicated and uncomfortable looking cast that was forcibly holding his wrist to his face. Connecting his wrist to the area of his nose was a pale tube of skin with a red row of sutures down the side. I felt totally repulsed and ashamed of my repulsion.
>
> After this patient had left, and not wanting to be rude, I calmly told the surgeon that I probably couldn't go through with the operations after all, because of the money involved. "Oh, don't let that worry you. You wait right here." He disappeared for a long fifteen minutes, leaving me alone in the office. I decided this was as good a time as any to see if I could have an out-of-body experience. Having read only in passing about out-of-body experiences, and these mostly in supermarket tabloids, I thought you were supposed to follow an actual physical route, so I closed my eyes and tried to imagine what the air duct over my head would look like if I were inside it.
>
> Eventually, the surgeon returned with a hospital finance officer who outlined a payment plan for the three major operations and the minor follow-up as well as the extended inpatient stays. When he had finished his calculations, he assured me that with payments of only $100 a month, I could pay off the original bill and all the accumulated interest by the time I was 42. He was very affable and I shook his hand, telling him I'd think about it
>
> I stayed calm until I reached the street where I broke into a run and didn't stop until I got home four miles away. There I started to hyperventilate. There was no way I was going to put myself through those operations, let alone have the pleasure of paying them off just when I should be rightfully starting my midlife crisis along with everybody else.
>
> I felt I had been shown a mirror of what my life really was, what I really was, and I did not want to look. I was someone whom the doctors talked to about sewing her hand to her face. I was trying to believe there really wasn't all that much wrong with me, but here were my worst suspicions confirmed [20].

Grealy's account is filled with such granular detail interspersed with a record of deep personal emotion that is only rarely encountered in a clinical consultation settings, even if a clinician or the patient may sense that it is there. It is very difficult for surgeons to assume a self-righteous attitude about their work after reading about how it might be perceived and remembered in such accounts. Like the silent weeping in the second toilet stall, these moments occur in private, unseen, deeply felt, remembered. Humility would seem a more desirable quality while being attentive to the technical demands of the work, striving ever to center them on the needs of the patient, by which we should mean, the needs of the patient as a complete human being.

Encounters with surgeons and other treating physicians are remembered in great detail and tell professionals something about themselves that they may be unaware of as they provide information which is often taken to be equivalent to communication, but can be far from the mark of understanding the person towards whom it is directed.

Exploding Into Life tells the story of Dorothea Lynch, a young poet living in Boston who discovers a lump in her breast at the age of thirty-four. A biopsy of the lump reveals malignancy. She undergoes surgery, chemotherapy, and radiation. Her partner, Eugene Richards, a photographer who would become world renowned for his work, kept a visual record of the events. Dorothea, the poet, kept a journal. Gene made photographs. Dorothea's records provide a lyrical yet accurate description of what it's like, what happens, and how it is remembered, combined with the acceptance of the final outcome.

We first meet Dorothea when the lump appears, when it "explodes into life":

> I am stunned.
>
> Right under my finger, as big as a wad of bubble gum, only harder, like the cap on a toothpaste tube. I feel it again, and my stomach jumps right up into my chest.
>
> No. Through the apartment, touching the leaves of plants. No. Feed the cats. Open the refrigerator. Close the refrigerator. I can't eat. I can't read, can't watch anymore of a television movie about a meteor falling straight into downtown Phoenix, people screaming and glass flying, a foolish movie that leaves me gasping. I am thinking of that thing, buried in my breast, breathing and nesting and eating like a fleshy mouth. I call Dr. Dragonas, "But maybe I'm just being silly," I say. "I'm only thirty-four. I don't even smoke anymore."
>
> I am supposed to cover a school committee for tomorrow's paper, but I just can't do it. I walk through the streets. It has begun to snow, sifting and hissing against the ground. I smell woodsmoke, someone's cozy fire. My father loved a fire, in all kinds of weather, but particularly in this kind of cold. Silver-haired, with his arm drawn back, snowball in hand, laughing – I have a photograph of him like that. His teeth were exactly like mine, very white and perfectly shaped. To share even the same mouth and nose and drooped eyelid. Martha, my cousin, died of cancer last year at thirty- three. Twelve years ago, I danced with her brother Bill in a little cafe, just before he landed in Vietnam and was killed. I remember dancing close, because neither of us felt like cousins, and laughing, and the lights turning blue with cigarette smoke.
>
> I sit on the examining table while Dr. Dragonas probes and tests. I would like to rest my head against his shoulder. Pressure against my left breast stirs the ache again, so like a toothache. In his waiting room I had felt diseased, a carrier among the pregnant women with their different sized stomachs. I am young enough to be having my first child. Dr. Dragonas discovers a second lump up high in my armpit that has been aching for the last few days like a strained muscle.
>
> What is it? What is it? But he will give nothing away except a shot of Metaxa brandy that he keeps for emergencies. He and the nurse with curly blonde hair take turns calling the hospital, looking for beds and an operating room.
>
> "Breast resection," they say into the beige telephone.
>
> Resection. It sounds like refashion, as if they are going to remake my breasts. No one says the word "malignant," or "tumor" or "cancer."
>
> "We'll just put you into the hospital for a few days and take a sampling of those tissues to find out what's going on." Dr. Dragonas says. "Don't worry, Dorothea. It's just a biopsy" [21]

The biopsy is positive and Dorothea is visited by several physicians to select treatment options. Her memories and descriptions of these visits should appear familiar to all who do or have seen this kind of work.

> Before dawn, a large man in a navy blue, three piece suit wakes me. In a voice so casual and so precise he could be talking about school budgets. Dr. Robert Shirley explains that a

modified radical mastectomy means removal of my left breast and the lymph glands under my arm. Or, I might choose to have primary radiation therapy instead – long needles with radium implants stuck into my breasts. "Maybe not the best thing," says Dr. Shirley, "what with the possible radiation spray effects that could generate tumor activity in the other breast."

A radiologist, Dr. Kinsella, visits my room next to tell me about the very same primary radiation therapy. Dr. Kinsella doesn't know what Dr. Shirley means by "spraying effect." Not in his experience, he says, has it ever happened. "We would give you twenty-five external radiation treatments, but we would use radiation shields to protect the rest of the body. The implant is a fairly low dosage and only remains in place for a few days."

I look at the doctors and I think of undertakers, straight and dark and inescapable. "Interstitial implant, morbidity, adjunctive chemotherapy." Listening to them is like trying to decipher the code in my Graham Greene spy stories where finding the answer means saving the hero's life. "Of course, it's your decision after all," each doctor tells me: "Radiation or surgery. You decide." [21]

Dorothea undergoes surgery—a radical mastectomy, complete breast removal with axillary lymph node dissection. We read on as she is recovering from her surgery in the hospital.

A lady with blonde hair pokes her head into my room, calling cheerfully, "hello there, Dorothea. Are you keeping busy? Want me to send the crafts card along for something to do? What are you writing?" I have no idea who she is. Someone is always walking into my hospital room, acting as if we have already met, old friends and all that. It is the medical professional's way of attempting to put a patient at ease. But it is disconcerting to me not to know to whom I am talking.

The woman eventually introduces herself as Helen. She's a psychologist. I show her my notebooks, explaining that I am writing about what it is like to have cancer. Why? Because writing is what I do. It helps me sort out ideas and emotions and find out what I really feel.

The hospital psychiatrist, Dr. Gates, makes me nervous when he visits later in the day, constantly jotting notes on a pad. He is conducting an independent study on the psychological reactions of breast cancer patients. Answering his questions I'm aware of sounding like a Pollyanna. What I mean to say twists away from me.

"Nothing is what I thought it would be," I tell him. "Getting cancer, not dying, not being alive. I feel I've been given a reprieve, like Lucky Lazarus, and have returned from the grave. The sound of my own heart is a miracle. The field of clean sheets against my skin a"…

Dr. Gage interrupts to say I'm experiencing a medical phenomenon called "euphoria," quite common after major operation. What I should expect, he says, is to have sexual difficulties, be shorter-tempered and more impatient with people.

After Dr. Gates leaves I close the door, do twenty five sit-ups and leg raises, careful not to crush my swollen arm, working against being a textbook cancer patient, I suppose. I keep wishing he would come back and catch me at it. Ah, one -two – three [21].

She undergoes chemotherapy, with the resultant nausea and vomiting that it so often induces. Gene's photographs conceal nothing of the visual details of these moments. The cancer returns to her chest wall, and she undergoes additional radiation therapy. In the end, it is clear that no other medical intervention will help her. We now reach the final pages of *Exploding Into Life* and read the last entry that Gene extracted from her journal when he assembled the book:

Mystery. What a mystery this life is. The plants are filling out. The garden outback of our house sprouts one-half-inch here, an inch there, and I am changing too; cancer

> plods on from node to node, remarkable and not remarkable at all, like summer itself. Just another growing season after all. Is this resignation? I hope not. I do not intend to give up without a struggle, but more and more I see myself as a thread in a huge and royal tapestry – important to the central design but having an end, a place, a physical destination.
>
> I think of the young daughter in Satyajit Ray's *Pather Panchali*, spinning, whirling in the rain, her hair flying out like a flag the night she died. I think of Sally Powers, who had just turned seventy. No one is special, are they, when all is said and done? And of course, each of us is very special, very singular, carrying weight. I matter. Sally mattered. I would like to open the window tonight and yell outside. I matter. Or go down and lie next to the grass and whisper it [21].

Combined with Gene's photographs, both powerful and unique in such a setting, the book provides immersion into the experiences of a single person with breast cancer who undergoes treatment, yet eventually succumbs to her disease. In medical terms, Dr. Gates or another physician like him might describe Dorothea as an index case, an" N of One" whose experience blends into an aggregate of statistical analyses, outcome measures, and Kaplan-Meier survival curves. Timothy Snyder, historian of events filled with death and execution that took place between 1932 and 1946 in the territories between central Poland in the West and Belarus in the East, what he called "Bloodlands," put it this way:

> Each record of death suggests, but cannot supply, a unique life. We must be able not only to reckon the number of deaths, but to reckon with each victim as an individual. The one very large number that withstands scrutiny is that of the Holocaust, with its 5.7 million Jewish dead, 5.4 million of whom were killed by the Germans. But this number, like all of the others, must be seen not as 5.7 million, which is an abstraction few of us can grasp, but as 5.7 million *times one* [italics by Timothy Snyder] [22].

Indeed, each record of illness, regardless of outcome, is the history of a present illness *times one,* as it is lived out in that one person. Rarely do we have time to hear it all or see it all, and even if we did, how would we go about generalizing? In a way, these stories we hear about the lives in medicine of patients, which are not limited to the way in which they present them but the way in which we see and hear them as witnesses, form a human side of medicine that, even if it does not consciously draw physicians in to the profession when they start out, will often keep them in it long after the technical demands of the craft have been mastered and become second nature.

25.4 The Physician's Voice

So far we have considered examples of how patients write their personal accounts from the perspective of the world of the sick. At some point, but not always, that world will overlap with the culture of medicine. Medical practitioners, whether doctors, nurses, rescue workers, military corpsmen, also write about their personal experience in medicine, revealing a human voice.

Although Hawkins concentrated her work almost entirely on patient narratives, she added a plea for authentic physician voices at the end of her book:

> Another voice we need to hear is that of the physician. This may seem a paradoxical statement at the end of a book that so insists on returning the patient to the medical enterprise and so often contrasts the patient's voice to that of medicine. But the "physician's voice" I am referring to [… is] the voice of the individual who is inevitably lost in that impersonal professional voice. We need to hear from them. […] …. We need more writing that conveys the inner reality of what it is to be a physician in today's technological medical system. Only when we hear both the doctor's and the patient's voice will we have a medicine that is truly human [4].

The library of physician life-writing is much larger than one might imagine, ranging from early experiences to final testaments at mature stages of life. Not all physician writers are the same. Some write ex cathedra, without really taking off their white coats, preserving their medical authority even as they take up the pen to write or expostulate what can be perceived as a blend of essay and anecdote. These writers often receive top billing and are often identified as "medical writers". I believe this is due to the public's respect for the profession and its insatiable hunger to know something, almost anything, about the inner workings of medicine and its inner sancta. But there are other physicians who write in a more personal and direct ways about their experience, writing as it were from "inside the whale" [23], a term used by George Orwell to compare the direct, personal, and sometimes chaotic writing of WW I soldiers who had served in the trenches, simply describing what really happened, not abstracting or idealizing from experiences as did some of the social champions writing and pamphleteering from the protected safety and comfort of their London clubs. It was the authenticity of these accounts from inside the whale that Orwell supported, having himself witnessed the duplicity and deceit concealed by socialist ideology he saw displayed while serving with the Republican forces during the Spanish Civil War. The reality of those experiences overcame his own earlier idealism and led him to write both *Animal Farm (1945)* and shortly after, *1984 (1949)*, criticizing the smugness and conceit of political dandies and demagogues.

One could argue that this kind of writing "inside the whale" by physicians is not medical writing at all, but closer to the kind of accounts that Porter described as "doing medical history from below," the kind of physician's voice to which Hawkins alluded in her conclusion. As Orwell directed our attention to the writing coming from the inside the whale, so this kind of writing comes from those actually caught up in lives in medicine, *thrown into* them (*geworfenheit*), as Martin Heidegger would say: these physician voices tell us something of what-it-is-like. For students and practitioners this is a treasury of medical experience that gives us a glimpse into what life in medicine might be like, or looking back, to share with colleagues we have never met their experiences and compare them to our own as if we had the amount of time we never seem to find when working, except in hallways or the corridors of conferences. And for the public, the presentation of the lives of physicians, in all their courage, fear and imperfections, shows that physicians can be not only expert technicians who understand illness, but people who understand illness in a deeper way than empirical medical science might suggest. Such work shows the human face of the medical profession to those who might long to see it.

When I was considering a surgical career in medical school, I came upon *The Making of a Surgeon* by William Nolen. His was a warm, welcoming and light-hearted invitation to follow him along during his training years at Bellevue Hospital in New York, an inner city teaching hospital filled with a wide variety of people and their maladies. Reading these pages, one felt like a companion going along with him on his surgical adventures. It drew me in completely, and although given time and my own experience I would come to view the surgical world differently, in some cases it was remarkably accurate. Consider this description of his first appendectomy.

> The patient, or better, victim, of my first major surgical venture was a man I'll call Mr. Polansky. He was fat, he weighed one hundred and ninety pounds and was five feet eight inches tall. He spoke only broken English. He had had a sore abdomen with all the classical signs and symptoms of appendicitis for twenty-four hours before he came to Bellevue.
>
> After two months of my internship, though I had yet to do anything that could be decently called an "operation," I had had what I thought was a fair amount of operating time.
>
> I'd watched the assistant residents work, I'd tied knots, cut sutures and even, in order to remove a skin lesion, made an occasional incision. Frankly, I didn't think that surgery was going to be too damn difficult. I figured I was ready, and I was chomping at the bit to go, so when Mr. Polansky arrived I greeted him like a long-lost friend. He was overwhelmed at the interest I showed in his case. He probably couldn't understand why any doctor should be so fascinated by a case of appendicitis: wasn't it a common disease? It was just as well that he didn't realize my interest in him was so personal. He might have been frightened, and with good reason….
>
> It went horribly. The wall of the cecum is not very thick – perhaps one eighth of an inch. The suture must be placed deeply enough in the wall so that it won't cut through when tied, but not so deep as to pass all the way through the wall.
>
> My sutures were alternately too superficial or too deep, but eventually I got the job done.
>
> "All right," said George, "let's get the appendix out of here. Tie off the base."
>
> I did.
>
> "Now cut off the appendix."
>
> At least in this, the definitive act of the operation, I would be decisive. I took the knife and with one quick slash cut through the appendix-too close to the ligature.
>
> "Oh oh, watch it," said George. "That tie is going to slip."
>
> It did. The appendiceal stump lay there, open. I felt faint.
>
> "Don't panic," said George. "We've still got the purse string. I'll push the stump in-you pull up the stitch and tie.
>
> "That will take care of it."
>
> I picked up the two ends of the suture and put in the first stitch. George shoved the open stump into the cecum. It disappeared as I snugged my tie. Beautiful.
>
> "Two more knots," said George. "Just to be safe."
>
> I tied the first knot and breathed a sigh of relief. The appendiceal stump remained out of sight. On the third knot for the sake of security pulled a little tighter. The stitch broke; the open stump popped up; the cecum disappeared into the abdomen. I broke out in a cold sweat and my knees started to crumble. Even George momentarily lost his composure. "For Christ's sake, Bill," he said, grasping desperately for the bowel, "what did you have to do that for?" The low point of the operation had been reached.
>
> By the time we had retrieved the cecum, Mr. Polansky's peritoneal cavity had been contaminated. My self -confidence was shattered. And still George let me continue. True, he all but held my hand as we retied and resutured, but the instruments were in my hand.

> The closure was anticlimactic. Once I had the peritoneum sutured, things went reasonably smoothly. Two hours after we began, the operation was over. "Nice job," George said, doing his best to sound sincere.
>
> "Thanks," I answered, lamely.
>
> The scrub nurse laughed.
>
> Mr. Polansky recovered, I am happy to report, though not without a long and complicated convalescence. His bowel refused to function normally for two weeks and he became enormously distended. He was referred to at our nightly conferences as "Dr. Nolen's pregnant man." Each time the reference was made, it elicited a shudder from me.
>
> During his convalescence I spent every spare moment I could at Mr. Polansky's bedside. My feelings of guilt and responsibility were overwhelming. If he had died I think I would have given up surgery for good [24].

Nolen's self-effacing, humorous account of his first appendectomy is so realistic, that even now, fifty years after I first read it, I find it as valid, truthful, and vivid an account as could be imagined.

Compare Nolen's account to that of Francis Moore, who would become one of the most distinguished academic surgical leaders and investigators in America. Here is the account of his first appendectomy.

> At some point in the spring of 1940, fully scrubbed and suitably attired, I stood a few paces back from the operating table on which lay a naked boy of about 10, anesthetized. One of my colleagues was sponging off the patient's abdomen with little gauze sponges soaked in iodine solution. The drapes were then firmly set in place, with a small opening over the bare skin where I planned to make the incision. I can remember thinking how remarkable it was that institutions in our society could set things up so all the pieces would fall in place…and I, then less than a year out of medical school and only 26 years of age, might have the immense privilege of relieving the pain, anguish, and threat to a wonderful small boy by making an incision in the right lower quadrant of his abdomen and taking out an appendix skillfully and safely. Only five years previously I had greeted the smelly collection of organs in the laboratory. Now here I was, with skilled nurses and an experienced anesthetist, shiny sterile instruments in hand, ready to operate, with all the protection given the patient by a venerable institution. I felt that this was both a miracle and a privilege. I still do [25].

Later in his professional life Moore conducted laboratory studies of fluid and electrolyte management of patients subjected to trauma and stress, advancing knowledge and saving countless lives through his discoveries [26]. Nolen would go on to write several more books about the surgical life. The tone, manner, and conduct of the two accounts could not be more different. No one outside of the operating room would have seen or known the difference, but as the anatomy dissecting room is a rite of passage for all medical students, the appendectomy is often a rite of passage for many surgeons in early training. For me, as an experienced surgeon, there is much to be learned and appreciated from each of these, though the differences speak for themselves.

Nolen's account, and to a certain extent Moore's, can be considered examples of what Donald Pollock called *Training Tales: U. S. Medical Autobiography*. Pollock's article is one of very few scholarly considerations of this kind of life-writing I have found [27]. Pollock considered a variety of such accounts along with the fictional *The House of God* [28], a satirical tour de force of internship by Samuel Shem (pen name of Dr. Steven Bergman) whose trench humor was successful enough to result in three million copies of the book being sold since its release, the largest number of medical memoir biographies ever sold [29]. Pollock argued that many of these training tales described the struggle of young physician to overcome the inhumanity of the system into which they had been thrown and forced to survive in their efforts to help patients who were sometimes themselves seen as the enemy. Despite this, many of these physicians somehow emerged as humane and decent people, having run and survived the challenges of the training gauntlet. It was a successful description of physician survival but it told only part of the story, a part which even today remains part of the hidden curriculum of medical education even if it cannot be spoken about in official settings. Pollock's collection of tales also, and perhaps unintentionally, focuses on modern hospital training as the primary venue for such maturation. Perhaps without meaning to, his account supports the trend of considering the modern hospital the epicenter of medicine, and the physicians as a form of human resource that is "passing though". When the business magazine, U. S. News and World Report, began producing lists of America's "best hospitals," it coincided with the gradual takeover of private practices by corporate structures in America. The public was being supplied an image of "the great hospital" as a shrine of technology, or a "temple of science," as the anthropologist and psychiatrist Melvin Konner called it [30], that provided medical care, while physicians and other health care practitioners, currently called "providers," served as their expendable employees. In this sense, the hospital can very much be seen as the "whale" within whose "inside" the narrator of personal accounts fulfills Orwell's criteria for authenticity and graphic detail.

Orwell himself has left us with an account of his own hospitalization for pneumonia in Paris, and it would seem very consistent with his preference for writing from the inside of the whale rather than providing learned reports ex cathedra. Here is a fragment from his essay describing how he was treated with "cupping" shortly after his admission for pneumonia.

> The cold air outside had probably lowered my temperature, and I watched this barbarous remedy with detachment and even a certain amount of amusement. The next moment, however, the doctor and the student came across to my bed, hoisted me upright and without a word began applying the same set of glasses, which had not been sterilized in any way. A few feeble protests that I uttered got no more response than if I had been an animal. I was very much impressed by the impersonal way in which the two men started on me. I had never been in the public ward of a hospital before, and it was my first experience of doctors who handle you without speaking to you or, in a human sense, taking any notice of you. They only put on six glasses in my case, but after doing so they scarified the blisters and applied the glasses again. Each glass now drew about a dessert-spoonful of dark-coloured blood. As I lay down again, humiliated, disgusted and frightened by the thing that had been done to me, I reflected that now at least they would leave me alone. But no, not a bit of it. There was another treatment. coming, the mustard poultice, seemingly a matter of routine like the hot bath [31].

He survived this and other forms of treatment and describes it all with a certain ghoulish humor that might be the corollary of the physician's perspective presented in House of God, but presented from the patient's perspective.

> During my first hour in the Hôpital X I had had a whole series of different and contradictory treatments, but this was misleading, for in general you got very little treatment at all, either

good or bad, unless you were ill in some interesting and instructive way. At five in the morning the nurses came round, woke the patients and took their temperatures, but did not wash them. If you were well enough you washed yourself, otherwise you depended on the kindness of some walking patient. It was generally patients, too, who carried the bedbottles and the grim bedpan, nicknamed *la casserole*. At eight breakfast arrived, called army-fashion *la soupe*. It was soup, too, a thin vegetable soup with slimy hunks of bread floating about in it. Later in the day the tall, solemn, black-bearded doctor made his rounds, with an interne and a troop of students following at his heels, but there were about sixty of us in the ward and it was evident that he had other wards to attend to as well. There were many beds past which he walked day after day, sometimes followed by imploring cries. On the other hand if you had some disease with which the students wanted to familiarize themselves you got plenty of attention of a kind. I myself, with an exceptionally fine specimen of a bronchial rattle, sometimes had as many as a dozen students queuing up to listen to my chest. It was a very queer feeling — queer, I mean, because of their intense interest in learning their job, together with a seeming lack of any perception that the patients were human beings. It is strange to relate, but sometimes as some young student stepped forward to take his turn at manipulating you he would be actually tremulous with excitement, like a boy who has at last got his hands on some expensive piece of machinery. And then ear after ear — ears of young men, of girls, of negroes — pressed against your back, relays of fingers solemnly but clumsily tapping, and not from any one of them did you get a word of conversation or a look direct in your face. As a non-paying patient, in the uniform nightshirt, you were primarily *a specimen*, a thing I did not resent but could never quite get used to [31].

Orwell's description of the rounds and the enthusiasm of the early trainees so closely resembles the description of similar situations in Margaret Edson's Pulitzer Prize winning play *WIT* [32], that one begins to wonder if it is only the technical dimensions of medicine that have been changing, and the human dynamics have remained the same. Vivian Bearing, the ill-fated protagonist of WIT, describes the "Grand Rounds" in which she is presented as an example of her type cancer and its treatments by Jason Posner, the oncology fellow, Dr. Kelekian, the attending oncologist, and a host of followers. As if taken directly from Hawkins' side-by-side comparison of the patient's perspective and the doctor's perspective, Jason, the oncology fellow, is describing the patient's condition, while Vivian, in a soliloquy delivered to the audience through a "a fourth wall" describes what she is going through. Here is a fragment from the text of the play, imagine VIVIAN and JASON alternating their lines, as if singing a duet of alternating lyrics of a libretto in an opera

VIVIAN: Grand Rounds. The term is theirs. Not "Grand" in the traditional sense of sweeping or magnificent. Not "Round" as in a musical Canon, or a *round* of applause (though either would be refreshing at this point). Here "Rounds" seems to significantly dart around the main issue… Which, I suppose would be the struggle for life… My life… With heated discussions of side effects, other complaints, additional treatment.
JASON: Very late detection. Staged as a four upon admission. Hexamethophosphacil with Vinplatin to potentiate. Hex at 300 mg per meter squared. Vin at 100. Today is cycle two, day three. Both cycles at the full dose. (The FELLOWS are impressed)
The primary site is here (he put his finger on the spot on her abdomen) behind the left ovary. Metastases are suspected in the peritoneal cavity—here. And - here (*he touches these spots*)
VIVIAN: Grand Rounds, there's not a grand opera, but compared to lying here it is positively dramatic.
JASON: Full lymphatic involvement. (*He moves his hands over her entire body.*)

VIVIAN: Full of subservience, hierarchy, gratuitous displays, sublimated rivalries—I feel right at home, it's just like a graduate seminar.
JASON: At the time of the first look surgery, a significant part of the tumor was developed, mostly in this area, here (*he points to each organ, poking her abdomen*). Left, right ovaries. Fallopian tubes, uterus. All out.
VIVIAN: With one important difference. In Grand Rounds, they read me like a book. Once I did the teaching, now I am taught.
JASON: Evidence of primary site shrinkage. Shrinking and metastatic tumor has not been documented. Primary less frankly palpable in pelvic exam, frankly all through here—*here*. (*Some FELLOWS reach and press where he is pointing.*)
VIVIAN: This is much easier. I just hold still and look cancerous. It requires less acting every time. Excellent command of detail.
KELEKIAN: Excellent command of detail.
VIVIAN: (To herself) I taught him, you know.

Later in the play, Jason comes to see Vivian in her hospital room during a more advanced stage of her illness. She is recovering from a septic episode brought about by her immunosuppression. Vivian asks him about what matters to him, and in response, he displays more enthusiasm for the disease than the person affected by it.

VIVIAN: I was just wondering why Cancer?
JASON: Why cancer?
VIVIAN: Why not open-heart surgery?
JASON: Why yeah, why not plumbing.? Why not run a lube rack, for all that surgeons know about *Homo sapiens*. No way. Cancer is the only thing I ever wanted.
VIVIAN: (Intrigued) Huh.
JASON: No, really. Cancer is… (*Searching*)
VIVIAN: (Helping) Awesome.
JASON: (Pause) Yeah. Yeah, that's right. It is. It is awesome. How does it do it? The intercellular regulatory mechanisms—especially for proliferation differentiation—the malignant neoplasia just don't get it. You grow normal cells and tissue culture in the lab, and they replicate just enough to make a nice, confluence monolayer. They divide 20 times, or 50 times, but eventually they conk out. You grow cancer cells, and they never stop. No contact inhibition whatsoever. They just pile up, just keep replicating forever. (Pause) That's got a funny name. Know what it is?
VIVIAN: No, what?
JASON: Immortality in culture
VIVIAN: Sounds like a symposium

Vivian goes on to ask about whether he ever misses people when they she avoids saying the word "die" and asks what he does to comfort people when they are frightened, Jason displays the clueless, emotional vacuity that has characterized his persona throughout the play. And it is important to remember that it is a play, and it is fictional with a portrayal of stereotypes, and yet, I have seen this behavior demonstrated all too often in my own clinical experience in real life. So it may be a fictional account, but as the writer and educator John Gardner would say, it is plausible, displaying the "moral truth of fiction" [33].

A century before our current "modern" hospital era, we can find earlier "training accounts". Mikhail Bulgakov's (1891–1940) "Notebook of a Country Doctor" (1926) [34] provides several such training tales, which display Bulgakov's immense ability as a writer and an observer of life and people. Despite taking place in a provincial setting, there are qualities of these tales that speak directly to any surgeon who has been faced with performing an operation that had been observed, but perhaps not performed before. Shortly after completing his medical training at the Sechenov University in Moscow, he recounts some scenes of his earliest operations performed in a rustic setting outside of Moscow where he was first assigned after graduation. First comes the amputation which he had never performed, expressing a hope that the patient would die of her wounds before she would die under his hands. Then comes a chapter entitled "Baptism by Version" in which he is called upon to deliver a transverse lie in an emergency setting having only read about it in books.

> To the accompaniment of the groaning and shrieks, Anna Nikolayevna told me how my predecessor – an experienced surgeon – used to do version. I listen to her avidly, trying not to miss a word. And those ten minutes were more help to me than everything I had read on obstetrics for the state exams, in which I had been awarded a top mark for that very obstetrics. From fragmentary words, unfinished phrases, hints dropped in passing, I learned those most essential things that are never in any books. And by the time I began wiping my ideally white, clean hands with sterile gauze, resolution had taken hold of me, and in my head there was an absolutely definite, firm plan. Combined or non-– combined, I didn't even need to think about that now. All those technical terms with no use at that moment. One thing was important: I had to introduce one hand, assist version from the outside with the other, and relying not on books, but on a sense of proportion, without which a doctor is unfit for anything, cautiously, but firmly bring one foot down, and by that foot extract the baby. I have to be calm and cautious and at the same time, boundlessly resolute, unafraid....
>
> The bloodied sheets are thrown aside, and the mother is hastily covered with a clean one, and the Feldspar and Aksinya carry her off to the ward. The swaddled baby rides off on a pillow. The wrinkled little brown face looks out from a white frame, and there is an uninterrupted, thin, piteous, squealing
>
> Water runs from the taps of the washbasins. Anna Nikolayevna draws greedily on a cigarette, screws up her eyes at the smoke, coughs.
>
> "You did the version well, Doctor., with real confidence."
>
> It was just after 1 o'clock when I got home. In a patch of lamplight on the desk in the study, Döderlein [obstetrics textbook] lay peacefully open at the page "The Dangers of Version". I sat with it for another hour or so, gulping tea that had grown cold, leafing through the pages. And now something interesting happened: all of the formerly obscure bits became completely comprehensible as though they had filled with light, and there, in the light of the lamp, at night, in the back of beyond, I realized what real knowledge means. "There's a great experience to be gained in the country – side," I thought, falling asleep, "only I have to read, read a lot... Read..." [34]

To consider training tales a full description of physician life-writing or experience would be too limited. After the laughter brought on by the trench humor and dramatic presentations of some of these tales grows quiet, one needs a sense of balance and something that more fully reflects the experience of training. There are many thoughtful and intelligent physicians who have described their experiences in non-satirical ways, in ways that a mature physician who has survived the "gauntlet" would understand and compare to their own experiences. They have described the emotional transformation that occurs during training, and the personal development that takes place, all against a background of human suffering and illness, a genuine landscape of the physician portrayed vividly and humanely. When I seek out titles to give to pre-medical students or student who wish to know "what it's like" I consider Bulgakov's account, vividly life-like in its depiction, and do not hesitate to offer it to pre-medical students. I will likewise prefer other more realistic accounts to more imperious or cynical ones. Students will be exposed to them sooner or later anyway.

Claire McCarthy began writing about her medical experiences as a first-year medical student after a privileged education at Princeton and Harvard, where she completed the medical school and remained in the residency programs to train in pediatrics, compiling a collection of clinical vignettes that chronicled her experiences from her first days in medical school to the completion of her residency, the birth of her first child and its effect on how she viewed her work and decision to become a primary care pediatrician. Many times in her book, *Learning How the Heart Beats: The Making of a Pediatrician,* she faces the question of identity. Is she who she wants to be, or is she supposed to become something that "they," the representatives of the system, her peers and professors, want her to be. The challenge of retaining her humanity while understanding that there are things she needs to learn to become "a doctor" is clearly foretold in one of the earliest vignettes, "Mrs. Asgarian". As a first-year medical student, she was sent on a home visit as part of her clinical skills course, writing about her experiences in the evenings after her assignments were completed. In this fragment, she visits an elderly widow to learn something of her heart disease, but along the way, she spends more time hearing the story of her patient's marriage and life after her husband died.

> "Nothing was the same after he was gone," she said. Her voice was so soft, I could barely hear it.
>
> "I found work as a secretary, and I read lots of books and had many friends, but nothing was ever the same."
>
> "I'm sorry," I said
>
> She was quiet. There was no sound except the sound of an occasional car going by outside, but the silence was very full.
>
> "Don't be sorry," she said finally. "I'm not sorry. I had Adam, and I could never ask anything more of life. But the days, the days are long."
>
> I looked at her, and I thought, I could never be her doctor. I couldn't hear the stories, I couldn't know these things about her and be her doctor, too. How did doctors do it? Was it better not to find out things about people? I wouldn't be able to lecture her about taking her medicines. I wouldn't be able to ask her to take off her clothes and then examine her, see her naked and touch her and ask her to breathe deeply while I listened to her lungs. I could never have enough distance; it would feel like a violation
>
> And, I realized as I looked at the old woman wrapped in the shadows, it would be too hard to know that I could do nothing to treat the real disease of her heart [35].

The title of her memoir, *Learning How the Heart Beats*, takes deliberate advantage of a double meaning of the word "heart" as both a mechanical pump whose intricacies we know so well, especially now due to achievements of empirical science of the last several hundred years. But the heart in the title is also a symbol of the emotional life, once referred to as "the seat of the soul" as it was viewed by Aristotle and the ancients. Such double meanings are seen in other medical memoirs as well. The title of Louse Aronson's *History of the Present Illness* [36] is drawn from the technical term used to structure a formal medical history, but in her writerly approach, it implies something far deeper, richer, and more complex that looks into the life of a person, and not just the medical details. Aronson's HPI (the abbreviation commonly used for this part of the history) is much closer to the kind of personal account of experience that Hawkins uses in her description of how a pathography differs from a clinical account. Henry Marsh's *Do No Harm* [37] adapts a term from the Hippocratic oath that is often recited in passing and turns it into a powerful statement that seems to challenge him with its implicit irony about the inevitable failings of medical work that sooner or later can and do lead to the harm of others and the effect it has on the surgeon. Atul Gawande's *Complications* [38] uses a similar approach for a title, adapting a term that is commonly used in technical reports into a different context in which it takes on a deeper, human meaning.

Once outside of training, though, life goes on and doctors continue to mature, not always under the supervision of others, but further under the watchful eye of their own conscience. Nothing really can prepare a physician for what he or she will encounter in the world, neither school nor training, for these are but preliminary steps. Bulgakov's account of his version delivery so clearly describes the maturation of his technical skills. As Aristotle wrote in the Nichomachean Ethics, Book II, Chap. I:

> For the things we have to learn before we can do them, we learn by doing them, e.g. men become builders by building and lyre players by playing the lyre; so too we become just by doing just acts, temperate by doing temperate acts, brave by doing brave acts [39].

We learn them by doing them. Abraham Verghese describes his emotional maturation after his fellowship in Infectious Disease at the Boston City Hospital that followed his internal medicine residency as an FMG (foreign medical graduate), often relegated to the B-list of training programs and positions in the United States. Verghese, born into the Indian diaspora, completed the necessary exams to be licensed in America and then completed his training in the U.S. But America remained an incompletely known territory to him and he wondered if he could ever belong here as he returned to Johnson City to begin his first professional appointment in Infectious Disease at the very beginning of the AIDS epidemic. At this time, the sons of prominent families were returning from the coasts to their home towns where the stigma of AIDS at that time would preclude their welcome. Verghese became their doctor while carrying on with his "day job" at the Veterans Administration hospitals. In the following passage, he described his growing sense of belonging to the community as his work pulled him ever deeper and closer into its people, both welcome and rejected:

> I suppose this is when you know the town has become your town: where others see brick, a broken window, all boarded up storefronts, you feel you are moved to tears or to joy. The map of the town becomes a map of your memories, the grid on which you play out your obsessions, on which you mark your great loves and your enmities; its geography becomes your destiny....That night, and for every night I lived in Johnson City, the town became the geography in which my dreams were set.

> I loved the old men; I loved their sounds; I loved the way they let us take care of them and the way they and their wives bonded to us, seeking us out on every visit. And when finally oat-cell cancer of the lung or a fatal variceal bleed would claim them, I would hear from the wives for years; cards on Memorial Day, a surprise visit to my office with the present of a giant hug and a homemade cornbread. I cannot tell you whether Johnson City actually made a place for me, a brown skinned man, among its own or whether I, like some of my patients, was forever outside its real heart. I can only say that in the strange times when it seemed death was everywhere, I thought of this place as a kind of safe haven, and when I dreamed of falling, as I often did, there were gentle hands waiting to break my fall [40].

This is not the cynical distance portrayed in *The House of God*, even if that was the best way by which the author was able to indicate his care for the patients and the profession. Later he would write an article entitled "Fiction As Resistance" describing his efforts against what he saw as the lack of humanity in medicine as he was exposed to it [29]. Verghese's account, by contrast, is a warm and perhaps idealistic expression of caring and compassion, a view of life that much more clearly coincides with the impressions of William Branch, who has studied professional development in medical education for many years, working with students as well as residents. He concluded, on the basis of group discussions and their personal writing of critical incident reports (accounts of meaningful experiences), that:

> The initial qualitative analysis of the critical incident reports concluded that students' acculturation into medicine was the theme that underlay the largest number of narratives [41]. A ubiquitous sub-theme was the powerful empathy that pervaded third year students' relationships with patients [42]. Medical students' empathic feelings clashed with the more dispassionate care displayed by the residents. Hence, the students resisted socialization when it seemed to demand relinquishing empathy. They often described wishing and sometimes struggling to comfort suffering and dying patients … A separate analysis of critical incident reports applied the philosophy of caring to the third year experiences [42]. This analysis concluded that caring was the natural philosophy of medical students as they ministered to patients [43].

Preserving one's self and finding one's self in medical work while becoming acculturated to professional demands are matters of great importance to medical students and young doctors, yet their voices are not often heard; rather, they are spoken of by others who seek to provide them with "formation". Branch's work is an exception to other approaches to the formation of medical students, often subsumed under the goal of "professionalism". Works, such as *The Soul of a Doctor* [44] at Harvard and the JAMA (*Journal of the American Medical Association*) *Piece of My Mind*, are a kind of "poet's corner" in which sentimental moments are welcomed, but rarely given the sort of undivided attention that a reader will give a full length book such as that by McCarthy or Verghese. But these shorter items are at least that: short. In a curriculum where every minute must be accounted for, time management is essential. One can hardly afford the luxury to spend time reading a sustained account of someone's experience unless they do so on their own time, which often means also "on their own dime". But while shorter pieces are suitable for shorter sessions, one-time-only seminars or group meetings, they offer a starting place. But there is no substitute for the deeper immersion made possible by reading a single work or pursuing the collected works of a single writer.

Robert McCrum, for example, wrote a companion to *My Year Off* entitled *Every Third Thought* [18] some twenty years after his stroke, after falling in the street due to his impaired gate and requiring a period of hospitalization. The title of the book is taken from Prospero's final soliloquy in Shakespeare's *The Tempest* in which he says: *And thence retire me to my Milan, where / Every third thought shall be my grave*. McCrum had already broadened our awareness of the literature of ailment by including John Donne's *Devotions on Emergent Occasions* (1624) in *My Year Off*. Here, he extends the literary references to show how much they are part of our life today, and indeed, how little some things have changed despite major advances in medicine.

John Donne had experienced an unidentified illness which had come upon him suddenly to leave him prostate with a fever from which he nonetheless recovered. But during the time of his illness and convalescence, he had time to think of his own mortality and seek reconciliation with God, exploring questions regarding his immortal soul. In the first Meditation of the first Devotion (prayer, in modern English) Donne comments on the suddenness of his ailment, and how all our attempts to prevent it seem abruptly overwhelmed.

> We study health, and we deliberate upon our meats, and drink, and air, and exercises, and we hew and we polish every stone that goes to that building; and so our health is a long and a regular work: but in a minute a cannon batters all, overthrows all, demolishes all; a sickness unprevented for all our diligence, unsuspected for all our curiosity; nay, undeserved, if we consider only disorder, summons us, seizes us, possesses us, destroys us in an instant. O miserable condition of man! [45]

It is striking to read such words written four hundred years ago. Seeing them expands greatly our sense of possible resources about the human condition of illness.

Longer personal accounts from physicians also take us out of the modern training environment. Sheila Cassidy gave up her training to become a plastic surgeon in Great Britain in Chile as a volunteer surgeon. After treating a member of a rebel group, she was imprisoned by the Pinochet government, tortured, and kept in solitary confinement. The British government eventually negotiated her release. At first she went to a Benedictine monastery as a nun, but eventually found her needs could not be fully met there. She returned to practice medicine, not as a surgeon, but rather as a palliative care and hospice physician, caring for the dying. In her memoir, *Sharing the Darkness*, she describes how she writes and why she writes:

> Is it right, I wonder, for me to write about my own experience of darkness? Would it not be better to write dispassionately about the problems of stress and depression in general outlining the causes and suggesting a few remedies such as counseling, support groups, regular exercise, relaxation and a healthy diet? Oh that would be safer all right. Then I would be seen as a calm knowledgeable professional, fully in control of my life and job and people would say, "Isn't she marvelous? So strong and capable.

> But it is my experience that people are hungry for personal testimony: they want to know how you do it. Whereas years ago I thundered eloquently from the platform and pulpit about the needs of the Third World, I now sit and talk more gently of the yawning gulf between my ideals and the actual realities of how I live my life. I have learned to laugh at myself in public and share my weaknesses with others so that they may be encouraged, rather than impressed [46].

Norman Bethune was a thoracic surgeon in Toronto who developed new surgical techniques for the treatment of tuberculosis in the 1930s, becoming famous for his surgical innovations introducing air into the pleural cavity to permit collapse of the infected lung, depriving the tubercle bacillus of the oxygen it needed to survive. In his experience with patients with the disease he wrote that he learned there were two forms of tuberculosis: that of the rich and that of the poor. He became politically radicalized and alienated from the medical elite in Toronto. He became a Communist, traveling to Spain to provide battlefield help during the civil war, developing mobile blood banking units. He was a painter and poet. In 1937, he wrote:

> And this same pallid moon tonight,
> Which rides so quietly, clear and high,
> The mirror of our pale and troubled gaze,
> Raised to a cool Canadian sky.
> Above the shattered mountain tops,
> Last night, rose low and wild and red,
> Reflecting back from her illumined shield,
> The blood bespattered faces of the dead.
> To that pale disc, we raise our clenched fists,
> And to those nameless dead our vows renew,
> "Comrades, who fought for freedom and the future world,
> Who died for us, we will remember you."
> [47]

After the Spanish civil war, Bethune volunteered to serve with Mao Tse-tung's (now Mao Zedong) Liberation Army in China, eventually dying of sepsis from infection acquired from cuts to his fingers by sharp bone fragments that he was removing from a soldier's battlefield injuries. He remained persona non grata in Canada until relations with China thawed. He had been revered there by the Maoist government. Only later would he become a celebrated Canadian figure, whose books were published and whose face appeared on postage stamps.

Other war memoirs offer striking glimpses into medicine practiced by doctors and surgeons forced to work under extraordinary circumstances, often struggling themselves merely to survive. In *Token of a Covenant: The Diary of an East Prussian Surgeon 1945–1947* by Hans Graf von Lehndorff [48], we follow the aristocratic Lehndorff, trained as a surgeon, desperately keeping his own countrymen as well as his Russian captors alive under conditions of starvation and lack of medicines to support wound healing, working under freezing temperatures, lack of bandages and surgical instruments, and the constant threat of being killed by Russian soldiers who succeeded in executing his mother and brother by firing squad while he watched. In *Doctor at Stalingrad*, Hans Dibold [49] writes of his experience as a German surgeon with the Wehrmacht at Stalingrad, one of the most brutal battles of World War

II. We follow him as one of the few survivors at the end of the battle, imprisoned by the Russians, treating and operating on his own countrymen as well as Russian wounded and sick with limited resources. In *Hiroshima Diary: The Journal of a Japanese physician, August 6–September 30, 1945* by Michihiko Hachiya [50], we follow Dr. Hachiya's experiences as he survives the blast to attend to burn injuries and acute radiation sickness of others affected by fire and radiation, a condition no one had ever seen before, in a landscape ravaged by vaporization of most resources, plastic tarps blowing in the wind to provide a roof to keep rain off the wounded, and absence of food or supplies. Such accounts go far beyond training tales, reaching into mature medical experience of physicians after formal training has stopped. In the absence of personal experience, few medical students would ever imagine that such medicine could exist anywhere. Most recently, Dr. David Nott, a British surgeon caring for civilian trauma in zones of conflict, describes his early work in *War Doctor* [51], providing a vivid description of this kind of work with graphic depiction of injuries and treatment, social conditions and the plight of civilians. And there are many, many more such accounts. They can be abstracted, they can be summarized, but nothing can quite replace the value of reading any one in greater detail, as nothing can quite substitute for hearing the extended tales of patients when presented as lengthy narratives. To find time in a busy schedule to hear these tales is nearly impossible, and it is almost as impossible for the tellers of these tales to stop telling them.

Alexis Carrel, recipient of the 1912 Nobel Prize for his work on vascular anastomosis and organ transplantation, struggled all his life to reconcile a desire to believe in miracles, the power of faith, and the quest for the simplicity of prayer with a brilliant analytical and experimental mind. He claimed to have witnessed an unexplained healing at the shrine of Lourdes in 1902 that led to his dismissal from a promising career in Lyons and exile to America. He described his experience as a doctor at the shrine in a manuscript discovered posthumously entitled *A Voyage to Lourdes* [52]. Despite his numerous writings and contributions to science and his protection of the French population during the war in France, post-war revisionism sought to discredit him for accepting working conditions under the Vichy government and earlier supporting what were commonly accepted social views on positive eugenics in his masterpiece *Man The Unknown* [53], second only to Margaret Mitchell's *Gone With The Wind* as the best-selling book of 1935. Carrel's world and writings expose us to a brilliant mind struggling to understand the many dimensions of human experience that medicine brought him to, combining these with the mysteries of wound healing, one of the cardinal interests of any surgeon, and the mysteries of prayer and the spiritual life.

Finally there is Axel Münthe, who trained in obstetrics and gynecology as a young man, cared for the poor as well as the privileged among the Italian immigrants of Paris, served with the British on the battlefields of World War I, argued with Charcot over the treatment of hypnotic subjects whom he considered to be little more than Charcot's guinea pigs, country girls flattered and removed from their home surroundings for medical "demonstrations". He eventually left Paris after these disagreements with Charcot, moving to Rome to live in John Keats's former rooms on the Spanish Steps, from where he provided medical care to the wealthy, including the crown princess of Sweden, his ancestral home, and also care for the poor of the city and his adopted island of Capri, on which he built his famous villa from where he wrote his masterpiece *The Story of San Michele* [54], translated into some forty languages. He wrote extensively about his life and work, depicting patients and others with a humane and reverent attitude, but also one that was realistic, and never romanticized. At one time, he was one of the most widely known, read, and beloved physicians in the world. No one fragment could begin to provide a sense of his humanity or love and acceptance of people, his respect for their silent decency, or his tolerance of their foibles. For those seeking alternative ways of being a physician in today's noisy, over-industrialized world in which questions of identity and belonging are still relevant, exploring the life and writings of Axel Münthe may be a place to start. Although his life took place nearly a century before our own time, his lessons and experiences still resonate with anyone who has looked upon the face of the sick with clarity, concern, and sympathy.

25.5 Summary

"Understanding the disease" is a goal that may be approached differently by patients and practitioners. For the patient, it may be a once in a lifetime experience understood not in medical terms, but in very personal ones, as Robert McCrum put it: "I've been given a story that made most of what I've written previously pale and uninteresting by comparison." For Joseph Conrad, it was the memory of a nightmare, for Jean-Dominique Bauby "…it had the ring of a life sentence. In one flash I saw the frightening truth. It was as blinding as an atomic explosion and keener than a guillotine blade." And for Lucy Grealy, it was her moment of weeping in the toilet stall in which "Be Here Now" was inscribed on the handle.

Nolen, Cassidy, Carrel, Münthe, Bulgakov, McCarthy, Verghese, and other physicians and surgeons whose works have been cited here all provide the kinds of voice that Anne Hawkins asked for, even if some of them predated her 1993 monogram, *Reconstructing Illness.* All of them have written from "inside the whale" to provide authentic accounts of what it is like for real doctors working in a real world. These are not noble sentiments or pronouncements ex cathedra, but granules of reality, which taken together form a rich sense of what doctors' lives are like.

At the same time, the accounts of the patients, who are providing us with "medical history from below" as Roy Porter put it, are also writing from inside the whale of their illness or the situations in which their illnesses have trapped them. For Orwell, it was in the hands of the students and trainees of hospital X; for Lucy Grealy, it was in the hands of Dr. Woolf or the toilet stalls in which "God is Near" and "Be Here Now" were inscribed, and in which she sat quietly to weep. In Bauby's case, it was the body itself that was his trap, and his inability to speak or react to the pronouncement of his attendants who might just as well have been described as his captors. For Murphy and McCrum, though somewhat authoritative about their experience, it was being brought to a common denominator of humanity by the illnesses which each of them saw as revelatory of the human condition. Though not discussed above, Henning Mankell, creator of the Kurt Wallander series of detective novels, wrote about his experiences with lung cancer in a memoir entitled *Quicksand: What It Means to Be a Human Being* [55], in which he speaks to us in a quiet voice meditating about eternity and the span of time. Faced with incurable cancer, standing somewhere with one foot in each dimension of the time we know, and the time we can only imagine, he forgoes all forensic detail about his illness and treatment and speaks only with an ethereal, single voice: a literary artist, reflecting on eternity as Dorothea Lynch did at the time of acceptance of the inevitable, reminding us that "I matter. I matter".

We have reviewed a handful of examples, and yet the richness and extent of this sample already seems overwhelming. In exploring the world's libraries using modern internet search methods, we have already found some 16,000 titles of physician and patient life-writing accounts. These stand in comparison to the 250 or so titles examined by Hawkins, collected before that internet era. Many of these recently discovered titles have been unread and remain unknown, a true frontier waiting to be explored. Are they of value? With regard to patient memoirs, I've heard them referred to them as "misery memoirs" in the U.K., and an American medical librarian with whom I spoke on the topic referred to them as "diseases of the month," received regularly in boxes from publishers, and just as regularly often returned unread. When I mentioned these numbers at a presentation, a senior faculty colleague commented "Why not just read one?" Indeed, to immerse oneself in only one such memoir could provide remarkable insight into one life. But, which one? Or again, why stop at one? Are they all the same? Indeed, when have we read enough to understand them all? Or perhaps we simply go about all this alone, then find a quiet place of our own, like Lucy Grealy's toilet stall, where we too might sit in silence and possibly weep.

Life-writing in all its various forms provides us a rich theater of Lives in Medicine. But what do we gain from entering such a theater and attending to its presentations? Does it make a difference in how medicine is taught or practiced? Hugh Jewett told me that he had been treating prostate cancer all his life but did not understand it until he developed it. That statement meant something to him, enough that he would relate it to a junior colleague of no special significance, his chauffeur, as it were, to a regional meeting of privileged physicians. Would he have been a better doctor treating prostate cancer had he "understood" it as he did when he developed it?

One has to experience life to really understand it, but insofar as the accounts themselves are concerned, we can extend the dictum of William Osler: "He who studies medicine without books sails an uncharted sea, but he who studies medicine without patients does not go to sea at all". Perhaps we can end by remembering the comments of Michael Bulgakov after he learned the hard way about version and then returned to his books: "and there, in the light of the lamp, at night, in the back of beyond, I realized what real knowledge means."

Bibliography

1. Didusch WPDCfUH. Hugh Jusge Jewett, MD (1903–1990). Available from: Hugh Judge Jewett, MD (1903–1990) – Didusch Museum. 2024.
2. Haines R. The Doctor. United States: Buena VistaPictures Distribution; 1991. p. 122 minutes.
3. Rosenbaum EE. A Taste of My Own Medicine: When the Doctor Is the Patient. 1st ed. New York: Random House; 1988.
4. Hawkins AH. Reconstructing Illness: Studies In Pathography. West Lafayette, Ind: Purdue University Press; 1993.
5. James W. The Varieties of Religious Experience; A Study In Human Nature. New York: Longmans, Green, and Co; 1902.
6. Conrad J. Twixt Land and Sea. New York: Hodder & Stoughton: George H. Doran Co; 1912.
7. Bauby J-D. The Diving Bell and the Butterfly. 1st ed. New York: A.A. Knopf: Distributed by Random House; 1997.
8. Woolf V, Lee H, Hussey M, Charon R, Stephen JD. On Being Ill. Ashfield, Mass: Paris Press; 2012.
9. Charon R. The patient-physician relationship. Narrative medicine: a model for empathy, reflection, profession, and trust. JAMA. 2001;286(15):1897–902.
10. Porter R. The patient's view: doing medical history from below. Theory Soc. 1985;14:175–98.
11. Condrau F. The Patient's view meets the clinical gaze. Soc Hist Med. 2007;20(3):525–40.
12. Risse GB. Mending Bodies, Saving Souls: a History of Hospitals. New York: Oxford University Press; 1999.
13. Frank AW. The Wounded sStoryteller: Body, Illness, and Ethics. Chicago: University of Chicago Press; 1995.
14. Ariès P, Duby G. A History of Private Life. Cambridge, Mass: Belknap Press of Harvard University Press; 1987.
15. BBC BN. How John Hersey's Hiroshima revealed the horror of the bomb. In: BBC News [internet]; 2016. Available from: How John Hersey's Hiroshima revealed the horror of the bomb - BBC News.
16. Clough AH. Plutarch's Lives: Modern Library; 2001.
17. OCLW. What is Life-Writing? 2024. Available from: What is Life-Writing? | The Oxford Centre for Life-Writing.
18. McCrum R. My Year Off. 1st ed. New York: W. W. Norton; 1998.
19. Murphy RF. The body silent,1st ed. New York: H. Holt; 1987.
20. Grealy L. Autobiography of a Face. Boston: Houghton Mifflin; 1994.
21. Lynch D, Richards E. Exploding Into Life. New York, N.Y: Aperture in association with Many Voices Press; 1986.
22. Snyder T. Bloodlands: Europe Between Hitler and Stalin. New York: Basic Books; 2010.
23. Orwell G. Inside the whale. In: Carey J, editor. Orwell: Essays: Introduction by John Carey (Everyman's library contemporary classics Series): everyman; 2002.
24. Nolen WA. The Making of a Surgeon. 1st ed. New York: Random House; 1970.
25. Moore FD. A Miracle and a Privilege: Recounting a Half Century of Surgical Advance. Washington, D.C.: Joseph Henry Press; 1995.
26. Moore FD. Metabolic Care of the Surgical Patient. Philadelphia: Saunders; 1959.
27. Pollock D. Training tales: U. S medical Autobiography. Cuktural Anthropology. 1996;11(3):339–61.
28. Shem S. The House of God: A Novel. New York: R. Marek Publishers; 1978.
29. Shem, S. Fiction as resistance. Ann Intern Med. 2002;137(11):934–7.
30. Konner M. Medicine At the Crossroads: The Crisis In Health Care. 1st ed. New York: Pantheon Books; 1993.
31. Orwell G. How the poor die. Now [Internet] 1946. Available from: Fifty Orwell Essays.
32. Edson M. Wit. New York: Dramatists Play Service; 1999. p. 68.
33. Gardner J. On Moral Fiction. New York: Basic Books; 1978.

34. Bulgakov M, Glenny M. A Country Doctor's Notebook. Brooklyn: Melville House Publishing; 2013.
35. McCarthy C. Learning How the Heart Beats: the Making of a Pediatrician. New York: Viking; 1995.
36. Aronson L. A History of the Present Illness: Stories. 1st ed. New York: Bloomsbury; 2013.
37. Marsh H. Do no harm: stories of life, death, and brain surgery. 1st ed. New York: Thomas Dunne Books/St. Martin's Press; 2015.
38. Gawande A. Complications: A Surgeon's Notes On An Imperfect Science. 1st ed. New York: Metropolitan Books; 2002.
39. Aristotle, Nichomachean Ethics. Scotts Valley: CreateSpace Independent Publishing Platform; 2016.
40. Verghese A. My Own Country: A Doctor's Story. 1st Vintage Books ed. New York: Vintage Books; 1995.
41. Branch W, Pels RJ, Lawrence RS, Arky R. Becoming a doctor. Critical-incident reports from third-year medical students. N Engl J Med. 1993;329(15):1130–2.
42. Branch WT Jr, Pels RJ, Hafler JP. Medical students' empathic understanding of their patients. Acad Med. 1998;73(4):360–2.
43. Branch WT Jr. The road to professionalism: reflective practice and reflective learning. Patient Educ Couns. 2010;80(3):327–32.
44. Pories S, Jain SH, Harper G. The Soul of a Doctor: Harvard Medical Students Face Life and Death,1st ed. Chapel Hill, N.C: Algonquin Books of Chapel Hill; 2006.
45. Donne J. Divine Poems, Devotions, Prayers. Mount Vernon, N.Y: Peter Pauper Press; 1953.
46. Cassidy S. Sharing the Darkness: the Spirituality of Caring. Maryknoll, N.Y: Orbis Books; 1991.
47. Bethune N. Red moon 1936 [poem]. Available from: Poetry—Friends and Veterans.
48. Lehndorff H. Token of a Covenant; Diary of An East Prussian Surgeon, 1945–47, Chicago: H. Regnery Co.; 1964.
49. Dibold H. Doctor at Stalingrad; the Passion of a Captivity. London: Hutchinson; 1958.
50. Hachiya M. Hiroshima Diary: the Journal of a Japanese Physician, August 6–September 30, 1945. Chapel Hill: University of North Carolina Press; 1995.
51. Nott D. War Doctor: Surgery On the Front Line. New York: Abrams Books; 2020.
52. Carrel A. The Voyage to Lourdes. 1st ed. New York: Harper; 1950.
53. Carrel A. Man the Unknown. New York, London: Harper & Brothers; 1935.
54. Münthe A. The Story of San Michele.London: J. Murray; 1929.
55. Mankel H. Quicksand: What It Means To Be a Human Being. New York City: Vintage; 2017.

Epilogue

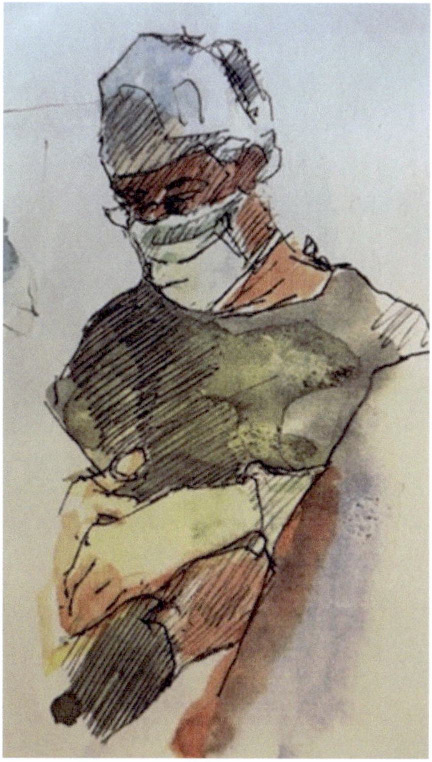

John McFarland operating in the Royal Liverpool University Hospital. The image of the surgeon operating the original painting by Janina Cerbetowitz

J. McFarland et al. (eds.), *Humanism in Surgery*, New Paradigms in Healthcare,
https://doi.org/10.1007/978-3-031-86018-8

May each day dawn clear
for you,
May each noon's repose
repose you.
May the softness of each evening
gentle you.
May each night your dreams
bless you. (JB. McFarland)

Acknowledgements

This book has been a labour of love, and in all such undergoings there are many people involved, and many people who we would wish to acknowledge and thank. Nevertheless, firstly we would like to thank all those surgeons past and present who have cared for their patients with unrelenting humanity. The act of the surgeon *per se* is harmful but a good surgeon operates with dedication and love.

Many have been involved in this book and we wish to thank all the authors of the chapters who have dedicated a lot of their time working on and writing up their ideas. Moreover, as we believe that this book is exceptional for the fact that not only are there chapters dedicated to different topics of humanism in surgery and medicine, but these chapters are complemented by interviews with living surgeons. We wish to thank all those surgeons who agreed to be interviewed. Their contributions shed light on the chapters as do the chapters intertwine with and enhance the interviews; the relationship between the two is fundamental to the working of this book, which we hope will benefit many. Each one of the Co-editors (interestingly half are surgeons, Jacek Mostwin and the René Génadry, and the other half non-surgeons, Susanna Magalhaes and Jonathan McFarland) also wish to make their individual acknowledgements and thanks.

I, Jonathan McFarland, wish to thank the other co-editors, Jacek, Susanna and Rene, for helping so much in this task, which was considerable. Along the way, however, our conversations and meetings were fun, informative and productive. Collaboration was, and is always the key. It goes without saying that I am very indebted to both Maria Giulia Marini, my co-editor in the series, and Donatella Rizza, from Springer, for without them this series would not be possible. I would also like to thank my wife, Polimnia, and my two daughters, Aina and Bianca, for always inspiring and supporting me in this endeavour, and everything I do. Two retired surgeons, Professors Sir John Temple and Dame Averil Mansfield helped me considerably in putting together the chapter of my family connections with surgery, both of whom worked with my father, and I am extremely indebted to them. I also wish to thank Manuel Pera for he and I had many interesting debates and

J. McFarland et al. (eds.), *Humanism in Surgery*, New Paradigms in Healthcare,
https://doi.org/10.1007/978-3-031-86018-8

conversations on the philosophy of surgery while we were writing and editing our chapter. It was, and, is always a delight to work with him. I would also like to thank all the members of The Doctor as a Humanist NPO since each in their own way have also made the writing of this book possible for me. I also wish to thank Janina Cebertowitzc for allowing me to use her beautiful painting of my father operating in the Royal Liverpool Hospital in the 1980s, and for helping me get the copyright permission for Don Mckinlay's painting 'Goose Girl'. Thanks also to Josephine Hughes for her continual support and advice in the wording of the text. And finally, this book is about the surgeons in my family, so I wish to thank my father and my two grandfathers.

I, René Génadry, would like to thank my co-editors Susanna and Jonathan who accepted my contributions and suggestions and particularly Jacek who got me involved in this project and the enlightening numerous online and personal meetings. Also, my wife Mona for her unwavering and continued support during this endeavour. Special thanks to the fistula surgeons that I was honoured to interview and their willingness to share their time and their insights as a clear indication of their commitment to improving the humanistic approach to the surgery of the patient with obstetric fistula, most in need of their support, dedication and humanity.

I, Jacek, wish to thank you, Rene, for your generous comments and for being a friend and colleagues for over 50 years since we first met in the corridors of the Johns Hopkins teaching hospitals. Over the years we've developed a friendship and shared collaboration between our specialties based on our personalities and mutual interests in education and patient welfare that offers a model to our colleagues on how our specialties can work together for a common good. To Susana, my appreciation for the patience, thoughtfulness and commitment to literary and ethical dimensions of medicine. Scholars like yourself working with clinicians offer a model for integration of approaches that will serve medical education well. Finally, to Jonathan, the glue that has brought us together and kept us going, whose vision grew out of his genealogy and reverence for the surgeons in his family: a father and two grandfathers, respected and successful surgeons with stories of their own, but above all, remembered by a loving son and grandson for their human qualities, doctors who remind us that in the end it is the person that matters.

I am also grateful to the many colleagues at Hopkins with whom I have interacted over the years both in clinical work and education, the medical and undergraduate students who have endured the presentation of my ideas as they took shape, my earlier experiences at Oxford University under the direction of Drs. Alison Brading and Edith Bülbring who allowed me to find my own way in the study of smooth muscle, develop scholarly skills and a respect for precision and accuracy, and above all an appreciation for perseverance, teaching by their example that no adversity is large enough to resist the determination and resolve of a committed spirit. To Dame Hermione Lee, who welcomed me back as then president of Wolfson College many years later to expand scholarship on life-writing to medicine and the illness experience. The project on Lives in Medicine continues at Wolfson under the direction of Drs. Elleke Boehmer and Kate Kennedy. I am grateful for many years of participation in the Harvard Macy Programs for medical educators and for Dr

Patricia Thomas who first directed me to them before leaving Hopkins to become Vice Dean of Medical Education at Case Western Reserve University. Many individuals at Macy, and the institution itself they have created, have provided a sustained platform that first taught me that there is more to teaching than being a content expert, and that there is no limit to learning about learning: classroom teaching and curriculum formation are arts in themselves and higher education can make a difference and has rules and theory of its own, that if grounded in human nature and understood, can make this possible. Finally, many of my ideas were forged slowly during years of experience in the clinic and at the operating table, all made possible by the support and under the direction of Dr Patrick Walsh who, as chairman of the Department of Urology, would ask us assistants and observers in the operating room before the case began, when we were all gowned and masked and focused on the work about to be done: 'Who is the most important person in the room?' As we looked around to see who in the room that might be, seeking the answer to his question, finally pausing, uncertain, he would slowly respond. 'The most important person in the room is… the patient' Then the case could begin.

Susana Magalhães would like to thank Jonathan McFarland, Jacek and Rene for having made this book a true work of Art and a tribute to all the health professionals and humanists who believe in Person Centred Care, Compassion and Creativity as the roots of meaningful Care. I would also like to thank all the speakers of the first Symposium on Humanism in Surgery organized by The Doctor as a Humanist and the Institute of Research and Innovation in Health, i3S-University of Porto, for having made this event come true. I am especially grateful to the speakers who have also accepted the invitation to contribute to this book, with their insights and their unique experience.

All my gratitude to José Poças and Ana Filipa Cardoso, for their commitment to preserving the essence of human care in their daily life and for being good friends of Literature and Art.

I also wish to thank Manuel Pera for having me on board in his effort to change the paradigm of medical curricula and for being a guiding light in the field of Medical Humanities.

A final word to Jonathan McFarland: without your wisdom and perseverance this book would not have been what it is today: a work that is made up of time lived by generations, starting in the past of your own family history throughout the present and flowing to the future of surgeons, health professionals, caregivers and patients.

Biographies of Surgeons

Prof Sohier Elneil is the first Professor of Urogynaecology at University College London and is a leading Consultant in Urogynaecology and Uro-neurology. Her career spans several decades looking after women with incontinence and prolapse, but specifically in those with complications following childbirth trauma, including fistula, female genital mutilation (FGM), mesh complications, chronic pelvic pain and neurological/ageing of the pelvic floor. She has chaired multiple Charities including FORWARD UK and Fistula Foundation. Elneil has a sustained track record of excellence in both clinical and scientific research, knowledge transfer, global reach, student personal and professional development and empowering the voices of women globally in their own health care.

Manuel Pera is active as the Professor of Surgery at the Hospital Clinic in Barcelona Spain. Growing up in a medical family, his education and training took him to many countries in Europe, the UK and the United States. His surgical specialization is the treatment of upper gastrointestinal malignancies. As an educator he has advanced programmes in early surgical opportunity and education for students, and the role of humanities and humanism in medicine. He is a member of the steering Committee of DASH, The Doctor As A Humanist. Our conversation was conducted between Baltimore and Barcelona over Zoom, recorded, then transcribed and slightly edited for ease of reading.

William Reiner trained in urology at the Brady Urological Institute of the Johns Hopkins School of Medicine in the 1980s. He then practised with a focus on paediatric urology in California for 15 years. He returned to Hopkins to train in paediatric and adolescent psychiatry, specifically to address the psychological need of children and adolescents with major paediatric birth defects for whose question she was unable to find answers. He then became Professor of Pediatric and Adolescent Psychiatry at the University of Oklahoma, having recently retired. He now lives in

J. McFarland et al. (eds.), *Humanism in Surgery*, New Paradigms in Healthcare,
https://doi.org/10.1007/978-3-031-86018-8

his original home state, California. Our conversation was conducted and recorded over Zoom then transcribed and slightly edited for ease of reading.

Christopher Wolfgang is currently active as Professor in the Department of General Surgery at the Langone School of Medicine of the New York University where he specializes in the surgical treatment of hepato-biliary disease, especially pancreatic cancer. After training in general surgery at Pennsylvania State University, he came to the Department of General Surgery at Johns Hopkins and remained there on faculty until his moving to NYU. In addition to extensive clinical experience, he directs scientific research on the basic biology of pancreatic cancer in his laboratories, teaches and continues to develop newer methods for treating pancreatic. I met with Dr Wolfgang at his offices in New York for an in-person conversation that was recorded, transcribed and slightly edited for ease of reading.

Jeffrey P. Wilkinson, MD, is the Jennifer and Wil Van Loh Professor of Global Women's Health and Surgery at Baylor College of Medicine and Texas Children's Hospital (BCM/TCH). He leads the global women's health initiatives for BCM and TCH and has lived and worked full time for most of the last 13 years in Malawi. He has helped establish the Freedom from Fistula Foundation Fistula Care Centre in Lilongwe, Malawi, in 2011.

John Tarpley entered the Halsted Residency in General Surgery at the Johns Hopkins School of Medicine in the early 1970s. He had extensive additional experience in orthopaedics and cancer chemotherapy, then shortly after completing this residency began a lifelong career as a medical educator and builder of programmes in sub-Saharan Africa, combined with regular extended returns to Hopkins and to Vanderbilt, his medical school alma mater. He maintained academic appointments at both institutions. He is retired from performing operations but remains active in medical education and programme development for African countries, in medical ethics, education and the religious and spiritual dimensions of medicine. The conversation took place in person at a private home in Lutherwville, MD. It was recorded, transcribed and edited for ease of reading.

James T. Handa, MD, is the Robert Bond Welch Professor and Chief of the Retina Division, the Wilmer Eye Institute, Johns Hopkins University. As an academic Vitreoretinal surgeon, he has split his energies on clinical care including caring for patients with age-related macular degeneration (AMD) as well as surgical problems and malignancies, and research. Beside clinical work and research, Dr Handa is passionate and dedicated to mentoring. He has established a regular volunteer mission to the island of Palau to care for patients with eye problems for the past 27 years.

Prof Judith Goh, MD, is a urogynaecologist, practicing in Brisbane (privately at the Greenslopes Private Hospital, publicly at QEII Hospital) and at the Qld Pelvic Mesh Service at the Gold Coast. Since 1995, Judith has been a self-funded medical volunteer, working mainly in the area of obstetric fistula, particularly in the field of fistula surgery, and the promotion of the rights of women and children in developing countries.

Michael Breen, MD, is an Ob/Gyn who trained in Ireland and for the last 30 years has worked in several African countries. Currently, he is based at the Fistula Care Centre in Tamatave, Madagascar, working as a surgeon for Freedom From Fistula Foundation. This allows him to improve the outcome for women with fistulas and to train local surgeons.

Steven Arrowsmith, MD, is a urologist by training in his fourth decade of fistula work. He helped to establish three African fistula centres, has performed repairs in 17 countries and mentored dozens of fistula surgeons. He was Co-Investigator on Fistula Care/WHO's clinical trial on catheter management after fistula repair and lead author of UNFPA/WHO's newly published global guidance on fistula. His most important mentors have been women with fistula, from whom he has drawn many life lessons and much personal strength.

Ana Pastor, head of Neurosurgery at the CHU of Ourense, in Spain, and Head of the Clinical Neurosciences group of Galicia Sur, has travelled to Africa to train local doctors in the health centre of Niamey, capital of Niger. Her work has focused on helping and training doctors to treat polytraumatized patients.

John Varallo, MD, MPH, FACOG, is Team Lead for Women's Health at the Global Surgery Foundation. He is a board-certified Ob/Gyn, based in Washington, DC, with over 20 years of clinical and surgical experience working in low-resource settings on three continents, and continues working clinically in Alaska.

MIX
Papier aus verantwortungsvollen Quellen
Paper from responsible sources
FSC® C105338

If you have any concerns about our products,
you can contact us on
ProductSafety@springernature.com

In case Publisher is established outside the EU,
the EU authorized representative is:
Springer Nature Customer Service Center GmbH
Europaplatz 3, 69115 Heidelberg, Germany

Printed by Libri Plureos GmbH
in Hamburg, Germany